T0344482

Computational Intelligence Aided Systems for Healthcare Domain

This book covers recent advances in artificial intelligence, smart computing, and their applications in augmenting medical and healthcare systems. It will serve as an ideal reference text for graduate students and academic researchers in diverse engineering fields including electrical, electronics and communication, computer, and biomedical.

This book

- Presents architecture, characteristics, and applications of artificial intelligence and smart computing in healthcare systems.
- Highlights privacy issues faced in healthcare and health informatics using artificial intelligence and smart computing technologies.
- Discusses nature-inspired computing algorithms for the brain–computer interface.
- Covers graph neural network application in the medical domain.
- Provides insights into the state-of-the-art artificial intelligence and smart computing enabling and emerging technologies.

This book discusses recent advances and applications of artificial intelligence and smart technologies in the field of healthcare. It highlights privacy issues faced in healthcare and health informatics using artificial intelligence and smart computing technologies. It covers nature-inspired computing algorithms such as genetic algorithms, particle swarm optimization algorithms, and common scrambling algorithms to study brain–computer interfaces. It will serve as an ideal reference text for graduate students and academic researchers in the fields of electrical engineering, electronics and communication engineering, computer engineering, and biomedical engineering.

Computational Intelligence Aided Systems for Healthcare Domain

Edited by
Akshansh Gupta
Hanuman Verma
Mukesh Prasad
Jyoti Singh Kirar
C. T. Lin

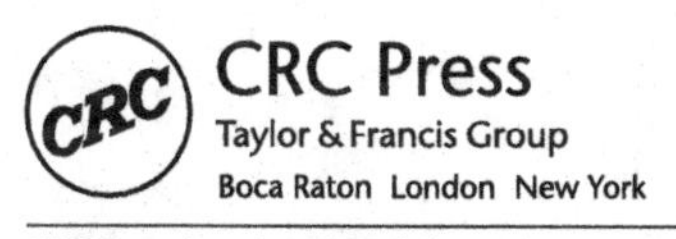

CRC Press is an imprint of the
Taylor & Francis Group, an informa business

Front cover image: elenabsl/Shutterstock

First edition published 2023
by CRC Press
6000 Broken Sound Parkway NW, Suite 300, Boca Raton, FL 33487-2742

and by CRC Press
4 Park Square, Milton Park, Abingdon, Oxon, OX14 4RN

CRC Press is an imprint of Taylor & Francis Group, LLC

ISBN: 978-1-032-21033-9 (hbk)
ISBN: 978-1-032-43665-4 (pbk)
ISBN: 978-1-003-36834-2 (ebk)

DOI: 10.1201/9781003368342

Typeset in Sabon
by codeMantra

Our Beloved Family Members,
Our Relatives & Friends

Contents

Preface

"Augmenting Medical & Health Care system using Artificial Intelligence and Smart Computing" will be a comprehensive and authoritative presentation of the current development of Artificial Intelligence (AI), Smart Computing, and applications of these techniques in augmenting Medical & Health Care Systems. The book is a convenient reader for an undergraduate and postgraduate level person knowing the various discipline of humanity, primarily related to health hospitality, and the students of multidisciplinary science, mathematics, and engineering and aimed to pursue their research in the field of health care and health informatics. The book has covered various computational intelligence methods in Machine learning and Deep learning algorithm. It aims to highlight the new advancement of machines & deep knowledge and advanced computing in the field of Medical & Health Care systems. Chapters of this book have been written by experts of their respective areas. The book's goal is to provide a diverse range of readers with a wide range of knowledge needed to interact productively with others from many different disciplines involved in health care and health informatics. The book has covered a wide range of physiological disorders such as cancer, heart stroke, brain stroke, skin disease, breast cancer, and many more, which can be easily diagnosed and cured with the help of a computer-aided system.

The structure of the proposed as follows: Chapter 1 throws light on basic concepts of computational intelligence methods related to Machine learning and Deep learning. Chapter 2 covers a comprehensive review of applications of Deep learning methods in the health sector. Chapter 3 discusses various dimensions of the application of deep multi-view learning in the field of health organization and medical practices, whereas Chapter 4 deals with applications of IoT and Big data in precision health care and self-care activities. Chapter 5 enriches the knowledge of readers about the application of machine learning algorithms in stroke patient classification. Chapter 6 puts a review on various Fuzzy C-means algorithms applicable to image segmentation. Chapter 7 contains a bibliometric analysis of the role of IoT, AI, blockchain, and network analysis during COVID-19. Chapter 8 throws light on Biomedical Named Entity Recognition using Natural Language Processing. Chapter 9 focuses on image segmentation using deep learning algorithms for skin disease, while Chapter 10 is informative on the utility of deep learning algorithms for dementia disease using multi-modality techniques. Chapters 11 and 12 focus on the application of machine learning algorithms and data exploratory analysis on the heart and diabetic diseases respectively. Chapter 13 keeps a glimpse of the deep learning techniques for fundus image classifications in the field of diabetic retinotopy.

Chapter 14 focuses on the emerging role of AI in precision oncology with the development of sequencing technologies, genomics and computation that identified thousands of cancer-causing genetic, epigenetic, and phenotypic abnormalities. And, further, the present and future trends of AI in precision oncology are presented in the Chapter 15. Chapter 16, through the light on computer-aided Breast Cancer (BrC) diagnosis, discusses the basics of BrC, Deep Learning, Machine learning, and the respective data sets used to evaluate the systems. Finally, Chapter 17 focuses on understanding the complex dynamical evolution and interplay of health, climate and conflicts, using a data-driven approach, which enables to assess of information, captures the underlying relational patterns between variables and provides deep insight into the systems.

Acknowledgements

The successful completion of this book, "Computational Intelligence Aided Systems for Healthcare Domain", could be possible with several individuals' help and unconditional support. We will take this opportunity to thank all who helped us directly or indirectly during this book. Without the experience and support from our peers and colleagues, this book would not exist.

First, we express our sincere gratitude and respect to Prof. Anirban Chakraborti, School of Computational and Integrative Sciences, Jawaharlal Nehru University, New Delhi, India, for encouraging us to draft this book proposal. We are very grateful to him for his support and guidance in initiating this book.

We express my sincere gratitude to CRC Press, Taylor & Francis Group publisher and their entire team, especially Gauravjeet, Isha and Shashi, for their continuous support and quick reply. We appreciate him for always showing keen interest in our queries related to proposal completion and editing works.

We want to thank our working institutes: CSIR-Central Electronics Engineering Research Institute, Pilani, Rajasthan, India (Dr Akshansh Gupta); Bareilly College, Bareilly, Uttar Pradesh, India (Dr Hanuman Verma); DST-CIMS, Banaras Hindu University, Varanasi, Uttar Pradesh, India (Jyoti Singh Kirar); Centre for Artificial Intelligence, University of Technology, Sydney, Australia (Dr Mukesh Prasad and Dr C. T. Lin) for providing us with ample computational facilities to complete this book in stipulated time.

Our special thanks to all the authors for contributing their chapters and support whenever we required. We could make this book a grand success with the mere cooperation, enthusiasm, and spirit of the authors and reviewers. The contributors have been a real motivation and key in establishing this book as one of the best books for publication in the area of computational artificial intelligence in healthcare. We thank them all for considering and trusting the book as the platform for publishing their valuable work. We also thank all authors for cooperating during the various stages of processing the chapters.

We owe a lot to our family members and friends for their constant love and support in this book's pursuits. Their support has been essential for us over the studies which matter in our lives. We want to thank them very much and share this moment of happiness with them. We would also like to thank all persons who have directly or indirectly helped us complete our edited book series.

Akshansh Gupta
Hanuman Verma
Mukesh Prasad
Jyoti Singh Kirar
C. T. Lin

About the editors

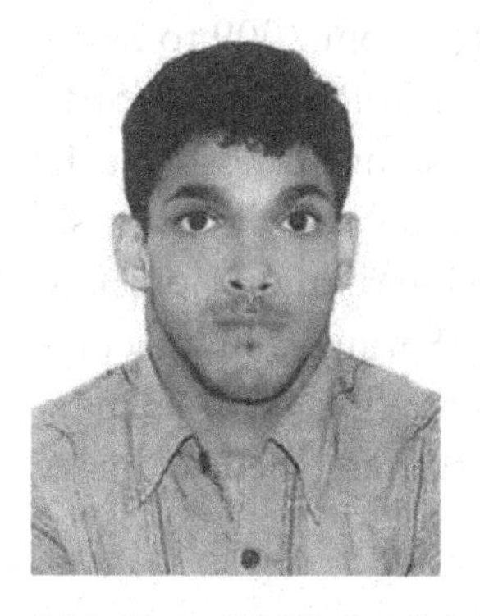

Dr Akshansh Gupta is a scientist at CSIR-Central Electronic Engineering Research Institute Pilani Rajasthan. He has worked as a DST-funded postdoctoral research fellow as a principal investigator under the scheme of the Cognitive Science Research Initiative (CSRI) from the Department of Science and Technology (DST), Ministry of Science and Technology, Government of India, from 2016 to 2020 in School of Computational Integrative and Science, Jawaharlal Nehru University, New Delhi. He has many publications, including Springer, Elsevier, and IEEE Transaction. He received his master's and a PhD degree from the School of computer and systems sciences, JNU, in 2010 and 2015, respectively. His research interests include Pattern Recognition, Machine Learning, Data Mining Signal Processing, Brain Computer Interface, Cognitive Science, and IoT. He is also working as CO-PI on a consultancy project named "Development of Machine Learning Algorithms for Automated Classification Based on Advanced Signal Decomposition of EEG Signals" ICPS Program, DST Govt. of India.

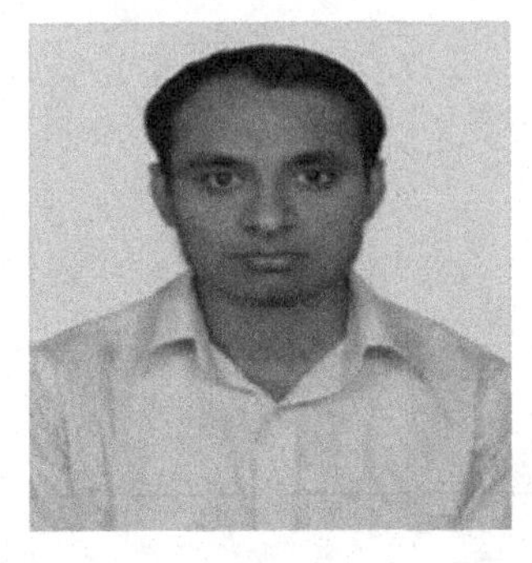

Dr Hanuman Verma received the PhD and M.Tech degrees in Computer Science and Technology from the School of Computer and Systems Sciences (SC& SS) at Jawaharlal Nehru University (JNU), New Delhi, India, in 2015 and 2010, respectively. He also did his master of Science (M.Sc.) degree in Mathematics & Statistics from Dr R. M. L. Avadh University, Ayodhya, Uttar Pradesh, India. He has worked as a junior research fellowship (JRF) and senior research fellowship (SRF) from 2009 to 2013, received from the Council of Scientific and Industrial Research (CSIR), New Delhi, India. Currently, he is working as Assistant Professor at the Department of Mathematics, Bareilly College, Bareilly, Uttar Pradesh, India. He has published research papers in reputed international journals, including Elsevier, Wiley, World Scientific, and Springer, in machine learning, deep learning and medical image computing. His primary research interest includes machine learning, deep learning, medical image computing, and mathematical modeling.

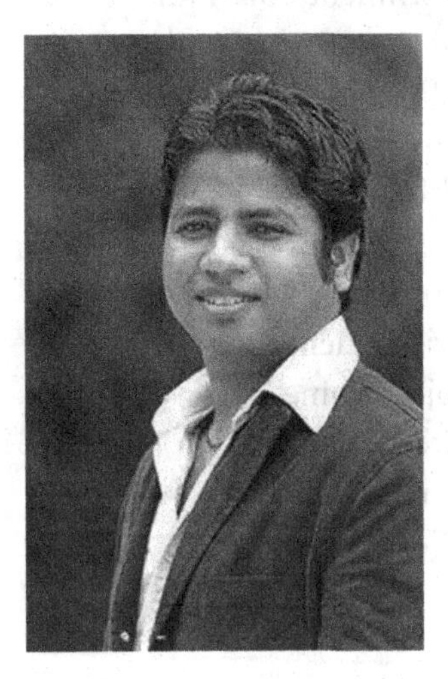

Dr Mukesh Prasad (SMIEEE, ACM) is a Senior Lecturer in the School of Computer Science (SoCS), Faculty of Engineering and Information Technology (FEIT), University of Technology Sydney (UTS), Australia. His research expertise lies in developing new methods in artificial intelligence and machine learning approaches like big data analytic, and computer vision within the healthcare domain, biomedical research. He has published more than 100 articles, including several prestigious IEEE Transactions and other Top Q1 journals and conferences in the areas of Artificial Intelligence and Machine Learning. His current research interests include pattern recognition, control system, fuzzy logic, neural networks, the internet of things (IoT), data analytics, and brain-computer interface. He received an M.S. degree from the School of Computer Systems and Sciences, Jawaharlal Nehru

University, New Delhi, India, in 2009, and a PhD degree from the Department of Computer Science, National Chiao Tung University, Hsinchu, Taiwan, in 2015. He worked as a principal engineer at Taiwan Semiconductor Manufacturing Company, Hsinchu, Taiwan, from 2016 to 2017. He started his academic career as a Lecturer with the University of Technology Sydney in 2017. He is also an Associate/Area Editor of several top journals in the field of machine learning, computational intelligence, and emergent technologies.

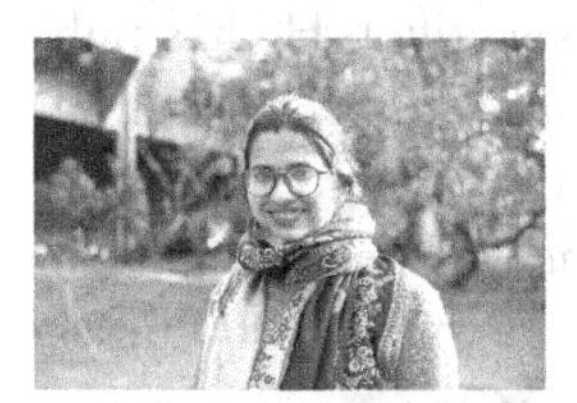

Dr. Jyoti Singh Kirar is currently as an Assistant Professor in DST-CIMS, BHU VARANASI. She has completed her Ph.D in Computer Science from Jawaharlal Nehru University, New Delhi. Her Research areas include Brain Computer Interfaces, Machine Learning, Signal Processing and Artificial Intelligence.

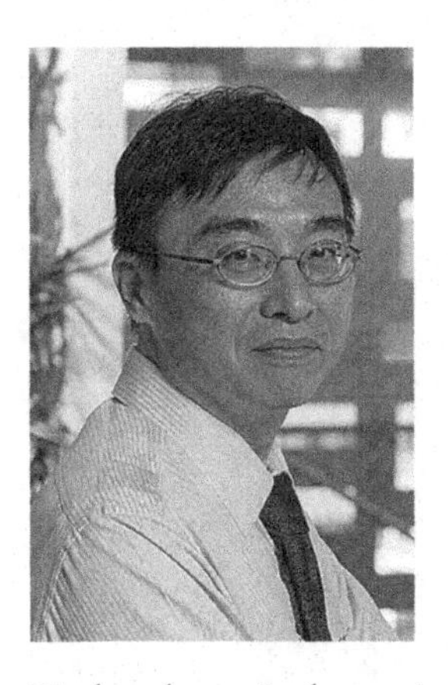

Prof. C. T. Lin Distinguished Professor. Chin-Teng Lin received a Bachelor's of Science from National Chiao-Tung University (NCTU), Taiwan, in 1986, and holds Master's and PhD degrees in Electrical Engineering from Purdue University, USA, received in 1989 and 1992, respectively. He is currently a distinguished professor and Co-Director of the Australian Artificial Intelligence Institute within the Faculty of Engineering and Information Technology at the University of Technology Sydney, Australia. He is also an Honorary Chair Professor of Electrical and Computer Engineering at NCTU. For his contributions to biologically inspired information systems, Prof Lin was awarded Fellowship with the IEEE in 2005 and the International Fuzzy Systems Association (IFSA) in 2012. He received the IEEE Fuzzy Systems Pioneer Award in 2017. He has held notable positions as editor-in-chief of IEEE Transactions on Fuzzy Systems from 2011 to 2016; seats on the Board of Governors for the IEEE Circuits and Systems (CAS) Society (2005–2008), IEEE Systems, Man, Cybernetics (SMC) Society (2003–2005), IEEE Computational Intelligence Society (2008–2010); Chair of the IEEE

Taipei Section (2009–2010); Chair of IEEE CIS Awards Committee (2022); Distinguished Lecturer with the IEEE CAS Society (2003–2005) and the CIS Society (2015–2017); Chair of the IEEE CIS Distinguished Lecturer Program Committee (2018-2019); Deputy Editor-in-Chief of IEEE Transactions on Circuits and Systems-II (2006–2008); Program Chair of the IEEE International Conference on Systems, Man, and Cybernetics (2005); and General Chair of the 2011 IEEE International Conference on Fuzzy Systems. Prof Lin is the co-author of Neural Fuzzy Systems (Prentice-Hall) and the author Neural Fuzzy Control Systems with Structure and Parameter Learning (World Scientific). He has published more than 400 journal papers, including over 180 IEEE journal papers in neural networks, fuzzy systems, brain-computer interface, multimedia information processing, cognitive neuro-engineering, and human-machine teaming, that have been cited more than 30,000 times. Currently, his h-index is 82, and his i10-index is 356.

List of contributors

Prem Shankar Singh Aydav
Department of Information Technology, Km. GGP,
Uttar Pradesh, India

Sumneet Kaur Bamrah
Department of Computer Science and Engineering,
Sri Venkateswara College of Engineering
Sriperumbudur, India

Syed Raza Bashir
Ryerson University Toronto
Ontario, Canada

Sujit Bebortta
Department of Computer Science,
Ravenshaw University Cuttack
Odisha, India

Adarsh Kumar Bharti
DST-CIMS, Banaras Hindu University
Varanasi, India

Bharti Rana
Department Computer Science, University of Delhi
Delhi, India

Pawan Kumar Chaurasia
Department of Information Technology,
Babasaheb Bhimrao Ambedkar University
Uttar Pradesh, India

Ashish Kumar Das
DST-CIMS, Banaras Hindu University
Varanasi, India

Pinki Dey
University of New South Wales
Sydney, Australia

Amit Doegar
National Institute of Technical Teachers
Training & Research (NITTTR)
Chandigarh, India

Sabiya Fatima
National Institute of Technical Teachers
Training & Research (NITTTR)
Chandigarh, India

Goldie Gabrani
VIPS-TC College of Engineering
Delhi, India

K. S. Gayathri
Department of Information Technology,
Sri Sivasubramaniya Nadar College of Engineering
Kalavakkam, India

Udita Goswami
Banaras Hindu University
Varanasi, India

Aaryan Gupta
Department of Applied Mathematics,
Delhi Technological University
Delhi, India

Syed Shariq Husain
Center for Complexity Economics, Applied Spirituality and
Public Policy,
Jindal School of Government and Public Policy,
OP Jindal Global University
New Delhi, India

Md. Rafiqul Islam
Department of Computer Science, University of Delhi
Delhi, India

Anwesha Kar
Banaras Hindu University
Varanasi, India

Ranjeet Kaur
National Institute of Technical Teachers
Training & Research (NITTTR)
Chandigarh, India

Inder Khatri
Department of Applied Mathematics,
Delhi Technological University
Delhi, India

Parul Khurana
School of Computer Applications,
Lovely Professional University
Phagwara, India

C. Rama Krishna
National Institute of Technical Teachers
Training & Research (NITTTR)
Chandigarh, India

Kushagra Krishnan
Jawaharlal Nehru University
New Delhi, India

Dhirendra Kumar
Department of Applied Mathematics,
Delhi Technological University
Delhi, India

Sumit Kumar
Kurukshetra University
Haryana, India

Vipin Kumar
Department of Computer Science and Information Technology,
Mahatma Gandhi Central University
Bihar, India

Monika Mokan
Department of Computer Science and Engineering,
BML Munjal University
Gurgaon, India

Ibrahim Momin
Department of Computer Science & Information Technology,
Mahatma Gandhi Central University
Motihari, India

Usman Naseem
The University of Sydney
Sydney, Australia

Prashant Prabhakar
Department of Computer Science & Information Technology,
Mahatma Gandhi Central University
Motihari, India

Shaina Raza
University of Toronto
Toronto, Canada

Devanjali Relan
Department of Computer Science and Engineering,
BML Munjal University
Gurgaon, India

Dilip Senapati
Department of Computer Science,
Ravenshaw University Cuttack
Odisha, India

Soharab Hossain Shaikh
Department of Computer Science and Engineering,
BML Munjal University
Gurgaon, India

Kiran Sharma
School of Engineering and Technology,
BML Munjal University
Gurugram, India

Manbir Singh
Punjabi University
Patiala Punjab, India

Maninder Singh
Punjabi University
Patiala Punjab, India

Ritika Singh
Department of Computer Science & Information Technology,
Mahatma Gandhi Central University
Motihari, India

Suyash Singh
All India Institute of Medical Sciences (AIIMS)
Raebareli, India

Vinod Kumar Singh
School of Computational and Integrative Sciences,
Jawaharlal Nehru University
New Delhi, India

Shruti Srivatsan
Department of Computer Science and Engineering,
Sri Venkateswara College of Engineering
Sriperumbudur, India

Vidhi Thakkar
University of Victoria
Victoria, Canada

Yashaswa Verma
Banaras Hindu University
Varanasi, India

Ravi Vishwakarma
DST-CIMS, Banaras Hindu University
Varanasi, India

Chapter 1

Introduction to computational methods

Machine and deep learning perspective

Hanuman Verma
Bareilly College

Akshansh Gupta
CSIR-Central Electronics Engineering Research Institute

Jyoti Singh Kirar
Banaras Hindu University

Mukesh Prasad and C. T. Lin
University of Technology Sydney

CONTENTS

DOI: 10.1201/9781003368342-1

1.1 ARTIFICIAL INTELLIGENCE

Artificial intelligence (AI) is a term used commonly in the current era. Here the term intelligence has a history way back a million year. Since the beginning of the life of Homo sapiens on earth, we are learning step by step with our experience to get a better solution in search of ease of human civilization till today (Figure 1.1). Intelligence and cognition are the two words used interchangeably with each other. However, they are different in their natural capacity. Acquiring knowledge and experience through the thought process is called the cognition process. Initially, the intelligence word comes from Latin word "Intelligere," which means pick-up. Encyclopedia Britannica defines it as "a mental quality that consists of the abilities to learn from experience, adapt to new situations, understand and handle abstract concepts, and use knowledge to manipulate one's environment." Thus, intelligence is applying the acquired knowledge in demanding situations.

Intelligence is the ability to perceive or deduce information and retaining it to be applied toward adaptive behaviors within an environment. Intelligence is defined in many ways, such as logic, learning, planning, creativity, critical thinking, reasoning, emotional knowledge, problem-solving, and perception. Human intelligence is the intellectual capability marked by a complex cognitive that includes learning from the prior experiences, adapting to new situations, understanding and handling abstract concepts, and using knowledge to manipulate and

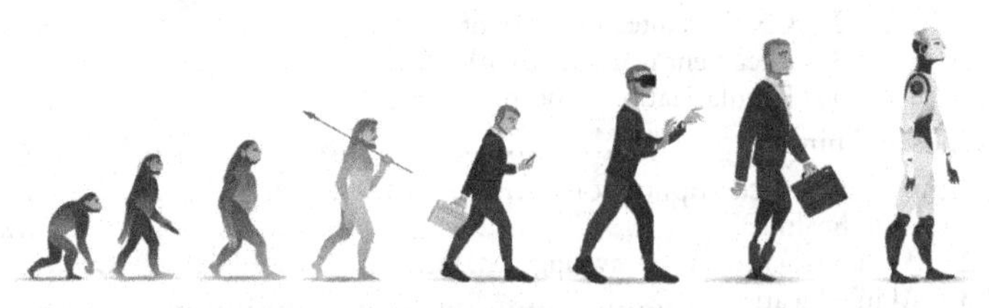

Figure 1.1 The evolution of artificial intelligence from ancient to present time. (Adopted from Google.)

analyze the social environment. The human brain, a very complex organ of the human body, can perceive, understand, predict, and manage various activities/actions happening in and out of the human body. Humans adapt to understand different activities by learning from their surroundings.

AI, on the other hand, is a wisdom that exhibited by computers or other machines compared to natural intelligence shown by humans or animals. The field of AI is building intelligent entities that can compute how to act effectively and safely in varying situations. AI has focused mainly on the following components of intelligence: learning, reasoning, problem-solving, and perception.

Learning is the process of adopting the new knowledge, abilities, concepts, attitudes, and preferences, among other things. Humans, animals, and some machines all have the ability to learn progressively. The recursive problem involves seeing the trend in previous data. Learning is skill and knowledge accumulated from repeated experiences and achieved by trial and error. Learning transforms people for a lifetime, and it is difficult to tell the difference between taught material that appears to be lost and material that cannot be retrieved. Human learning starts at birth and continues until death as a consequence of ongoing interactions between people and their environment.

The reasoning makes appropriate inferences depending on the situation. Deductive and inductive inferences have been used alternately. The primary distinction between these two modes of reasoning is that in deductive reasoning, the truth of the premises assures the validity of the conclusion, whereas in inductive reasoning, the reality of the premises lends support to the conclusion without providing total assurance. Programming computers to make conclusions, particularly deductive inferences, has seen enormous achievement. Machine learning is a learning process by the computing device; that is the study of computer algorithms that improve automatically through experience and by using input data [31]. Thus, the machine learning algorithms are processes that can learn from the data. This is accomplished with the minimum extent of human intervention without explicit programming like in abstraction form. The learning process in machine learning is improved based on the experiences of the machines throughout the execution process. It builds a model or map based on training data that can be used to make predictions or decisions. Machine learning is different from traditional

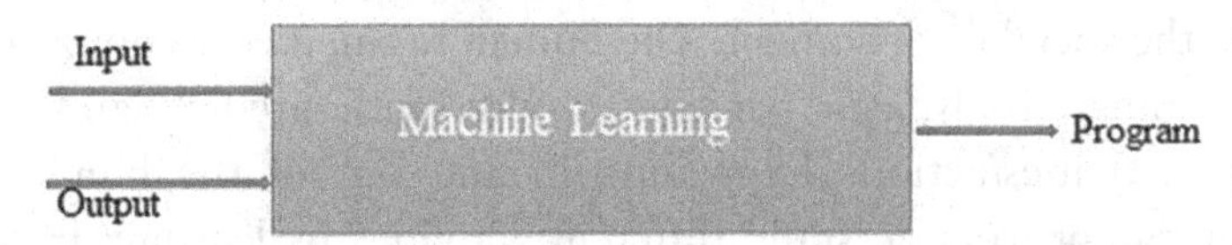

Figure 1.2 Architecture of modern machine learning. The inputs or queries and the expected output or answers are fed to a machine, shown in the above figure and it can deduce and extract the rules and map that is the program.

programming; in machine learning, the input data along with the output is passed into the machine during, the learning process. It gives out a program, presented in Figure 1.2, to better understand.

Data or data set (different sets of the data in a specific domain) plays an essential role in the building of a model in machine learning algorithms, as computationally intelligent technique is used in the algorithm to learn intrinsic properties of the data set from that data itself. Thus, learning and prediction performance are affected by the quality and quantity of the data set. In general, there are two types of data set, one is labeled data set $\{(x_i, y_i)\}_{i=1}^{N}$ and the other is an unlabeled data set $\{(x_i)\}_{i=1}^{N}$, where x_i denotes the feature vector with dimension D, represented as $x^{(j)}(j = 1, 2, \ldots, D)$. In the feature vector, each dimension represents a feature. And, y_i denotes the label or output vector corresponding to the feature vector x_i The transforming of raw data into a data set is called feature engineering [6]. Further, labeled data sets are divided into training and testing data sets. Training data sets are used to train the model, and testing data is used to examine the learning model's performance. For example, if a teacher assigns a pattern of problem set (samples) with corresponding solution set to their students for practice, then the problem set is known as training data set; if the teacher gives another pattern of the problem set without solution set for examining the performance of their students, then the set is known as a testing data. Machine learning can be taught using shallow or deep architecture.

1.2 TYPE OF LEARNING

On the basis of the problem domain and nature of the data set, learning techniques are categorized into three main categories, namely supervised, unsupervised, and reinforcement learning.

1.2.1 Supervised learning

The supervised learning technique deals with labeled data. These techniques build a mathematical model from the labeled data $\{(x_i, y_i)\}_{i=1}^{N}$ that contains the inputs variables $\{(x_i)\}_{i=1}^{N}$ and the corresponding outputs variables $\{(y_i)\}_{i=1}^{N}$ [36]. It tries to find the function $y = f(x)$ between the input and output variables; that is, it looks at a trend of data and defines a relationship. In this case, the learning is observed or supervised with the logic that output is known, and the algorithms are modified each time to optimize their results with the experience. The algorithm is trained and adjusted until it attains a suitable level of performance while measuring the error as well. In this way, supervised learning algorithms learn a function via iterative optimization of an objective function, which can then be used to predict the output associated with new inputs [32]. The types of supervised learning algorithms encompass classification (with discrete or predefined labels) and regression (with continuous labels) problems. The regression problem is used for the prediction with trend, and the model is trained with the prevalent data. In classification problems, a model is trained to categorize objects within a precise category. In this subsection, we discuss some of the most popular supervised machine learning algorithms that are utilized for the classification purpose.

1.2.1.1 Linear discriminant analysis

Linear discriminant analysis (LDA), as the name suggests, is a linear model for classification and dimensionality reduction. It is one of the most extensively used classifiers [17, 18], for classifying data into two or more categories. The fundamental theory of LDA in the scatter properties of the data set; it finds out the scatterness properties of within class and between classes data set. It maps a decision boundary using linear discriminant functions $h_i, \ \forall i = 1, \ldots, k$, if and only if, the sample $\mathbf{x}$ assigns to class c_i.

$$h_i(\mathbf{x}) \geq h_j(\mathbf{x}), \ \forall j \neq i \tag{1.1}$$

where $h_i(\mathbf{x})$ is measured in form of posterior probability function.

$$p(c_i|\mathbf{x}) = \frac{p(\mathbf{x}|c_i) * p(c_i)}{p(\mathbf{x})} \tag{1.2}$$

LDA considers the probability distribution $p(\mathbf{x}|c_i)$ and d-dimension normal distribution having mean vector μ_i and with equal covariance matrix, that is $p(\mathbf{x}|c_i) \sim N(\mu_i, \Sigma)$.

Under the assumption that covariance matrix Σ_i of all classes are identical but an arbitrary value of Σ then $h_i(\mathbf{x})$ can be expressed as:

$$h_i(\mathbf{x}) = \mathbf{w}_i^T \mathbf{x} + w_{i0} \tag{1.3}$$

where

$$\begin{aligned} \mathbf{w}_i &= \Sigma^{-1}\mu_i \\ w_{i0} &= \mu_i^T \Sigma^{-1}\mu_i + \ln p(c_i) \end{aligned} \tag{1.4}$$

Samples belonging to class c_i and class c_j are separated by a decision boundary $h_i(\mathbf{x}) - h_j(\mathbf{x}) = 0$, which is equation of a hyperplane. Sample will belong to class c_i if $h_i(\mathbf{x}) > h_j(\mathbf{x})$, otherwise belong to class c_j.

1.2.1.2 Support vector machine

Support vector machine (SVM) [9] is a well-known supervised learning classification technique, which is used for classification especially in biomedical field such as in Electroencephalography (EEG) classifications [17, 18], which has a solid statistical theoretical background. The primary goal of SVM is to find the decision boundary or best division that can separate n-dimensional space into the respective classes in order to put the new data point in the correct classes. This best decision boundary is called a hyperplane. The underlying idea of this algorithm lies in construction of a decision boundary for separating two or more classes by applying a nonlinear function to transfer an input vector from lower to higher dimension space. It applies a linear separating hyperplane to form a classifier with a maximal margin. Consider a binary classification task in which the matrix $X \in R^{l \times n}$ represents a linearly separable data set X of l points in real n dimensional space of features. The relevant target class of each data point X_i; $i = 1, 2, \ldots, l$ is represented by the diagonal matrix $D \in R^{l \times l}$ with entries $D_{ii} = +1$ or -1.

The expression of an optimal hyperplane is given as:

$$HP: \; d(\mathbf{x}) = \mathbf{w}^T \mathbf{x} + b, \tag{1.5}$$

where **x** employs a test data point in R^n that is $x \in R^n$ For linear separable data, there can be two parallel hyperplanes determined as:

$$HP1: \mathbf{w}^T\mathbf{x}_i + b = 1 \quad (1.6)$$

$$HP2: \mathbf{w}^T\mathbf{x}_i + b = -1 \quad (1.7)$$

The hyperplane defined by eq. (1.5) will lie midway between the bounding planes which are given as follows:

$$\mathbf{x}^T\mathbf{w}_{(1)} + b_{(1)} = 1, \quad \text{and} \quad \mathbf{x}^T\mathbf{w}_{(2)} + b_{(2)} = -1 \quad (1.8)$$

Here T demonstrates the transpose operation of the matrix. By a margin of $\rho = \frac{2}{||w||}$, the hyperplane will apart the two classes from each other. Belonging of the new sample point in +1 or −1 class will decide on the basis of the decision function $(w^T x+b)^*$, that values either has 1 or 0. The geometrical interpretation of this formulation is represented in Figure 1.3. SVM has the essential property of building nonlinear boundaries with relative ease.

The main objective of SVM is to maximize margin between the two hyperplanes, ρ which can be rewritten as minimization of the optimization function of SVM function

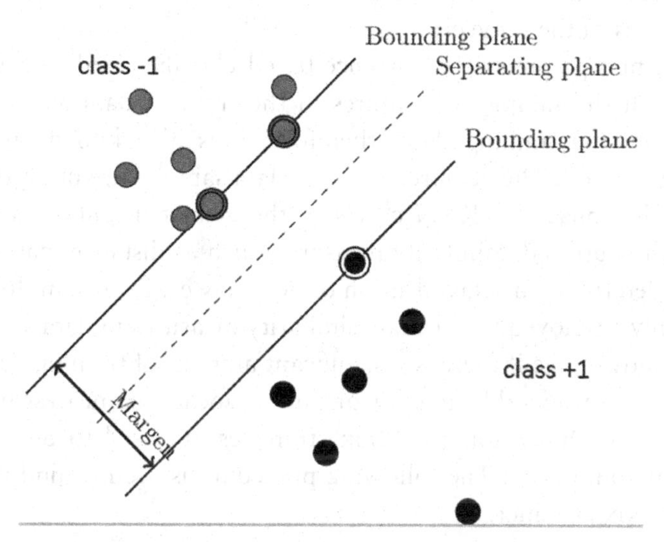

Figure 1.3 Geometrical interpretation of SVM.

$$\psi = \frac{1}{2}\|w\|^2 \tag{1.9}$$

subject to

$$c_i(\mathbf{w}^T\mathbf{x}_i + b) \geq 1, \text{ for } i = 1, \ldots, n \tag{1.10}$$

Using Lagrange's method of undetermined multipliers, the optimization problem can be solved to find optimal weights. For this optimization problem, Lagrange function is given by:

$$L(\mathbf{w}, b, \alpha) = \frac{1}{2}\|w\|^2 - \sum_{i=1}^{n} \alpha_i \left[c_i(\mathbf{w}^T\mathbf{x}_i + b) - 1\right] \tag{1.11}$$

where α_i are Lagrange multipliers.

1.2.1.3 K-nearest neighbor

K-nearest neighbor (KNN) is one of the essential classification algorithms widely used by the machine learning community. It is supervised machine learning and has various applications in data mining, intrusion detection, and pattern recognition. It has many applications such as classifications of two or more than two mental tasks [19]. The KNN is based on the premise that the features corresponding to distinct classes would typically form distinct clusters in the feature space, while their close neighbors will be members of the same class.

It is a non-parametric occurrence-based classifier [26]. It just accumulates all the samples of features in the training data and does not learn from the training data; therefore, it is also known as a lazy learning method. The acquired training data samples are utilized during the training phase. In KNN classifier, the closest neighbor estimation approach is utilized. Similarity measures, such as distance matrices, are used to determine the classification of new classes. Euclidean distance is commonly employed to calculate similarity measures in data sets. KNN has a disadvantage if there is a significant amount of training data, as it will take a considerable amount of time to locate the nearest neighbor nearest [12]. Dimension reduction strategies are used to decrease the temporal complexity. The following procedure is used to find the class of x in KNN classifier:

1. Based on the distance measure, determine the k instance to the nearest class x.
2. Now, the k instant is allowed to vote for finding the class x.

Regression analysis is the other sub-category technique in the supervised machine learning algorithms. It deals with continuous class labels rather than discrete class labels in classification algorithms. The fundamental goal of the regression analysis is to predict future patterns on the ground of past observations or seen data. It also determines the relevance of a variable to other variables in a non-deterministic manner [33] and can be used as a feature selection algorithm [18, 20]. In the subsequent sections, we discuss some of the basic regression algorithms.

1.2.1.4 Linear regression

Linear regression is a predictive analysis that determines future values of a dependent variable or variables using an independent variable or a set of independent variables in a linear manner. Regression with one independent variable is known as simple regression and regressions those contain more than one independent variable are referred to as multiple regression. If there are one dependent variable **y** and one independent variable **x**, then these variables relate to each other using the following mapping f:

$$\mathbf{y} = f(\mathbf{x}) \tag{1.12}$$

where f is a linear function.

$$f = \alpha + \beta.\mathbf{x} \tag{1.13}$$

Equation 1.13 can be referred as regression model. β depicts coefficient of slope and α stands for point of intercept. **y** denotes the continuous class label vector and **x** demonstrates a feature vector or a set of feature vectors. If y_i is an actual value instance of the **y**, and y_i^p is a corresponding predicted value, then sum of square error (difference between predicted and actual value) denoted as:

$$\text{SSE} = \sum_{i=1}^{n} (y_i^p - y_i)^2 \tag{1.14}$$

Sum of square total denotes summation of difference between actual values and mean value of actual values. It can be represented as:

$$\text{SST} = \sum_{i=1}^{n} (y_i - \bar{y})^2 \tag{1.15}$$

Here $\bar{y}$ denotes mean value of y. **Regression determination coefficient** R^2 demonstrates a strengthen of the regression analysis, and is represented as:

$$R^2 = 1 - \left(\frac{\text{SSE}}{\text{SST}}\right) \tag{1.16}$$

The higher value of R^2 indicates better regression model.

1.2.1.5 Artificial neural network

An artificial neural network (ANN), generally called a neural network (NN), is a sub-field of AI. An ANN is a computing system inspired by the human nervous system, found in the human brain that mimics the brain's decision-making ability [16]. The objective of the NN is to design a novel computer architecture and algorithm simulating a biological NN in comparison to conventional computers. Just as the human brain is used to identify patterns and categorize different types of information, NNs can perform similar tasks on given data. Like a neuron in the brain is interconnected to each other, ANN also has an artificial neuron, known as a node, which is linked to each other in a different layer of the networks, as demonstrated in Figure 1.4. These neurons are building blocks of NN. This ANN is obtained by combining two or more artificial neurons, which can solve a real complex problem by transferring information in the neurons. The connection between the neurons, known as edges, can transfer the signal to another neuron, as the synapses transfer the signal in a biological brain. The neurons and edges are associated with a weight (w_i) that adjusts as a learning process in ANN, with the associated weight optimizing the signal's strength at the edges. ANN accomplishes computations through a process of learning, where the network learns by adjusting the weights. The neurons are combined into layers, and information pass from the first layer (known as the input layer) to the last layer (known as the output layer) through some possible intermediate layers (known as the hidden layer), shown in Figure 1.5.

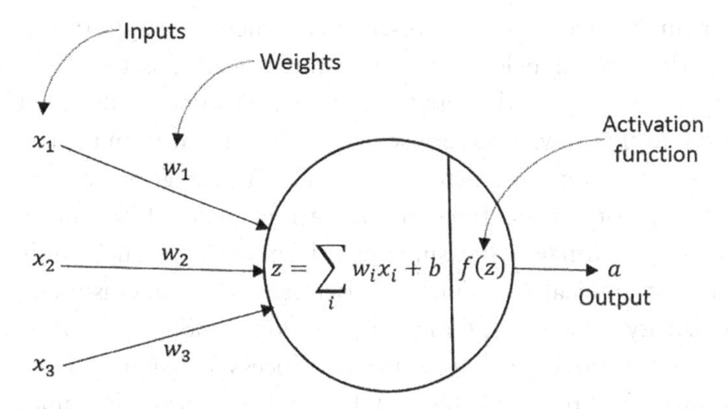

Figure 1.4 Architecture of a typical neural network node. The inputs (x_i) and weights (w_i) are multiplied and summed, and bias b is added and passed in the activation function f.

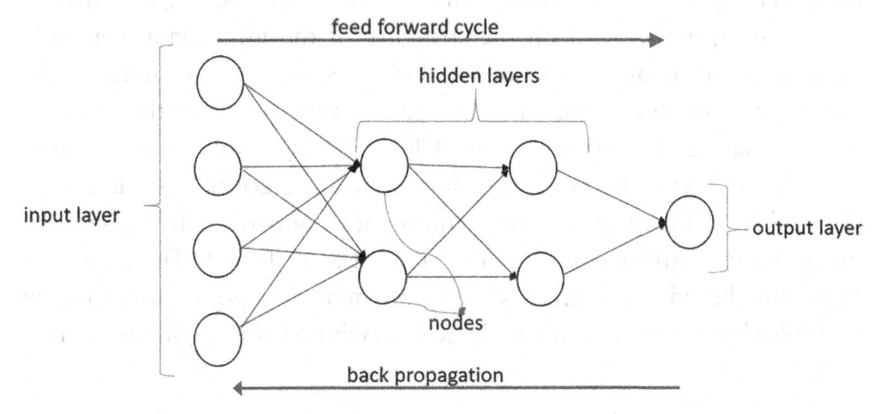

Figure 1.5 Architecture of neural network and forward and backward learning [11].

The output of a node is computed as a weighted (w_i) sum of its input (x_i), known as the net sum $z = \sum_i w_i\, x_i + b$, where b is the bias [13], the net sum, which is a linear sum passed into an activation function $f\,(z)$, is a nonlinear transformation, which enables to network to learn the complex patterns. The activation function determines whether a particular neuron in the network should be activated.

1.2.2 Unsupervised learning

The unsupervised learning technique deals with the learning process in the absence of available labeled data. This takes unlabeled data $\{(x_i)\}_{i=1}^{N}$, that comprises only inputs variables, then learn by itself, and determines structure in the given data. The discovered structure may be the grouping or clustering of unlabeled data. Here the objective is to interpret the primary distribution in the input data based on some similarity measure functions. In this way, unsupervised algorithms learn from the unlabeled data, and there is no instructor or teacher, and categorize the data in a different category. It identifies the similarities in the data and responds with some performance measures based on available such similarities. A significant application of unsupervised learning is in clustering, probability density estimation, finding associations among the features, and dimensionality reduction. Clustering is a process of assigning a set of data points into a group (called clusters). Data points within the same cluster are similar according to one or more predesigned measures (similarity measure). In contrast, data points in another cluster are dissimilar from those in the previous cluster. The different clustering techniques consider some assumptions based on the structure of the input data, generally defined and evaluated by some similarity metric. For example, in the fuzzy c-means algorithm, the similarity is measured via the distance between data and cluster centroids. Clustering algorithms may be based on a classical set or fuzzy set. The hard c-means algorithm is based on a classical set, which restricts each data point to only one cluster, with the membership degree (u_{ji}) of each data point to be 0 or 1. The clustering algorithm based on a fuzzy set allows each data point to belong to multiple clusters with membership degrees whose value lies in the interval $[0, 1]$.

1.2.2.1 Hard c-means algorithm

Hard c-means algorithm groups the unlabeled data points into the cluster, and it is based on the classical set theory that is data either belongs ($u_{ji} = 1$) to a set or does not belong ($u_{ji} = 0$) to a set [30]. Suppose we have to assign the unlabeled data $\{(x_i)\}_{i=1}^{N}$ in c number of clusters. In this each cluster is associated with a centroid and objective to minimize the sum of distances between the data point (x_i) and their corresponding clusters centroids (v_j), which is mathematically defined as:

$$\min\ J_{\text{HCM}} = \sum_{j=1}^{c} \sum_{i=1}^{N} u_{ji}\ d^2(x_i,\ v_j) \tag{1.17}$$

In the above minimization equation, $u_{ji} \in \{0,1\}$ along with constraints $\sum_{j=1}^{c} u_{ji} = 1$. To minimize the objective function of HCM, the membership and centroids are updated as:

$$v_j = \frac{\sum_{i=1}^{N} u_{ji}\ x_i}{\sum_{i=1}^{N} u_{ji}} \tag{1.18}$$

$$u_{ji} = \begin{cases} 1 & d^2\left(x_i,\ v_j\right) < d^2\left(x_i,\ v_r\right) \quad \forall\, j \neq r \\ 0 & \\ & \text{otherwise} \end{cases} \tag{1.19}$$

1.2.2.2 Fuzzy c-means algorithm

The fuzzy c-means (FCM) algorithm introduced by Bezdek [5] is a well-known unsupervised clustering algorithm based on fuzzy set theory [47] to handle the vague information in imprecise data and has been used in many applications successfully. In a fuzzy set, data points belong to their respective set with some degree of belongingness termed as membership degree ($u_{ji} \in [0,1]$), and the data point that does not belong to that set with some degree of non-belongingness is termed as non-membership degree $(1 - u_{ji})$. Suppose, we have to assign the unlabeled data $\{(x_i)\}_{i=1}^{N}$ in c number of classes which is the number of clusters. The FCM is an alternative nonlinear optimization problem formulated with an objective function J_{FCM} , mathematically defined as:

$$\min\ J_{\text{FCM}} = \sum_{j=1}^{c} \sum_{i=1}^{N} u_{ji}^{m} \left\| x_i - v_j \right\|^2 \tag{1.20}$$

In the above objective function, the term $\left\| x_i - v_j \right\|^2$ is Euclidean distance between the centroids (v_j) and data points (x_i), and $m\,(> 1)$ is the fuzzifier constant. To optimize the FCM objective function, it solved with the condition $\sum_{j=1}^{c} u_{ji} = 1$ using alternative optimization technique, and its extrema, that is centroids (v_j) and membership degree (u_{ij}) is obtained as:

$$v_j = \frac{\sum_{i=1}^{N} u_{ji}^{m}\ x_i}{\sum_{i=1}^{N} u_{ji}^{m}} \tag{1.21}$$

$$u_{ji} = \frac{1}{\sum_{r=1}^{c} \left(\frac{d(x_i, v_i)}{d(x_i, v_r)} \right)^{\frac{2}{m-1}}} \tag{1.22}$$

It can be observed that u_{ij} is a function of distance $\|x_i - v_j\|^2$ and data points which are near to centroid, more membership value is assigned, and which is far from the centroid, less membership value is assigned. The FCM is an iterative method that updates the centroids and membership degree to the data points and minimizes the objective function. Further, to improve the FCM clustering performance in various applications, many variants of FCM have been introduced [1, 8, 34, 39, 45].

1.2.2.3 Intuitionistic fuzzy c-means algorithm

With the development of the higher-order fuzzy set theory, the intuitionistic fuzzy c-means (IFCM) algorithm has been proposed by Xu and Wu [46] based on the intuitionistic fuzzy set (IFS) theory [3, 4] to handle the uncertainty in the real problem. The IFS theory is an extension of fuzzy set theory, and it is defined in terms of membership $(u_{ji} \in [0,1])$, non-membership $(\nu_{ji} \in [0,1])$, and hesitation degree $(\pi_{ji} = (1 - u_{ji} - \nu_{ji}) \in [0,1])$. In IFS theory, data points $\{x_i)\}_{i=1}^{N})$ are represented in intuitionistic fuzzification form as $x_i^{\mathrm{IFS}} = (u(x_i), \nu(x_i), \pi(x_i))$ in order to incorporate the qualitative information. Suppose we have to assign the unlabeled data $\{x_i)\}_{i=1}^{N}$ in c number of classes, and the data is represented in terms of an intuitionistic fuzzy set. The IFCM is a nonlinear optimization problem and is a variant of the FCM algorithm, where Euclidian intuitionistic fuzzy distance $\| x_i^{\mathrm{IFS}} - v_j^{\mathrm{IFS}}\|^2 = (((u(x_i) - u(v_j))^2 + ((\nu(x_i) - \nu(v_j))^2 + ((\pi(x_i) - \pi(v_j))^2)$ between data points $x_i^{\mathrm{IFS}} = (u(x_i), \nu(x_i), \pi(x_i))$ and centroids $v_j^{\mathrm{IFS}} = (u(v_j), \nu(v_j), \pi(v_j))$ is used to formulate the objective function. The objective function of IFCM is formulated as [46]:

$$\min\ J_{\mathrm{IFCM}} = \sum_{j=1}^{c} \sum_{i=1}^{N} u_{ji}^{m} \left\|x_i^{\mathrm{IFS}} - v_j^{\mathrm{IFS}}\right\|^2 \tag{1.23}$$

In IFCM, $m(>1)$ is fuzzifier constant and $u_{ji} \in [0,1] \subset U_{(c\times N)}$ is the membership value of ith data to the jth cluster. Using alternative optimization technique, the IFCM optimization problem has been solved with the condition $\sum_{j=1}^{c} u_{ji} = 1$. The membership function u_{ji} and centroids of clusters $v_j^{\mathrm{IFS}} = (u(v_j), \nu(v_j), \pi(v_j))$ are obtained as [46]:

$$u_{ji} = \frac{1}{\sum_{r=1}^{c} \left(\frac{\| x_i^{\text{IFS}} - v_j^{\text{IFS}} \|^2}{\| x_i^{\text{IFS}} - V_r^{\text{IFS}} \|^2} \right)^{\frac{2}{m-1}}} \quad (1.24)$$

$$u\left(v_j\right) = \frac{\sum_{i=1}^{N} u_{ji}^m \; u\left(x_i\right)}{\sum_{i=1}^{N} u_{ji}^m} \quad (1.25)$$

$$\nu\left(v_j\right) = \frac{\sum_{=1}^{N} u_{ij}^m \; \nu\left(x_j\right)}{\sum_{j=1}^{N} u_{ij}^m} \quad (1.26)$$

$$\pi\left(v_j\right) = \frac{\sum_{=1}^{N} u_{ij}^m \; \pi\left(x_j\right)}{\sum_{j=1}^{N} u_{ij}^m} \quad (1.27)$$

The IFCM is an iterative method that updates the centroids and membership degree to the data points, minimizes the objective function, and provides promising results in uncertain information. Further, to improve the IFCM performance in various applications, many variants of IFCM have been developed [7, 25, 41–43].

1.2.3 Reinforcement learning

This type of learning is one of the basic machine learning approaches besides supervised and unsupervised learning that interacts with the environment. In reinforcement learning, models are trained to make a series of decisions based on the feedback and rewards they receive for their actions. During the learning period, the machine is rewarded for achieving a goal in complex and uncertain situations. It is used to solve a particular type of problem requiring successive decision-making with a long-term objective such as game playing, robotics, resource management, or logistics.

1.2.4 Deep learning

Deep learning (DL) is a subarea of machine learning based on conventional ANN with representation learning [37], which attempts to mimic like the human brain. Representation learning is a set of techniques that allow a machine to be fed input with raw data and then automatically learn the representations required for classification or detection [28].

That kind of ML is motivated by the structure of a complex human brain with billions of neurons. DL is derived from the conventional ANN and uses the many-layered structure of NNs to design a structure like the human brain. It comprises many hidden layers to learn different features with more abstraction and perform complex operations. The first layer extracts the low-level features, whereas the last layer extracts the high-level features. In DL, the word deep refers to the use of many layers in the network, and these number of layers used to build the model for the data, determines the depth of the model. Machine learning is a subset of AI, and DL is a subset of machine learning that implies that DL is a subset of AI, represented by the Venn diagram in Figure 1.6.

One advantage of DL over the ML is that there is no requirement for feature engineering (feature generation, feature extraction, features selection) from the raw data in DL algorithms, unlike the utmost necessity of feature engineering in ML algorithms, shown in Figure 1.7. The feature engineering step is already part of the process in DL. This feature of DL encourages researchers to extract the relevant features using less human interaction and field knowledge [28]. The second advantage of DL is that it is powered by a vast amount of data. In the big data era, machines and humans generate vast amounts of data, an opportunity for

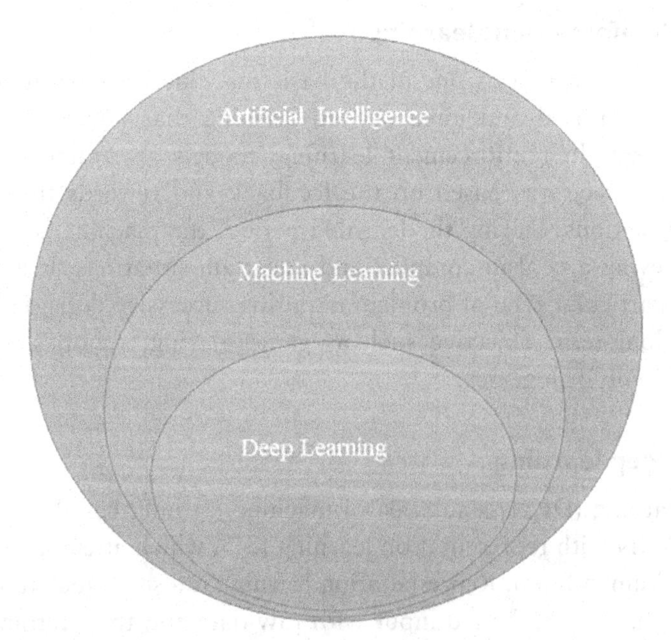

Figure 1.6 Relationship between deep learning, machine learning, and AI.

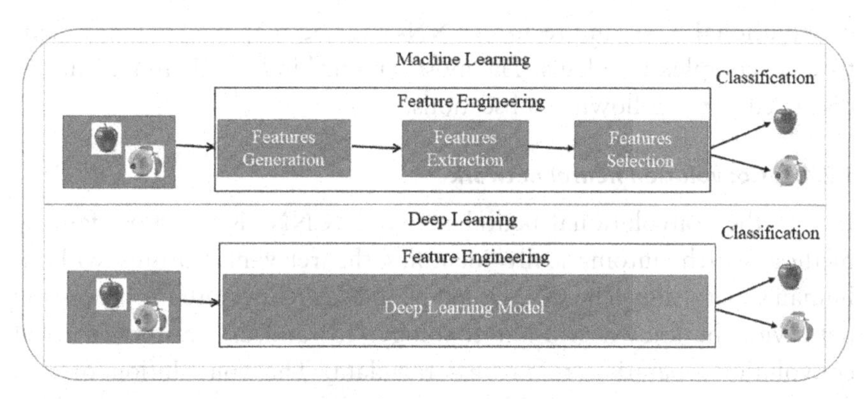

Figure 1.7 Feature engineering in deep learning and machine learning.

DL. Deep learning models' performance (prediction and classification) tends to increase as the amount of training data increases, whereas other machine learning models such as Naive Bayes Classifier and SVM stop improving after a certain point. There are some performance features that distinguish why DL is used over the ML [2]:

- *Universal learning technique:* DL has been used in many application domains generally where humans are unable to make decisions over the problem and give a promising performance; that is, it is sometimes called universal learning.
- *Robustness:* In DL, during the training under the consideration problem, the optimized feature engineering is automatically learned, which delivers the robustness of the model.
- *Generalization:* The pre-trained DL model that has been trained on similar kinds of data and applications that can be used is known as transfer learning. It uses the knowledge learned from the different data types or applications and uses the same DL on a new task as DL needs an enormous amount of labeled data to train the model and design a good performance model. However, in some cases, a large amount of labeled data is not available. The transfer learning approach is used where data is insufficient.

In recent years, the DL has become the most popular kind of learning with the considerable growth and evaluation of big data. Most scientific fields have felt the impact of the DL approach. The DL architectures such as deep NNs, deep reinforcement learning, deep belief networks, convolutional NNs, and recurrent NNs have been applied in many fields to solve complex problems. The most famous kind of DL architecture is discussed in the following subsections.

1.2.4.1 Convolution neural network

In DL, the convolutional neural network (CNN) is the most famous method which automatically identifies the relevant features without human supervision. The CNN is a type of DL architecture for processing data with the known grid-like topology [15] and uses a mathematical convolution operation to process the data. The convolution of two functions f and g is defined as $(f * g)\,(t) = \int f(a)\; g(t - a)\; da$, which yields a new function $(f * g)$ that demonstrates how the other function changes the shape of one function. It employed a convolution operation: hence, the network's name is the CNN. Three key features of CNN, such as sparse interactions, equivalent representations, and parameter sharing, are identified by Goodfellow et al. [15]. The weight sharing feature in CNN reduces the number of trainable network parameters. In general, used CNN, which is similar to the multi-layer perceptron (MLP), comprises mainly three types of layers: convolution, pooling, and fully connected layers.

- *Convolution layer:* In CNN architecture, the convolution layer is the core layer that uses convolution operation in general matrix multiplication, along with a set of learnable filters, also known as kernels which slide over the entire image and look for the pattern. The kernel is a gird of discrete value. The input data, represented as n–dimensional array, is convolved with the kernel filter and determines the feature map. It is the first layer in CNN architecture, mainly associated with identifying features from raw data, which is achieved by applying filters having a predefined size followed by a convolution operation. The first layer determines the simple features like edges in an image, and the second and higher layers begin to determine the higher-level features.
- *Pooling layer:* In CNN architecture, the pooling layer is a down-sampling of the feature map and applies a pooling operation, which reduces the dimension of feature maps while retaining the relevant information. In other words, the pooling approach reduces the large-size feature maps to smaller maps, which is the dimensional

reduction. It accepts each feature map output from the convolutional layer and down-samples it. Various pooling methods: max pooling, min pooling, gated pooling, tree pooling, average pooling, global max pooling, and global average pooling are available for utilization in pooling layers.

- *Activation function (or Transfer function):* In ANN, the activation function decides whether a neuron should be activated or not. The important feature of an activation function is to add nonlinearity in ANN, which gives the CNN ability to learn the complex pattern in the data. It takes in the output signal from the previous neurons, determines the net sum and converts it into some form based on an activation function that can be taken as input to the subsequent neurons. The following types of the activation function mainly used in CNN are summarized below:
  Sigmoid: The sigmoid activation function $f : R \rightarrow [0,1]$ is mathematically defined as:

$$f(z) = \frac{1}{(1+e^{-z})} \tag{1.28}$$

  Tanh: The Tanh activation function $f : R \rightarrow [-1,1]$ is mathematically defined as:

$$f(z) = \frac{e^{z}-e^{-z}}{e^{z}+e^{-z}} \tag{1.29}$$

  ReLU (rectified linear unit): It is the most commonly used activation function in CNN, which converts the input value to a positive number, and is mathematically defined as:

$$f(z) = \max(0, z) \tag{1.30}$$

  Other activation fucntions are leaky ReLU, noisy ReLU, softmax, parametric linear units, etc.
- *Fully connected layer (FC):* The FC layer is placed at the end of CNN architecture. Fully connected or dense layers associate each neuron in one layer with every neuron in another and so-called fully connected methods. Further, a flattened matrix converts 2–Dimensional arrays from the last pooled or convolution layer into a single long continuous linear vector. This input is in the

form of a vector created from the feature map with flattening is fed as input to the fully connected layer to classify the image or CNN output.

- *Loss function:* In CNN architecture, the loss function is used in the output layer to compute the predicted error created during training, which helps a network understand whether the learning is in the right direction. This error is the difference between the actual output and the predicted output by the model. Several types of loss functions are used in the various NNs are Mean Squared Error (MSE), Mean Absolute Error (MAE), Mean Absolute Percentage Error (MAPE), Cross-Entropy, or Softmax loss function, Euclidean loss function, and Hinge loss function.

1.2.4.2 CNN architecture variants

CNN is one of the best-supervised learning techniques for understanding and analyzing image processing. Many technology companies, such as Google, Microsoft, Facebook, etc., have established active research groups to explore the new CNN architectures. Many variants of CNN architectures have been introduced to solve complex real-life problems with time. The first CNN-based architecture was LeNet [29], which used backpropagation for training the network. The evolution of different variants of CNN is shown in Figure 1.8 [23]. Some famous CNN architectures: AlexNet, VGG-16, VGG-19, Inception and GoogLeNet, ResNet, Squeeze Net, DenseNet, Shuffle Net, boost deep learning [2]. Some of these models are contenders in the ImageNet Large Scale Visual Recognition Challenge (ILSVRC), trained on ImageNet data. These architectures are different in topology, the number of layers (this is the depth of the network), the types of optimizers used, and many more aspects. These models are available as pre-trained models on various deep learning frameworks such as Tensorflow, PyTorch, and many more. These deep learning models can be used as transfer learning for a similar type of data.

1.2.4.2.1 AlexNet

The development of deep CNN architecture began with the introduction of LeNet [29]. To achieve innovative results in the field of image recognition and classification, Krizhevsky et al. introduced the AlexNet [24] to increase the learning ability of CNN by increasing its depth and

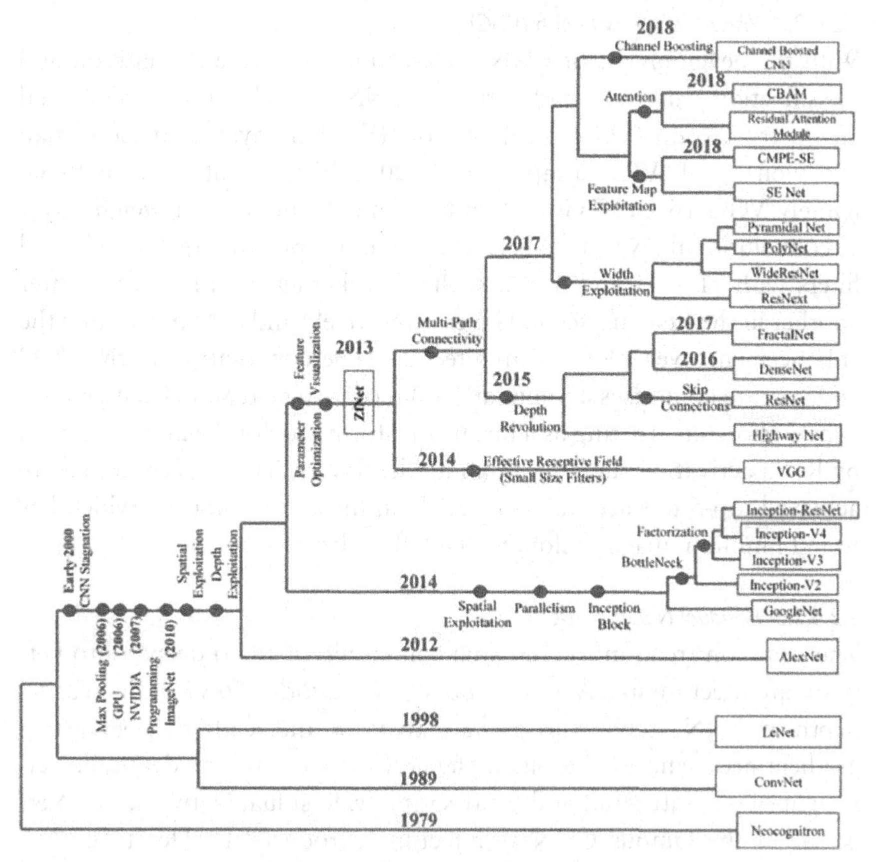

Figure 1.8 Evolutionary history of CNN architectures [23].

adding several parameters. The AlexNet model is trained and designed on the ImageNet data set to classify the 1.2 million high-resolution images into 1,000 different classes. The AlexNet architecture consists of eight layers, out of which five were convolutional layers with a combination of pooling layers, and the other three were fully connected layers with learnable parameters. The nonlinearity ReLU activation function is used in each of these layers except the output layer and found that ReLU accelerated the speed of the training process by almost six times. To avoid overfitting, the dropout layers and data augmentation are implemented. The AlexNet model has 60 million parameters with 650,000 neurons. It has 62.3 million learnable parameters and achieved top-1 and top-5 error rates of 37.5% and 17.0%; AlexNet architecture won the Imagenet large-scalez visual recognition challenge (ILSVRC) in 2012.

1.2.4.2.2 Visual Geometry Group (VGG)

With the development of CNN architecture for image recognition and classification, an easy and efficient CNN model, known as Visual Geometry Group (VGG) [38] proposed by Simonyan and Zisserman and won the ILSVRC competition in 2014. Two architecture of VGG, namely VGG-16 and VGG-19 with 16 and 19 number of weight layer in convolutional layer have been designed. It replaced large kernel-sized filters with 11×11 and 5×5, with 3×3 kernel-sized filters one after another in the first and second layer respectively and it demonstrated the enhancement over AlexNet architecture. The convolution in the VGG architecture comprises a minimal 3×3 receptive field and also uses 1×1 convolution filters acting as a linear transformation of the input followed by ReLu activation function in all hidden layers. The VGG architecture achieved top-5 test accuracy of 92.7% in ImageNet data set, which has over 14 million images belonging to $1,000$ classes.

1.2.4.2.3 Residual Network (ResNet)

The common trend in the research community is to go deeper into network architecture like AlexNet and VGG network. However, increasing depth in CNN architecture is hard to train and leads to a vanishing gradient problem. As a result, as the network increases its depth, its performance gets saturated or degrades rapidly. Residual Network (ResNet) is one of the famous CNN architecture introduced by He et al. [21]. The core idea of ResNet is introducing an identity shortcut connection in the residual block. In this architecture, 34-layer plain network in the architecture comprises that is inspired by VGG-19, and shortcut connections or skip connections are added to these layers. These skip connections or the residual blocks then convert the architecture into the residual network. Many variants of ResNet architectures: ResNet-18, ResNet-34, ResNet-50, ResNet-101, ResNet-110, ResNet-152, ResNet-164, ResNet-1202 etc have been designed, which have the same concept but with a different number of layers. The ResNet model is trained on the ImageNet data set with a depth of up to 152 layers, which is ResNet 152, and achieved a 3.57% error. This result won the ILSVRC competition in 2015 for the classification task.

1.2.4.3 Recurrent neural network

A recurrent neural network [35], abbreviated as RNN, is a deep learning architecture for processing sequential data such as time series, speech, text, and videos. It is designed with recurrence relations and so-called RNN. A recurrence relation, in mathematics, is the set of equation(s) that defines the next element of a sequence as a function of preceding elements of the same sequence. This relation is basically defined as a map, and it determines the next value from the initial value. For example, the Fibonacci series follows a recurrence relation. RNN is derived from the feed-forward NNs with no limitation of back loops that can use an internal state (memory) to process variable-length data sequences. The output of a particular layer is saved and further fed back to the input for determines the layer's output. Its architecture comprises an input layer, hidden layers, and an output layer, where the updated weights and bias of all the hidden layers are the same, and hence these hidden layers can be rolled in together in a single recurrent layer.

Bidirectional recurrent neural networks (BRNN), long short-term memory (LSTM), and gated recurrent unit (GRU) are the variants of the RNN which overcome the issues in the general RNN. In BRNN, the information is pulled in the future to improve accuracy. LSTM is a famous RNN architecture introduced by Hochreiter and Schmidhuber [22] and overcomes the vanishing and exploding gradient problem of RNN architecture. It worked to handle the problem of long-term dependencies and proved to be very promising for modeling sequential data. A standard LSTM unit comprises a cell, an input gate, an output gate, and a forget gate. These three gates in LSTM control the flow of information and transmit needed information to determine the output in the network. GRU is similar to LSTM and also works to address the short-term memory problem of RNN, which uses hidden states, a reset gate, and an update gate to process the data. The RNN, GRU, and LSTM have supervised learning techniques. Moreover, the RNN, which includes the LSTM and GRU methods, has also been used for unsupervised learning in many applications.

1.2.4.4 Regularization in deep learning

In the process of developing and training a model, generally, there is a scenario where the trained model well performed on training data but does not succeed on the test data (unseen data). This scenario is called overfitting, is the model is overfitted for the data. Overfitting is a central issue during the generalization of the training model. Another scenario, where the model does not learn a sufficient amount from the training data and does not generalize well on the test data, is termed underfitting. The underfitting can be very easily identified by the performance metrics. If training performance is not good, try other models tuning hyperparameters for better results. Regularization is a set of tactics used to reduce overfitting or generalization error. There are various regularization techniques in deep learning, and some most popular are: $L1$ and $L2$ regularization, dropout, data augmentation, and early stopping, discussed below.

- *$L1$ and $L2$ regularization:* It is the most common types of regularization, which update the cost function by adding regularization term in the loss function and reducing the weight (w), defined as:

$$L1 \text{ regularization} : \text{cost function} = \text{loss} + \frac{\lambda}{2\,m}\sum \|w\|$$

$$L2 \text{ regularization} : \text{cost function} = \text{loss} + \frac{\lambda}{2\,m}\sum \|w\|^2$$

- *Dropout:* This technique is mostly used for generalization. In this method, the training model randomly dropped or deactivated some neurons for a layer in each training epoch based on the defined percentage. Furthermore, the dropped neurons are not part of forward-propagation and backward-propagation during the training.
- *Data augmentation:* The easiest way to avoid overfitting is to expand the size of the training data. To achieve this goal, one technique, data augmentation, is used. In data augmentation, several methods such as flipping, scaling, shifting, rotation, cropping, color space, and noise injection are used to artificially generate the data and expand the training data's size.
- *Early stopping:* In the training process, too many epochs can result in overfitting, whereas too few may result in an underfitting issue. To obtain the optimal number of epochs, in the training model, the validation error on validation data is recorded, and when there is no improvement on the validation error, the epochs stopped, rather than going through all the epochs fixed. This technique of stopping early is called Early Stopping.

1.3 INTERNET OF THINGS

Internet of Things (IoT) is a network of networked computing devices, mechanical and digital machinery, products, animals, and people with unique identities (UIDs) and the capability to transfer collected data without human-to-computer or human-to-human interaction. The human with a heart monitor implant, the animal with a biochip transponder, the automobile and others with built-in sensors to alert the driver when tire pressure is low, and any other artificial or natural object that can be assigned an Internet Protocol (IP) address and transfer data over a network are examples of things in the IoT. Organizations are rapidly turning to IoT to improve operational efficiency, better understand customers to deliver better customer service, enhance decision-making, and increase corporate value.

The utility of IoT has been found in many areas: medical and health care, consumer applications such as smart home and elder care, transportation, buildings and home automation, vehicle-to-everything communication (V2X), manufacturing, agriculture, and maritime. In the health care system, an IoT-based medical system is sometimes referred to as the Internet of Medical things (IoMT) [10, 14, 40]. The primary purpose of the IoMT is remote health monitoring and an emergency health alarm system. The monitoring parameters can vary from simple measurement of the blood pressure to observations of some specific biomedical signals (brain, heart, muscles, and others) [27].

1.4 ARTIFICIAL INTELLIGENCE APPLICATIONS

The intelligence in AI is demonstrated via the machine that tries to mimic a human brain, which has become very popular in today's world. It can solve complex real-world problems more efficiently and make our daily lives more comfortable and fast. AI has various applications in many fields. Some applications of AI are summarized in the following subsections.

1.4.1 AI in healthcare

Computational intelligence has many applications in the healthcare system and helps patients with diagnosis and treatment. AI builds the tools with existing medical data that can be used in the early detection of diseases and identify cancer cells. It uses historical medical data and intelligence for the discovery of new drugs. Through medical imaging such as MRI, CT scan, ultrasound, etc., the medical image used for computing and analysis identify the tumors and other malignant growths faster than radiologists with a considerably lower margin of error. The robot-assisted surgery is less invasive and has faster recovery than traditional approaches that reduce hospital stay. Telemedicine allows medical professionals to check, diagnose, and treat patients without physical visits and reduces the workload of hospitals. The computational intelligence systems help day-to-day administrative tasks minimize human errors and maximize efficiency in the health care system. The iWatch or Fitbit device collects many data such as sleep pattern, calories burnt, heart rate, and more from the individual that helps early detection. In the coronavirus disease 2019 (COVID-19) outbreak, AI is used to understand the dynamic trend of COVID-19 outbreaks and for ahead prediction [44], processing healthcare claims to identify the person with COVID-19 positive or negative by analyzing the data.

1.4.2 AI in navigation and traveling

GPS technology using CNN and graph NN suggests accurate timing and details such as the number of lanes, turning points with distance, and road types behind obstructions on the roads. AI can also help users find available hotels, flights, and other traveling mediums for the users. Uber and many logistics companies use AI to analyze road traffic and optimize routes.

1.4.3 AI in education

AI helps educators in academic and non-teaching tasks such as preparing the report, tracking class attendance through the ERP system, conducting online examination, managing enrollment, courses, and other administrative tasks. These data are helpful in further analysis. It helps educators in teaching by creating digital content like video lectures, presentations, and some software to demonstrate more effectively, online classes, and textbook guides. This would help extend the reach of education in urban and remote areas.

1.4.4 AI in agriculture

Climate change, food security, and population growth concerns have pushed the world to seek more advanced approaches to a large amount of production. This is possible one way with computational intelligence in agriculture to reduce human resources and proper monitoring of crops. To achieve this goal, agriculture today uses AI for solid and crop monitoring, drones, and predictive analysis, which is very helpful for farmers.

1.4.5 AI in robotics

AI has an incredible role in robotics because it helps the robots learn the model and execute the tasks with complete autonomy without requiring any human intervention. The complete automation that is the technology not only performs the particular task but also observes, checks, and improves the process without any human intervention. This is achieved with the assistance of AI. Recently, developed Humanoid robots such as Sophia and Erica are the best examples of AI in the field of robotics that can talk and behave like humans.

1.4.6 AI in social media

Social media platforms, such as Telegram, Facebook, Twitter, and Snapchat, contain billions of personal user profiles and generate a huge amount of data from information through message posts, tweets, chats, etc. To manage this huge amount of data that is generated every moment, AI will help by learning from the data. AI in social media is used to identify hate speech, offensive content, the latest trends, hashtags, and requirement of different users by analyzing a considerable amount of data.

1.4.7 AI in automobiles

Some automotive companies are engaged in developing self-driving vehicles, which can make the journey safer by using AI along with radar, cloud services, cameras, GPS, and other control systems to operate the vehicle. Tesla's self-driving car is a famous example of an autonomous vehicle. The computer vision, deep learning, and image detection that is AI is used to develop cars that can automatically detect objects in the vehicle's vicinity and drive without human intervention.

1.4.8 AI in gaming

In the gaming field, the computer game system supported by AI is under exploration, in which AI is engaged to get responsive, intelligent behaviors mainly in non-player characters like human-like intelligence in video games. AI-leveraged machines are able to play tactical games such as chess, where the AI thinks and analyzes many possible choices.

1.4.9 AI in space exploration

A huge amount of data is required to explore the space, for which AI is the best way to process the data. The astronomers used AI to help discover galaxies, planets, stars, and, more recently, identify a distant eight-planet solar system. NASA and ISRO also use AI for space exploration like computerized image analysis and autonomous building spacecraft.

1.4.10 AI in banking and finance

The banking and finance industries are one of the early adopters of AI application that provides customer support, detect credit card frauds and anomalies, chatbot, adaptive intelligence, and trading. Thus, banking and finance services become more valuable and personalized experiences to customers and reduce risks. Through a huge amount of data, AI can learn to capture the complex trends in past data and predict how these trends might repeat in the future.

1.4.11 AI in everyday life

AI has much influence on our everyday life. A few of them are discussed below:

Online shopping: AI is helping the customer to find related products with recommended color, size, or even brand based on their previous searches and purchases during online shopping.

Digital personal assistants: Smartphones use AI, which provides personal services to the users and uses other particular apps.

Cyber security: Cyber-attacks can be recognized and resolved using AI, based on recognizing patterns and backtracking the attacks.

Surveillance: AI-based surveillance is automatic and works all time, and provides footage in real-time for security purposes and comparison to manual monitoring of CCTV cameras.

Entertainment: AI uses many platforms such as entertainment, e-commerce, social media, video YouTube, etc. These platforms use the recommendation system to provide required content to users to increase engagement.

REFERENCES

[1] Mohamed N Ahmed, Sameh M Yamany, Nevin Mohamed, Aly A Farag, and Thomas Moriarty. A modified fuzzy c-means algorithm for bias field estimation and segmentation of mri data. *IEEE Transactions on Medical Imaging*, 21(3):193–199, 2002.

[2] Laith Alzubaidi, Jinglan Zhang, Amjad J Humaidi, Ayad Al-Dujaili, Ye Duan, Omran Al-Shamma, J Santamaría, Mohammed A Fadhel, Muthana Al-Amidie, and Laith Farhan. Review of deep learning: Concepts, cnn architectures, challenges, applications, future directions. *Journal of Big Data*, 8(1):1–74, 2021.

[3] Krassimir Atanassov. Intuitionistic fuzzy sets. *International Journal Bioautomation*, 20:1, 2016.

[4] Krassimir T Atanassov. More on intuitionistic fuzzy sets. *Fuzzy Sets and Systems*, 33(1):37–45, 1989.

[5] James C Bezdek. *Pattern Recognition with Fuzzy Objective Function Algorithms*. Springer Science & Business Media: Berlin, Germany, 2013.

[6] Andriy Burkov. *The Hundred-Page Machine Learning Book*, volume 1. Andriy Burkov: Quebec City, Canada, 2019.

[7] Tamalika Chaira. A novel intuitionistic fuzzy c means clustering algorithm and its application to medical images. *Applied Soft Computing*, 11(2):1711–1717, 2011.

[8] Songcan Chen and Daoqiang Zhang. Robust image segmentation using fcm with spatial constraints based on new kernel-induced distance measure. *IEEE Transactions on Systems, Man, and Cybernetics, Part B (Cybernetics)*, 34(4):1907–1916, 2004.

[9] Corinna Cortes and Vladimir Vapnik. Support-vector networks. *Machine Learning*, 20(3):273–297, 1995.

[10] Cristiano André Da Costa, Cristian F Pasluosta, Björn Eskofier, Denise Bandeira Da Silva, and Rodrigo da Rosa Righi. Internet of health things: Toward intelligent vital signs monitoring in hospital wards. *Artificial Intelligence in Medicine*, 89:61–69, 2018.

[11] Sanjiv R Das, Karthik Mokashi, and Robbie Culkin. Are markets truly efficient? experiments using deep learning algorithms for market movement prediction. *Algorithms*, 11(9):138, 2018.

[12] Belur V Dasarathy. *Nearest Neighbor (NN) Norms: NN Pattern Classification Techniques*. IEEE Computer Society Press: Washington, DC, 1991.

[13] Richard O Duda, Peter E Hart, et al. *Pattern Classification*. John Wiley & Sons: Hoboken, NJ, 2006.

[14] Arthur Gatouillat, Youakim Badr, Bertrand Massot, and Ervin Sejdić. Internet of medical things: A review of recent contributions dealing with cyber-physical systems in medicine. *IEEE Internet of Things Journal*, 5(5):3810–3822, 2018.

[15] Ian Goodfellow, Yoshua Bengio, and Aaron Courville. *Deep Learning*. MIT Press: Cambridge, MA, 2016.

[16] Daniel Graupe. *Principles of Artificial Neural Networks*, volume 7. World Scientific: Singapore, 2013.

[17] Akshansh Gupta, Ramesh Kumar Agrawal, Jyoti Singh Kirar, Javier Andreu-Perez, Wei-Ping Ding, Chin-Teng Lin, and Mukesh Prasad. On the utility of power spectral techniques with feature selection techniques for effective mental task classification in noninvasive bci. *IEEE Transactions on Systems, Man, and Cybernetics: Systems*, 51(5):3080–3092, 2019.

[18] Akshansh Gupta, RK Agrawal, and Baljeet Kaur. Performance enhancement of mental task classification using eeg signal: a study of multivariate feature selection methods. *Soft Computing*, 19(10):2799–2812, 2015.

[19] Akshansh Gupta, Riyaj Uddin Khan, Vivek Kumar Singh, Muhammad Tanveer, Dhirendra Kumar, Anirban Chakraborti, and Ram Bilas Pachori. A novel approach for classification of mental tasks using multiview ensemble learning (mel). *Neurocomputing*, 417:558–584, 2020.

[20] Md Abid Hasan, Md Kamrul Hasan, and M Abdul Mottalib. Linear regression–based feature selection for microarray data classification. *International Journal of Data Mining and Bioinformatics*, 11(2):167–179, 2015.

[21] Kaiming He, Xiangyu Zhang, Shaoqing Ren, and Jian Sun. Deep residual learning for image recognition. In *Proceedings of the IEEE Conference on Computer Vision and Pattern Recognition*, Las Vegas, NV, pp. 770–778, 2016.

[22] Sepp Hochreiter and Jürgen Schmidhuber. Long short-term memory. *Neural Computation*, 9(8):1735–1780, 1997.

[23] Asifullah Khan, Anabia Sohail, Umme Zahoora, and Aqsa Saeed Qureshi. A survey of the recent architectures of deep convolutional neural networks. *Artificial Intelligence Review*, 53(8):5455–5516, 2020.

[24] Alex Krizhevsky, Ilya Sutskever, and Geoffrey E Hinton. Imagenet classification with deep convolutional neural networks. *Advances in Neural Information Processing Systems*, 25:1106–1114, 2012.

[25] Dhirendra Kumar, Hanuman Verma, Aparna Mehra, and RK Agrawal. A modified intuitionistic fuzzy c-means clustering approach to segment human brain mri image. *Multimedia Tools and Applications*, 78(10):12663–12687, 2019.

[26] R Kumari and J Jose. Seizure detection in EEG using biorthogonal wavelet and fuzzy KNN classifier. *Elixir Human Physiology*, 41:5766–5770, 2011.

[27] Phillip A Laplante, Mohamad Kassab, Nancy L Laplante, and Jeffrey M Voas. Building caring healthcare systems in the internet of things. *IEEE Systems Journal*, 12(3):3030–3037, 2017.

[28] Yann LeCun, Yoshua Bengio, and Geoffrey Hinton. Deep learning. *Nature*, 521(7553):436–444, 2015.

[29] Yann LeCun, Lawrence D Jackel, Léon Bottou, Corinna Cortes, John S Denker, Harris Drucker, Isabelle Guyon, Urs A Muller, Eduard Sackinger, Patrice Simard, et al. Learning algorithms for classification: A comparison on handwritten digit recognition. *Neural Networks: The Statistical Mechanics Perspective*, 261(276):2, 1995.

[30] James MacQueen et al. Some methods for classification and analysis of multivariate observations. In *Proceedings of the Fifth Berkeley Symposium on Mathematical Statistics and Probability*, Oakland, CA, vol. 1, pp. 281–297, 1967.

[31] Tom M Mitchell et al. *Machine Learning*. McGraw-Hill Education: New York, 1997.
[32] Mehryar Mohri, Afshin Rostamizadeh, and Ameet Talwalkar. *Foundations of Machine Learning*. MIT Press: Cambridge, MA, 2018.
[33] Douglas C Montgomery and George C Runger. *Applied Statistics and Probability for Engineers*. John Wiley & Sons: Hoboken, NJ, 2010.
[34] Nikhil R Pal and Kaushik Sarkar. What and when can we gain from the kernel versions of c-means algorithm? *IEEE Transactions on Fuzzy Systems*, 22(2):363–379, 2013.
[35] David E Rumelhart, Geoffrey E Hinton, and Ronald J Williams. Learning representations by back-propagating errors. *Nature*, 323(6088):533–536, 1986.
[36] Stuart Russel, Peter Norvig, et al. *Artificial Intelligence: A Modern Approach*. Pearson Education Limited: London, 2013.
[37] Jürgen Schmidhuber. Deep learning in neural networks: An overview. *Neural Networks*, 61:85–117, 2015.
[38] Karen Simonyan and Andrew Zisserman. Very deep convolutional networks for large-scale image recognition. arXiv preprint arXiv:1409.1556, 2014.
[39] László Szilagyi, Zoltán Benyo, Sándor M Szilágyi, and HS Adam. Mr brain image segmentation using an enhanced fuzzy c-means algorithm. In *Proceedings of the 25th Annual International Conference of the IEEE Engineering in Medicine and Biology Society (IEEE Cat. No. 03CH37439)*, Cancun, Mexico, vol. 1, pp. 724–726, IEEE, 2003.
[40] Eric Topol. *The Patient Will See You Now: The Future of Medicine Is in Your Hands*. Basic Books: New York, 2015.
[41] Hanuman Verma and RK Agrawal. Possibilistic intuitionistic fuzzy c-means clustering algorithm for mri brain image segmentation. *International Journal on Artificial Intelligence Tools*, 24(05):1550016, 2015.
[42] Hanuman Verma, RK Agrawal, and Aditi Sharan. An improved intuitionistic fuzzy c-means clustering algorithm incorporating local information for brain image segmentation. *Applied Soft Computing*, 46:543–557, 2016.
[43] Hanuman Verma, Akshansh Gupta, and Dhirendra Kumar. A modified intuitionistic fuzzy c-means algorithm incorporating hesitation degree. *Pattern Recognition Letters*, 122:45–52, 2019.
[44] Hanuman Verma, Saurav Mandal, and Akshansh Gupta. Temporal deep learning architecture for prediction of covid-19 cases in india. *Expert Systems with Applications*, 195:116611, 2022.
[45] Hanuman Verma, Deepa Verma, and Pawan Kumar Tiwari. A population based hybrid fcm-pso algorithm for clustering analysis and segmentation of brain image. *Expert Systems with Applications*, 167:114121, 2021.
[46] Zeshui Xu and Junjie Wu. Intuitionistic fuzzy c-means clustering algorithms. *Journal of Systems Engineering and Electronics*, 21(4):580–590, 2010.
[47] Lotfi A Zadeh. Fuzzy sets. In: Lotfi A Zadeh (Ed.), *Fuzzy Sets, Fuzzy Logic, and Fuzzy Systems: Selected Papers*, pp. 394–432. World Scientific: Singapore, 1996.

Chapter 2

Machine learning applications in healthcare

Kushagra Krishnan
Jawaharlal Nehru University

Sumit Kumar
Kurukshetra University

Pinki Dey
University of New South Wales

CONTENTS

DOI: 10.1201/9781003368342-2

2.1 INTRODUCTION

Proper treatment in time is tremendously valuable for saving human lives when diseases are diagnosed. What matters is the efficiency of the plan of treatment. Artificial intelligence is an umbrella that embraces machine learning as a sub-domain. Artificial intelligence is dominating the world right now as it is being used to make technology smarter. Machine learning methods enhance the decision-making capacity of machines, and the healthcare industry is also not unaffected by this tremendous tool. It has enormous potential, and there can be huge alterations in the medical field including the development of improved procedures and efficient handling of medical records. The two essential components of the healthcare industry are patient care and administrative processes, which can largely benefit from the use of AI. Diagnosis of disease can be revolutionized; for example, with the help of AI, there can be faster spotting of a malignant tumour than the radiologist. Precision medicine can be generated for individuals by healthcare professionals. Algorithms with self-learning neural networks can be proven capable of increasing the quality of treatment. Moreover, the quality of treatment can be enhanced by analysing the data of the patient's condition, X-rays and CT scans, screenings and tests. This has led to the increasing use of machine learning and AI-based methods in healthcare over the years. There are even more applications which we will cover one by one in this chapter.

Machine learning technically means training the model with available data. A regular healthcare professional does 25% of work as administrative and regulatory responsibilities. This includes processing of claims, management of revenue cycles, clinical documentation and management of records for dozens of patients, and this is where ML-based techniques come into play.

Application of machine learning comprises the following tasks:

Classification: Identify the disease and type of specific stage based on the classification of disease data.

Recommendation: Recommending the necessary information without the requirement of searching.

Clustering: Grouping similar cases to analyse the disease patterns so that there can be faster research in future.

Forecasting: Using the previous and current data, forecasting on how future events are going to unfold for a particular patient.

Spotting anomaly: Detection of the patterns which are not earlier identified and requirement of action based on the level of severity.

Automation: Repetitive procedures can be handled efficiently which will eventually reduce the workload of administrative staff.

Ranking: Showing the relevant information first is very important, so here ranking comes in picture.

Machine learning algorithms have three components: Representation, Evaluation and Optimization. Representation is done by using decision trees, set of rules, graphical models, neural networks and support vector machine methods. Evaluation is based on accuracy and error, precision, recall, likelihood and probability, entropy and divergence. Optimization can be further categorized into three types- combinatorial, convex and constrained optimization. Combinatorial optimization consists of finding for maxima or minima of an objective function with discrete and large domain. Greedy search algorithm is an example of solving combinatorial optimization. Convex optimization consists of studying the problems of minimizing convex functions over convex sets. Convex optimization problems can be solved by using bundle methods, sub-gradient descent, interior-point methods, ellipsoid methods and cutting-plane methods. Constrained optimization is defined as the process of optimization of objective function with constraints on variables. Solution methods of constraint programming consist of linear programming, nonlinear programming and quadratic programming, etc. (Ban et al., 2018).

Machine learning approaches are broadly categorized (Kang and Jameson, 2018) into four types based on the nature of signal and feedback of learning systems-

1. *Supervised learning*: Training data given to model given as input includes desired outputs in supervised learning and the aim is to learn mapping inputs to outputs.
2. *Unsupervised learning*: Training data given to model as input does not include desired outputs in unsupervised learning and the aim is to discover hidden patterns in the data.

3. *Semi-supervised learning*: training data given to model as input includes a few desired outputs in semi-supervised learning and aim can be both to find new patterns and mapping input to output.
4. *Reinforcement learning*: training data in a dynamic environment in which feedback is provided analogous to rewards which the programme then attempts to maximize.

2.2 USE CASES OF MACHINE LEARNING IN HEALTHCARE

2.2.1 Imaging analytics and diagnostics

Computational tools and methods, currently developed and employed in machine learning, offer novel methods to take advantage of the exponentially growing volume of medical imaging data. Machine learning approaches can now address and resolve data-related problems whether it is an analytical query related to existing measurement data or the even more complex and challenging task of analysing raw images. Automation of tasks and the generation of clinically important new knowledge resources are both required for the success of machine learning techniques in healthcare.

2.2.1.1 Use cases of machine learning in CT scans and MRI

Active studies using machine learning methods on computer-aided diagnosis (CAD) for medical-related images have also been actively conducted in the case of COVID-19. However, machine learning requires a huge amount of training data with proper annotations to train the model. But it is a tedious task for radiologists to label a large number of images as normal and abnormal (Mabu et al., 2020). Globally, this pandemic situation has enormously impacted human beings and medical systems. However, computer-aided tomography images can excellently balance RT-PCR testing (Zhao et al., 2021).

Machine learning is repeatedly used for quick examination of individuals with internal injuries due to trauma. Doctors may use CT scans to assess the brain, spine, neck, chest and whole abdomen. Scans produce clear images of both hard and soft tissues. The pictures produced by the scans allow doctors to quickly make a medical decision as per the requirement. Because of this calibre, CT scans are generally done for the patients in hospitals and diagnostic and imaging centres. CT scans assist physicians in detecting injuries and diseases that could previously only be detected through an autopsy or surgery. CT scans use low doses of radiation and are regarded as relatively non-invasive and safe. Nowadays, for COVID-19, CT scan testing is being recommended in severe cases where RT-PCR is unable to detect the infection. Scientists also refer to a CT scan as "cat scan." This test amalgamates a string of X-ray scans or images taken from numerous angles. The machine learning-based tool then produces many cross-sectional images of blood vessels and soft tissues inside the human body. CT scans may furnish a more thorough picture as compared to standard X-rays, and machine learning is a very successful approach to detect the medical problem from the scanned images.

Machine learning methods include a class of algorithms named "neural networks". Data from neural network is often alternating between linear and nonlinear transformations. Neural networks, comprising hundreds and millions of stacked layers, have made a quantum leap in text, image and speech processing. The current methods are considered the gold standard to forecast using the imaging data. Specifically, convolutional neural networks (CNNs) can be employed for improving upon the regulation in radiology practices through the determination of the protocols that are based on short-text classification (Lee, 2018). CNNs can also be used to decrease the gadolinium dose in contrast-enhanced MRI of the brain by an order of desired magnitude (Gong et al., 2018) without significant reduction in image quality for MRI. Machine learning is also applied in various therapy-based techniques such as radio therapy (Meyer et al., 2018).

One more significant application area of machine learning in image analytics is advanced deformable image registration, which results in the quantitative analysis across various imaging sensory systems e.g., elastic registration between transrectal ultrasound and 3D MRI for leading targeted prostate biopsy deformable registration for brain MRI where a "cue-aware deep regression network" trains from an available set of images (Cao et al., 2018; Haskins et al., 2019). In the case of MRI, valuation of noise and image denoising is a very important research field employing a number of methods for many years e.g., field models, Bayesian Markov random and rough set theory, etc. Recently machine learning approaches have been introduced for denoising of images to make implicit learning of brain MRI (Huang et al., 2017; Xie et al., 2017).

2.2.1.2 Use cases of machine learning in breast cancer

Breast cancer is the most common cancer in women as compared to other types. Early detection of breast cancer is clinically significant and beneficial to improve the survival rate of the patients. A CT scan generally acts according to the myelogram procedure to assist in better description of the possible issues in the human body. Integrated with CT technology, myelograms can provide in-depth information to doctors than they can get with X-rays alone. Imaging analytics such as contrast-enhanced CT may also be prescribed to differentiate the tissues and suspicious nodules in the body. When detected nodules are found to be highly suspicious by the examining CT scan, a follow-up pathology examination is prescribed to confirm the malignancy. In the 1980s, researchers proposed computer-aided diagnostic methods for molybdenum target images. Most of the algorithms of the diagnostic methods are based on traditional CAD algorithms only. Over the last 10 years, machine learning has gradually come into the picture of mainstream methodology of computer-based visions. At first, the multi-level convolution and pooling of mammograms are performed which results in automatic feature extraction followed by feature maps used as input for regional proposal network (RPN) which further extracts the regions of interest (ROI). The regions of interest, further, are mapped to feature maps to confirm the cancer (Girshick, 2015).

2.2.1.3 Use cases of machine learning in cardiovascular recognition

To date, a large number of cardiovascular imaging studies have been focused on task-oriented problems, but recently more studies have involved algorithms directed at generating novel clinical insights from cardiovascular data. Continuing development in the size and dimensionality of cardiovascular imaging data is the driving force behind the impregnable interest in the application of machine learning methods in cardiovascular recognition. Collectively, the most efficient approaches with the larger impact necessitate resource investment which is explicitly required to prepare large data sets for analysis in a pertinent manner.

The machine learning methods, available currently, have garnered the interest of scientists due to their capability of getting new insights from images and image-related data. Given the expanding size of cardiovascular data, it will be required to also multiply the resources to create high-quality labelling methods resulting in efficient analyses of images.

Therefore, the progress in this field will largely depend on thoughtful commitment and strategic investment. Despite current technical and logistical challenges, machine learning methods have more to offer and will significantly impact the future medical practice and science of cardiovascular imaging (Henglin et al., 2017).

2.2.2 Drug discovery and AI-based precision medicine

Conventional drug discovery process is a highly laborious and very expensive process. The journey of developing a new drug consists of the identification and validation of a target, assay development and screening followed by hit identification, lead optimization and finally the selection of a molecule for clinical development (Hughes et al., 2011). Each of these development stages marks a significant time-consuming and expensive milestone in the whole drug development process. Although this process aims to identify potential drugs against selective targets along with ADME (absorption, distribution, metabolism, and excretion), it mostly disregards patient diversity. In addition, traditional drug discovery in large pharmaceutical companies is a risk-averse discipline with slow adaptation to rapidly changing external innovation in healthcare and data science (Hartl et al., 2021). Despite all these efforts, novel drugs record a low success rate of ~66% in Phase I clinical study about tolerability and side effects, ~48% in Phase II clinical study regarding dosage and efficacy, and ~59% in Phase III clinical study concerning efficacy and toxicology (Wong et al., 2019; Boniolo et al., 2021). However, to mitigate the bottlenecks in the research and development (R&D) process, large leaps are being taken towards the direction of precision medicine.

The principal tenet of precision medicine is to integrate different technologies to collect and interpret personalized data of individuals for the only purpose of diagnosis and treatment. In simpler terms, its main objective is to provide the right treatment to the patients at the right dose and at the right time based on the patient's characteristics rather than average-patient one-size-fits-all approach (Dugger et al., 2018; Seyhan and Carini, 2019). The concept of precision medicine was made possible due to the rapid development in the next-generation sequencing (NGS) technologies combined with advances in information technology and computational biology. This recent pathway of precision medicine employs numerous cutting-edge technologies in multiple ways to enhance the productivity of healthcare workers. Among them, artificial intelligence (AI), deep learning (DL) and machine learning (ML) technologies provide a great aid in the progress of precision medicine in healthcare.

The recent availability of high-performance computing (HPC) systems and large biological datasets helps to bridge the gap between these data science technologies and treatment. At the core of these technologies is a set of computer algorithms that identify embedded information or patterns in noisy and multidimensional biological data to predict appropriate diagnosis and treatment based on similar data of the individual patient. AI-based drug development technologies have been successfully used in the progress of some precision medicine (Muller et al., 2018; Schubert et al., 2018; Zhavoronkov et al., 2019; Stokes et al., 2020). Not only can AI-based technologies improve the success rate of clinical trials by identifying key biomarkers for including in the trials (Bai et al., 2020), but they can also help to unravel novel mechanistic insights into the disease pathogenesis and underlying molecular processes (Dugger et al., 2018). Over the years, many AI algorithms have been developed that are broadly classified as supervised or unsupervised. Examples of some of the commonly used AI methods are support vector machines, neural network, random forest, linear/logistic regressions and evolutionary algorithm.

These technological advances make AI particularly popular in healthcare where it has led to radical changes in patient care (Nemati et al., 2018), biomedical image processing (Litjens et al., 2017), clinical decision-making (Shortliffe and Sepulveda, 2018), etc.

Despite all the developments in AI-based technologies, they are not immune to obstacles and pitfalls. The use of limited and inconsistent training data has led to erroneous predictions for patients (Miller, 2013). In addition, most of the AI algorithms share the same working principles, and there is still potential scope to develop the most robust algorithms. However, this doesn't mean the failure of AI in healthcare but suggests the need to put greater effort into the collection of more comprehensive and accurate data from a more diverse population (Figure 2.1).

2.2.3 Clinical decision support and predictive analysis

Clinical trial is an essential stage of drug discovery procedure which takes several years and constant supervision which certainly costs substantially. In spite of drug discovery being a prime focus among researchers, on average only one-tenth of the molecules are successful. This makes a

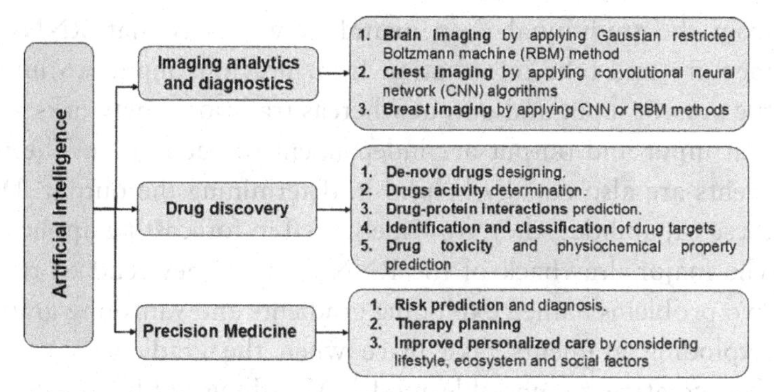

Figure 2.1 The applications of Artificial Intelligence in different sectors of the healthcare industry.

huge loss of industry in terms of money and time. During trials, multiple factors influence the failure i.e., wrong selection of patients, scarcity of technical requirements and poor infrastructure. Patient selection is very important in clinical trials. The therapeutic responses vary from patient to patient and are uncertain. Establishing the protocols to investigate the relationship between in-vitro phenotypes and appropriate biomarkers is extremely essential for successful, accurate and quantifiable prediction assessment of the response data. The recruitment of patients for phase 2 and phase 3 trials can be aided by AI-based approaches which involve the identification of the appropriate biomarkers of human diseases (Peiffer-Smadja et al., 2020). The ideal efficient AI tool must have the capability to identify the gene target and predict the effect of the molecule designed in addition to recognition of disease in the patient. AI-based tools will enhance the success rate in clinical trials. Approximately one-third of clinical trials just fail due to the opting out of the patients from the trial. This amounts to huge waste of time and money. The quality of data also gets suffered. The cost gets increased further recruitment for completion of the trials is required. Patients' faithfulness can be increased by closely observing the patients and required methods can be developed to assist them to follow the assigned rules of necessary clinical trials.

Methods used in prediction:

1. *Recurrent neural networks (RNN)*: DL characteristic has a hierarchical model which is much more efficient as compared to shallow models. RNN uses time series data or the data which is in sequential order. These also utilize training data to learn. The difference

from the traditional deep neural networks is that RNNs have memory and take information from previous inputs to influence the present input and output whereas traditional networks assume that input and output are independent of each other. The future events are also equally helpful in determining the output. Due to these capabilities, they are widely used in forecasting applications. The major drawback of the RNNs is that they tend to run into two problems named exploding gradients and vanishing gradients. Exploding gradients take place when the gradient is too large thus creating an unstable model. Vanishing gradients occur due to smaller gradients thus resulting in no longer learning of the algorithm (Kong et al., 2019).

2. *Long Short-term Memory (LSTM)*: This is a special type of RNN capable of learning long-term dependencies. These techniques were introduced by Hochreiter and Schmidhuber and are the most efficient solutions for predictions. The knowledge is passed on by cell state elements and they can recollect or overlook details correctly. A means to calculate data value over progressive stretches of time from the time series data is done by LSTMs. The model converts the prior hidden state to the most relevant arrangements. The problem of RNNs is resolved in LSTMs. The memory blocks are replaced by hidden modules to overcome the problem in RNNs. There are two different types of LSTMs - Deep or stacked LSTM and Bidirectional LSTM. Moreover, the network depth is improved by multi-layer stackings with each layer having some details and transferring them to the next layer. For each step, a distinct output is produced whereas bidirectional LSTM has the capability of processing the inputs from both the directions as compared to single direction of traditional RNNs. Moreover, the previous and following information is taken into account in the Bi-LSTM approach (Kong et al., 2019).

2.2.4 AI in gene expression profiling

ML algorithms have been used to identify the most recurrence-predictive genes. Genes were used in a molecular signature to determine the risk of recurrence within 5 years duration of post-resection of bladder tumour. Gene scale profiling has been extensively used on large scale for characterizing biological states in response to different disease conditions, to decipher the underlying molecular mechanisms of various biological processes, and to identify the genetic perturbations, etc.

The price of genome expression profiling is getting lower day by day but compiling the huge data of millions of samples is still a tedious task from the cost angle. Linear regression-based computational approach was developed by NIH researchers to profile approximately 1000 landmark genes. Linear regression (LR) does not capture the complex nonlinear relationship between gene expression. A DL method was developed on microarray-based data was used to train the model and compare its performance vs. other methods. DL was proven better than the LR method.

Gene expression is primarily responsible for the adaptation, growth, development and reproductive success of living organisms. Understanding the regulatory code can be helpful in preparing cures for various diseases. Transcriptional regulation has been a focus of research in the previous decade. The technology advancement now allows us to measure the mRNA expression up to several thousand copies per cell.

One of the fundamental challenges in biomedicine is the requirement of establishing relationships between diseases, physiological processes and the role of small molecule therapies. A genomic signature with sufficiently high complexity is needed that can provide rich description for all biological stages whether physiological or related to disease or treatment condition with high throughput investing low-cost efficiency.

2.2.5 Reducing human medical errors and the use of AI in surgery

Medical human errors around the globe cost billions of dollars (Van Den Bos et al., 2011), many of which go unnoticed. This kind of error not only harms the patients but also leads to the prescription of drug services to patients to neutralize the side effects of the medical errors. Recent studies have estimated the measurable cost of human medical errors in the US at 17.8 billion dollars (Van Den Bos et al., 2011) with 2,500 deaths. Here, AI can play a major role in bringing down the cost of human medical errors. The primary research questions that motivated the use of AI in health care are: (i) What are the types of medical errors that can be addressed with the help of AI (ii) how AI can help medical staff and surgeons to make better real-time decisions and risk assessments (iii) how feasibly and precisely AI can perform complex surgeries by learning from the experience. Researchers and medical professionals are gradually incorporating the AI-based techniques to derive more accuracy and less cost of errors. As a result, ML and AI are increasingly being used in clinical and surgical practices.

In addition to AI medicine, AI surgeries have improved in recent years with developments in the field of robotics technology. The potential to use autonomous actions in carrying out complex medical procedures such as endoscopy, spinal surgery, etc. has gained momentum with more surgeons interested in cutting-edge technologies. Several studies on the use of AI in surgical procedures are available, many of them with a focus on performance evaluation, treatment decision-making, etc. Corey et al. evaluated risk assessment for surgical patients by using patient electronic health record data, medications, co-morbidities, demographics, surgeries, and other variables for the identification of high-risk patients (Corey et al., 2018). Similarly, a user-friendly ML based Predictive OpTimal Trees in Emergency Surgery Risk (POTTER) was designed by (Bertsimas et al., 2018) to predict postoperative mortality and morbidity. Comparing the 2014 ACS-NSQIP database and the American Society of Anaesthesiologists (ASA), Emergency Surgery Score (ESS), and performance of ACS-NSQIP calculators, the performance of POTTER emergency risk calculator was measured. Moreover, surgical performance is also measured and refined using the experience of the surgeons and their skills by using recorded surgical video clips and virtual reality scenarios, etc. Other studies where AI is used in surgeries include treatment decision-making (Maubert et al., 2019), estimations of case durations (Bartek et al., 2019), etc.

The primary thrust areas where AI is being increasingly used in health care include ML, artificial neural networks (ANN), natural language processing (NLP) and computer vision (CV). ML allows to intercept patterns in large datasets that are imperceptible to manual analysis by employing more complex nonlinear relationships than any traditional statistical analysis (Miller et al., 1982). ML techniques can be broadly classified into supervised learning, unsupervised learning, and reinforcement learning. In supervised learning, labelled data is used, whereas in unsupervised learning, unlabelled data is used and patterns are searched within the data itself. In reinforcement learning, the programmes train by learning from its successes and failures. These algorithms are used based on the type of data available or many ML algorithms can be used together (Ensemble ML) for high accuracy predictions than conventional statistical methods (Wang et al., 2000).

NLP emphasizes the ability of computing to understand human language which has potential in the large-scale analysis of electronic medical record (EMR). NPL has been used for the analysis of EMR data to infer meaning and detect adverse effects and complications from the documentation of the physicians (Melton and Hripcsak, 2005; Murff et al., 2011).

ANNs are inspired by the biological nervous system and have found great importance in AI. ANN works by processing signals in layers of computational units called as neurons which are connected and parameterized via weights that change as the network learns different inputs and outputs. These algorithms have been increasingly used in pattern/image recognition and data classification, etc. and work with significant accuracy as compared to other traditional risk assessing methods (Mofidi et al., 2007).

CV and DL involve the development of methods to process and analyse digital images and videos to localize and track the image of interest. These techniques have been increasingly used in medical image analysing, with potential applications in image-guided surgeries, virtual colonoscopy, etc. (Kenngott et al., 2015). While CV is still in its infancy, AI can be used to leverage a wealth of actionable data from video clips to predict adverse effects and possible complications in real-time clinical decision-making during crucial surgeries.

2.2.6 Smart record management

ML algorithms can be applied to unstructured texts in the documents and learn the formats of the content and information provided. Record management was a tedious task but thanks to ML, as it has become less arduous to classify the records. These algorithms simultaneously can be used to remove the documents which are no longer required or redundant. No worries even if there are millions of files; it is just a process of three steps, namely, identify, delete and remove. Ranking the relevant information in higher order is another attribute of the ML. Compliance is required in some cases, and ML algorithms can be trained to detect the keywords and patterns or labelling to identify the documents relevant for compliance purposes. Data quality is another aspect which is improved by many folds as the formatting errors and spelling mistakes

Table 2.1 Recent applications of AI in healthcare

AI in healthcare	*Applications*	*References*
Heart Rhythm and Respiration Module	ECG, vital signs, cardiac function	Larimer et al. (2021)
FibriCheck	Atrial fibrillation detection	Proesmans et al. (2019)
CNN in the IDx-DR diagnostic system (IDx Technologies Inc., Coralville, IA, USA)	diabetic retinopathy screening	Acemoglu et al. (2016)
Inf-Net based quantification of COVID-19	Assessment and Tracking of COVID-19 Pulmonary Disease Severity on Chest Radiographs	Li et al. (2020)
U-Net++ based diagnosis of COVID-19	CT image analysis of COVID-19	Wang et al. (2021)
Multivariate Functional Principal Component Analysis (MFPCA) based detection	Oropharyngeal Cancer	Barua et al. (2021)

can be stopped. Even the models can be trained to rectify the errors in the records. If a person goes to another country, he doesn't need to take all the documents in printed form because all the records can be retrieved where he is going for treatment. The general indicators before admitting the patients can also be clubbed with the history of the patient and thus making the scope for larger evaluation.

All these advantages have led to the increased application of AI in healthcare in recent times (Table 2.1).

2.3 CHALLENGES AND BARRIERS

Health care industry is regularly facing so many challenges in managing healthcare services using ML algorithms. We are highlighting important problems so that those can be resolved in future.

2.3.1 Computational data handling – data volume, superiority and temporality

The innovation of ML has enabled us to achieve a huge amount of computational success but in the case of healthcare sector, ML faces a different set of problems. As of September 2021, the population of the world is ~7.9 billion people, and a larger part is not having access to primary health care. Because of that, researchers can't reach to each and every person in the world and it becomes difficult to train the model for the medical information of all the people. In ML, it is required that a large quantity of data is available for generating highly accurate results. It is also required that the input data contains important features for the training purpose. But, sometimes the lack of labelling data that requires domain experts is restricted due to difficulties in acquiring or generating the data. Also, an important question that shapes the results is how much data is really enough and what is the information available in the large data (Xie et al., 2017; Yang et al., 2017). Effective and robust ML model is required to solve the problem of computational data volume.

Data superiority refers to the capability to generate new, data-driven insights that lead to new high value offerings. Healthcare data is much more noisy, huge and incomplete. Training people is also challenging. Missing values in the healthcare data have created the biggest problem.

Over time, diseases are always evolving in a nondeterministic way. However, the already existing ML models assume static vector-based inputs, including those proposed in the medical sector. Therefore, the accurate design of ML approaches capable of handling temporal health care data is an important measure required for the development of novel solutions.

2.3.2 Health care data representation and handling biomedical data stream

ML algorithms evaluate the effective prediction based on the quantity of data. Healthcare data currently is in disorganized formats such as trees, text data and unfortunately, ML techniques can only process numeric input data.

With a rapidly changing healthcare industry and generation of a large volume of healthcare data, ML faces major challenges in handling these fast changing data (Najafabadi et al., 2015). These data are generally obtained in thousands of terabytes from real-time signals such as monitoring of blood glucose levels, oxygen saturation level, neuronal activity, etc. and biomedical imaging from MRI, ultrasound, electrography for crucial insight into different health conditions (Hasan and Roy-Chowdhury, 2015).

2.3.3 Domain complexity and accountability

The problems in healthcare sector are more complicated than those in other application domains such as image and speech analysis. Moreover, the highly heterogeneous nature of the diseases adds to the problems and a complete knowledge on their causes and pathogenesis is still lacking. The problem is augmented by the limited number of patients in a practical clinical scenario.

Few application domains, in ML often dried as blue, black boxes. In healthcare system, quantitative algorithm is not working quite well but it's very important at the same time. In fact, the interpretability of such model is crucial for building confidence among the medical professionals about implementing the recommended actions from the predictive system, such as medication and potential risk for diseases.

2.3.4 Hardware requirements

Real-world healthcare data are exponentially increasing and demand computers with sufficient processing power to create and implement appropriate ML models. However, high-performing GPUs and similar processing units are developed to handle such requirements, as the regular CPUs are unsuitable to tackle such large-scale ML problems (Raina et al., 2009).

The other significant challenges are legal issues pertaining to the ethics of research, paucity of medical expertise, high cost of equipment that need to be deployed, poor data storage capacity, missing and limited data, inconsistent measurement scale across organizations and countries, low accuracy due to insufficient data at required time and limitation of disease-specific data of rare diseases. Problem is interpretability is also there which makes it like a black-box as not everyone can understand it (Lee and Yoon, 2017).

2.4 FUTURE PROSPECTS

Over the years, the applications of AI and ML are rapidly evolving in healthcare and clinical practices. This process is augmented with the availability of a large amount of patient data, data obtained from health wearable and other monitoring sensor devices. Despite all the advancements, the successful applications of AI and ML-based medical technologies are seen in very limited clinical practices such as the detection of hypoglycaemia, atrial fibrillation, or medical imaging, etc. (Briganti and Le Moine, 2020). The following factors are at the core of these limitations: (i) unreliable or lacking primary replication, i.e., the sources of samples that are used for validation of the AI algorithms are different from that of the training samples, (ii) over fitting of the AI models, i.e., the datasets are chosen such that the datasets can optimally fit to it, (iii) resistance from clinicians and doctors with different views resulting in their insufficient training in the use of AI in medicine and, (iv) ethical implications regarding data protection and ownership. However, with more responsible and transparent use of open data of larger communities and best practices in R&D, clinicians will be able to interact with AI models more efficiently for superior medical practices.

Also, with increased patient safety, AI will also lessen the economic burden of the patient. For example, in case of a patient with type 2 diabetes, AI can provide the patient with important risks and actions to take from the patient's previous clinical data rather than performing routine clinical appointments, blood checks, etc. (Buch et al., 2018). Moreover, the potential of AI in efficiently interpreting imaging data is a boon to the early identification and treatment of diseases such as skin cancer (Buch et al., 2018). This concept has the potential to expand to different clinical practices that can interpret diseases from image data such as ultrasound (Chen et al., 2017), radiographs (Lakhani and Sundaram, 2017), retinal scan, etc. These promising potentials are causing a huge surge in the market of AI in healthcare with companies such as Amazon and Google investing heavily in the concept. Amazon's Echo and Google's Home may soon be able to remotely connect doctors with patients and perform visual scans, where the patient's wearable can provide with sufficient data to the AI models to conduct necessary diagnosis. These techniques can not only improve the lifestyle of the patients but also lead to a better organized healthcare system. With the help of AI, the healthcare systems will be able to reduce the frequency of patients' visit and when to visit the medical centres. It can also help in reducing the medical journey time of the patient by providing real-time information on which queue is shorter or which test will take lesser time to complete. These steps will prevent physician burnout and help them maintain a better work-life balance.

AI not only reduces the ecological footprints of the patients, but it can also immensely help pharmaceutical companies to speed up the drug creation process, making it more cost-effective. For instance, an AI pharma start-up identified a new drug in only 46 days in 2019 by using hordes of already generated data. In 2015, Atomwise developed two drugs with significant efficiency against Ebola in just 1 day. This clearly indicates the huge potential of AI-based drug discovery in the pharmaceutical industry to provide more patient-friendly and personalized healthcare applications. And the first step towards this process is to tear down the prejudices against AI-based healthcare by making the general population understand the benefits of AI and how to use it to optimize its benefits.

2.5 CONCLUSION

Over time, AI based technologies are increasingly employed in the health care sector such as precision medicine, imaging analytics, diagnostics, drug discovery, etc. It has been extensively studied to improve the diagnosis and treatment of complex diseases such as various cancer and neurodegenerative diseases. Moreover, several reports are showing up on how DL and AI applications can efficiently predict the advanced stages of cancer progression. Recent advances in ML techniques allow the use of real-time data from previous surgeries to enhance the effectiveness of surgical medical tools, thereby reducing human errors. These techniques have also demonstrated their effectiveness in advanced personalized care for various diseases, ranging from cancer to depression. These advancements led to the increased usage of AI-based technologies by various life sciences companies, pharmaceutical companies, and private care providers all over the globe.

Despite the entire efficacy, AI technologies come with many ethical, occupational, and technological challenges. In fact, the greatest challenge will not be just the improvement in technological but ensuring their ethical adoption in daily clinical practices. To limit the negative implications, government regulations, standardization of clinical practices, training of clinicians, etc. will need to be addressed to protect key privacy issues responsibly. With responsible scientific and ethical changes, AI-based technologies and AI supplementing to patient care are expected to bring tectonic shifts in healthcare service in the coming years.

REFERENCES

Abramoff, M.D., Lou, Y., Erginay, A., Clarida, W., Amelon, R., Folk, J.C. and Niemeijer, M. (2016) Improved automated detection of diabetic retinopathy on a publicly available dataset through integration of deep learning. *Invest Ophthalmol Vis Sci*, 57, 5200–5206.

Bai, R., Lv, Z., Xu, D. and Cui, J. (2020) Predictive biomarkers for cancer immunotherapy with immune checkpoint inhibitors. *Biomark Res*, 8, 34.

Ban, G.-Y., El Karoui, N. and Lim, A.E.B. (2018) Machine learning and portfolio optimization. *Management Science*, 64, 1136–1154.

Bartek, M.A., Saxena, R.C., Solomon, S., Fong, C.T., Behara, L.D., Venigandla, R., Velagapudi, K., Lang, J.D. and Nair, B.G. (2019) Improving operating room efficiency: Machine learning approach to predict case-time duration. *J Am Coll Surg*, 229, 346–354 e343.

Barua, S., Elhalawani, H., Volpe, S., Al Feghali, K.A., Yang, P., Ng, S.P., Elgohari, B., Granberry, R.C., Mackin, D.S., Gunn, G.B., Hutcheson, K.A., Chambers, M.S., Court, L.E., Mohamed, A.S.R., Fuller, C.D., Lai, S.Y. and Rao, A. (2021) Computed tomography radiomics kinetics as early imaging correlates of osteoradionecrosis in oropharyngeal cancer patients. *Front Artif Intell*, 4, 618469.

Bertsimas, D., Dunn, J., Velmahos, G.C. and Kaafarani, H.M.A. (2018) Surgical risk is not linear: Derivation and validation of a novel, user-friendly, and machine-learning-based Predictive OpTimal Trees in Emergency Surgery Risk (POTTER) calculator. *Ann Surg*, 268, 574–583.

Boniolo, F., Dorigatti, E., Ohnmacht, A.J., Saur, D., Schubert, B. and Menden, M.P. (2021) Artificial intelligence in early drug discovery enabling precision medicine. *Expert Opin Drug Discov*, 16, 991–1007.

Briganti, G. and Le Moine, O. (2020) Artificial Intelligence in medicine: Today and tomorrow. *Front Med (Lausanne)*, 7, 27.

Buch, V.H., Ahmed, I. and Maruthappu, M. (2018) Artificial intelligence in medicine: Current trends and future possibilities. *Br J Gen Pract*, 68, 143–144.

Cao, X., Yang, J., Zhang, J., Wang, Q., Yap, P.T. and Shen, D. (2018) Deformable image registration using a cue-aware deep regression network. *IEEE Trans Biomed Eng*, 65, 1900–1911.

Chen, H., Wu, L., Dou, Q., Qin, J., Li, S., Cheng, J.Z., Ni, D. and Heng, P.A. (2017) Ultrasound standard plane detection using a composite neural network framework. *IEEE Trans Cybern*, 47, 1576–1586.

Corey, K.M., Kashyap, S., Lorenzi, E., Lagoo-Deenadayalan, S.A., Heller, K., Whalen, K., Balu, S., Heflin, M.T., McDonald, S.R., Swaminathan, M. and Sendak, M. (2018) Development and validation of machine learning models to identify high-risk surgical patients using automatically curated electronic health record data (Pythia): A retrospective, single-site study. *PLoS Med*, 15, e1002701.

Dugger, S.A., Platt, A. and Goldstein, D.B. (2018) Drug development in the era of precision medicine. *Nat Rev Drug Discov*, 17, 183–196.

Girshick, R. (2015) Fast R-CNN. In 2015 *IEEE International Conference on Computer Vision (ICCV)*, Santiago, Chile, pp. 1440–1448.

Gong, E., Pauly, J.M., Wintermark, M. and Zaharchuk, G. (2018) Deep learning enables reduced gadolinium dose for contrast-enhanced brain MRI. *J Magn Reson Imaging,* 48, 330–340.

Hartl, D., de Luca, V., Kostikova, A., Laramie, J., Kennedy, S., Ferrero, E., Siegel, R., Fink, M., Ahmed, S., Millholland, J., Schuhmacher, A., Hinder, M., Piali, L. and Roth, A. (2021) Translational precision medicine: An industry perspective. *J Transl Med,* 19, 245.

Hasan, M. and Roy-Chowdhury, A.K. (2015) A continuous learning framework for activity recognition using deep hybrid feature models. *IEEE Trans Multimedia,* 17, 1909–1922.

Haskins, G., Kruecker, J., Kruger, U., Xu, S., Pinto, P.A., Wood, B.J. and Yan, P. (2019) Learning deep similarity metric for 3D MR-TRUS image registration. *Int J Comput Assist Radiol Surg,* 14, 417–425.

Henglin, M., Stein, G., Hushcha, P.V., Snoek, J., Wiltschko, A.B. and Cheng, S. (2017) Machine learning approaches in cardiovascular imaging. *Circ Cardiovasc Imaging,* 10, e005614.

Huang, G., Liu, Z., Van Der Maaten, L. and Weinberger, K.Q. (2017) Densely connected convolutional networks. 2017 *IEEE Conference on Computer Vision and Pattern Recognition (CVPR),* Honolulu, HI, pp. 2261–2269.

Hughes, J.P., Rees, S., Kalindjian, S.B. and Philpott, K.L. (2011) Principles of early drug discovery. *Br J Pharmacol,* 162, 1239–1249.

Kang, M. and Jameson, N.J. (2018) Machine learning: Fundamentals. In: M. G. Pecht and M. Kang (Eds.), *Prognostics and Health Management of Electronics: Fundamentals, Machine Learning, and the Internet of Thing* (pp. 85–109). John Wiley & Sons Ltd: Hoboken, NJ.

Kenngott, H.G., Wagner, M., Nickel, F., Wekerle, A.L., Preukschas, A., Apitz, M., Schulte, T., Rempel, R., Mietkowski, P., Wagner, F., Termer, A. and Muller-Stich, B.P. (2015) Computer-assisted abdominal surgery: New technologies. *Langenbecks Arch Surg,* 400, 273–281.

Kong, W., Dong, Z.Y., Jia, Y., Hill, D.J., Xu, Y. and Zhang, Y. (2019) Short-term residential load forecasting based on LSTM recurrent neural network. *IEEE Trans Smart Grid,* 10, 841–851.

Lakhani, P. and Sundaram, B. (2017) Deep learning at chest radiography: Automated classification of pulmonary tuberculosis by using convolutional neural networks. *Radiology,* 284, 574–582.

Larimer, K., Wegerich, S., Splan, J., Chestek, D., Prendergast, H. and Vanden Hoek, T. (2021) Personalized analytics and a wearable biosensor platform for early detection of COVID-19 Decompensation (DeCODe): Protocol for the development of the COVID-19 decompensation index. *JMIR Res Protoc,* 10, e27271.

Lee, C.H. and Yoon, H.J. (2017) Medical big data: Promise and challenges. *Kidney Res Clin Pract,* 36, 3–11.

Lee, Y.H. (2018) Efficiency improvement in a busy radiology practice: Determination of Musculoskeletal magnetic resonance imaging protocol using deep-learning convolutional neural networks. *J Digit Imaging,* 31, 604–610.

Li, M.D., Arun, N.T., Gidwani, M., Chang, K., Deng, F., Little, B.P., Mendoza, D.P., Lang, M., Lee, S.I., O'Shea, A., Parakh, A., Singh, P. and Kalpathy-Cramer, J. (2020) Automated assessment and tracking of COVID-19 pulmonary disease severity on chest radiographs using convolutional Siamese neural networks. *Radiol Artif Intell,* 2, e200079.

Litjens, G., Kooi, T., Bejnordi, B.E., Setio, A.A.A., Ciompi, F., Ghafoorian, M., van der Laak, J., van Ginneken, B. and Sanchez, C.I. (2017) A survey on deep learning in medical image analysis. *Med Image Anal,* 42, 60–88.

Mabu, S., Kido, S., Hirano, Y. and Kuremoto, T. (2020) Opacity labeling of diffuse lung diseases in CT images using unsupervised and semi-supervised learning. In: Y.-W. Chen and L.C. Jain (Eds.), *Deep Learning in Healthcare, Paradigms and Applications* (vol. 171, pp. 165–179). Springer Nature: Berlin, Germany.

Maubert, A., Birtwisle, L., Bernard, J.L., Benizri, E. and Bereder, J.M. (2019) Can machine learning predict resecability of a peritoneal carcinomatosis? *Surg Oncol,* 29, 120–125.

Melton, G.B. and Hripcsak, G. (2005) Automated detection of adverse events using natural language processing of discharge summaries. *J Am Med Inform Assoc,* 12, 448–457.

Meyer, P., Noblet, V., Mazzara, C. and Lallement, A. (2018) Survey on deep learning for radiotherapy. *Comput Biol Med,* 98, 126–146.

Miller, A. (2013) The future of health care could be elementary with Watson. *CMAJ,* 185, E367–E368.

Miller, R.A., Pople, H.E., Jr. and Myers, J.D. (1982) Internist-1, an experimental computer-based diagnostic consultant for general internal medicine. *N Engl J Med,* 307, 468–476.

Mofidi, R., Duff, M.D., Madhavan, K.K., Garden, O.J. and Parks, R.W. (2007) Identification of severe acute pancreatitis using an artificial neural network. *Surgery,* 141, 59–66.

Muller, A.T., Hiss, J.A. and Schneider, G. (2018) Recurrent neural network model for constructive peptide design. *J Chem Inf Model,* 58, 472–479.

Murff, H.J., FitzHenry, F., Matheny, M.E., Gentry, N., Kotter, K.L., Crimin, K., Dittus, R.S., Rosen, A.K., Elkin, P.L., Brown, S.H. and Speroff, T. (2011) Automated identification of postoperative complications within an electronic medical record using natural language processing. *JAMA,* 306, 848–855.

Najafabadi, M.M., Villanustre, F., Khoshgoftaar, T.M., Seliya, N., Wald, R. and Muharemagic, E. (2015) Deep learning applications and challenges in big data analytics. *J Big Data,* 2, 1–21.

Nemati, S., Holder, A., Razmi, F., Stanley, M.D., Clifford, G.D. and Buchman, T.G. (2018) An interpretable machine learning model for accurate prediction of sepsis in the ICU. *Crit Care Med,* 46, 547–553.

Peiffer-Smadja, N., Rawson, T.M., Ahmad, R., Buchard, A., Georgiou, P., Lescure, F.X., Birgand, G. and Holmes, A.H. (2020) Machine learning for clinical decision support in infectious diseases: A narrative review of current applications. *Clin Microbiol Infect,* 26, 584–595.

Proesmans, T., Mortelmans, C., Van Haelst, R., Verbrugge, F., Vandervoort, P. and Vaes, B. (2019) Mobile phone-based use of the photoplethysmography technique to detect atrial fibrillation in primary care: Diagnostic accuracy study of the FibriCheck App. *JMIR Mhealth Uhealth,* 7, e12284.

Raina, R., Madhavan, A. and Ng, A.Y. (2009) Large-scale deep unsupervised learning using graphics processors. In *ICML*, pp. 1–8.

Schubert, B., Scharfe, C., Donnes, P., Hopf, T., Marks, D. and Kohlbacher, O. (2018) Population-specific design of de-immunized protein biotherapeutics. *PLoS Comput Biol,* 14, e1005983.
Seyhan, A.A. and Carini, C. (2019) Are innovation and new technologies in precision medicine paving a new era in patients centric care? *J Transl Med,* 17, 114.
Shortliffe, E.H. and Sepulveda, M.J. (2018) Clinical decision support in the era of artificial intelligence. *JAMA,* 320, 2199–2200.
Stokes, J.M., Yang, K., Swanson, K., Jin, W., Cubillos-Ruiz, A., Donghia, N.M., MacNair, C.R., French, S., Carfrae, L.A., Bloom-Ackermann, Z., Tran, V.M., Chiappino-Pepe, A., Badran, A.H., Andrews, I.W., Chory, E.J., Church, G.M., Brown, E.D., Jaakkola, T.S., Barzilay, R. and Collins, J.J. (2020) A deep learning approach to antibiotic discovery. *Cell,* 180, 688–702 e613.
Van Den Bos, J., Rustagi, K., Gray, T., Halford, M., Ziemkiewicz, E. and Shreve, J. (2011) The $17.1 billion problem: The annual cost of measurable medical errors. *Health Aff (Millwood),* 30, 596–603.
Wang, B., Jin, S., Yan, Q., Xu, H., Luo, C., Wei, L., Zhao, W., Hou, X., Ma, W., Xu, Z., Zheng, Z., Sun, W., Lan, L., Zhang, W., Mu, X., Shi, C., Wang, Z., Lee, J., Jin, Z., Lin, M., Jin, H., Zhang, L., Guo, J., Zhao, B., Ren, Z., Wang, S., Xu, W., Wang, X., Wang, J., You, Z. and Dong, J. (2021) AI-assisted CT imaging analysis for COVID-19 screening: Building and deploying a medical AI system. *Appl Soft Comput,* 98, 106897.
Wang, P.S., Walker, A., Tsuang, M., Orav, E.J., Levin, R. and Avorn, J. (2000) Strategies for improving comorbidity measures based on Medicare and Medicaid claims data. *J Clin Epidemiol,* 53, 571–578.
Wong, C.H., Siah, K.W. and Lo, A.W. (2019) Estimation of clinical trial success rates and related parameters. *Biostatistics,* 20, 273–286.
Xie, S., Girshick, R., Dollar, P., Tu, Z. and He, K. (2017) Aggregated residual transformations for deep neural networks. In 2017 *IEEE Conference on Computer Vision and Pattern Recognition, CVPR 2017*, Honolulu, HI, pp. 5987–5995.
Yang, J., Jiang, B., Li, B., Tian, K. and Lv, Z. (2017) A fast image retrieval method designed for network big data. *IEEE Trans Ind Inf,* 13, 2350–2359.
Zhao, W., Jiang, W. and Qiu, X. (2021) Deep learning for COVID-19 detection based on CT images. *Sci Rep,* 11, 14353.
Zhavoronkov, A., Ivanenkov, Y.A., Aliper, A., Veselov, M.S., Aladinskiy, V.A., Aladinskaya, A.V., Terentiev, V.A., Polykovskiy, D.A., Kuznetsov, M.D., Asadulaev, A., Volkov, Y., Zholus, A., Shayakhmetov, R.R., Zhebrak, A., Minaeva, L.I., Zagribelnyy, B.A., Lee, L.H., Soll, R., Madge, D., Xing, L., Guo, T. and Aspuru-Guzik, A. (2019) Deep learning enables rapid identification of potent DDR1 kinase inhibitors. *Nat Biotechnol,* 37, 1038–1040.

Chapter 3

Deep multi-view learning for healthcare domain

Vipin Kumar
Mahatma Gandhi Central University

Bharti
University of Delhi

Pawan Kumar Chaurasia
Babasaheb Bhimrao Ambedkar University

Prem Shankar Singh Aydav
Km. GGP

CONTENTS

DOI: 10.1201/9781003368342-3

3.1 INTRODUCTION

Multiple sourced data (multi-view data) is commonly available with different measuring methods in this digital era. Usually, the dataset analysis is performed by combining multiple source data (called single-view data), which decreases the comprehensive overall information of the data. Because the sources yield different characteristics of the data, the multi-view data can be understood with multiple examples [90], i.e., described as follows:

- In Figure 3.1a, the website web pages may be perceived as multiple views (distinct sources of information) such as images, texts, videos,

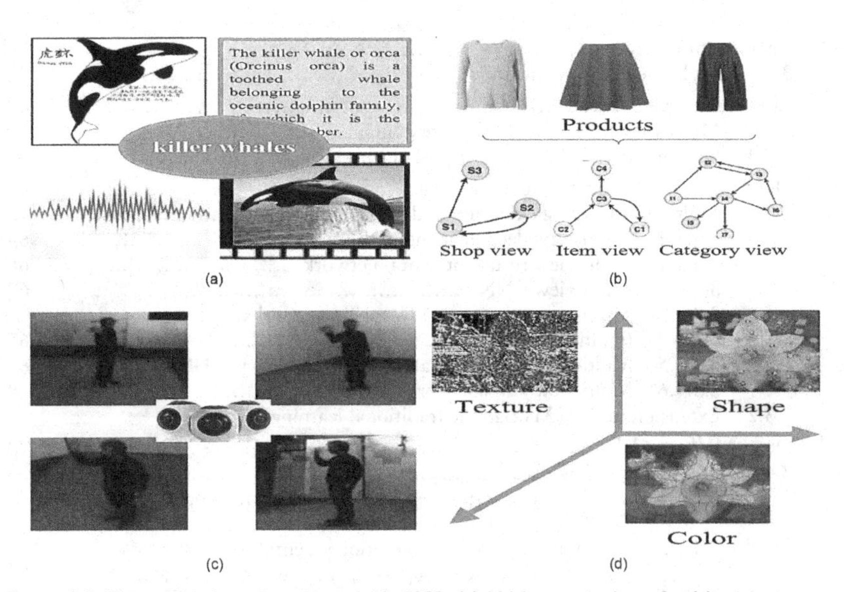

Figure 3.1 The multi-view data in real life [90]. (a) Webpage is described by image, text, audio, and video; (b) The multi-view graphs for a product; (c) Different cameras can capture the different viewpoints of one action; and (d) An image description by heterogeneous features such as texture, shape, color.

and audio available on the pages. Each has a distinct nature of the information to describe the type of webpage.

- In Figure 3.1b, a product may be considered with multiple views based on graph representation, such as shop view, item view, and category view.
- In Figure 3.1c, a person's single action can be captured using a camera from a different viewpoint, which can be perceived distinctly.
- Figure 3.1d shows that an image can be described with multiple features such as texture, shape, and colors.

Now, it can be observed that multi-view of the data has distinct characteristics that describe the same data, and combining them all will devalue the individual interpretation of data. Therefore, it is evident that distinct view information may be utilized to enhance performance. A classical machine learning approach utilizes single-view data (or merged multiple views as a single view) for supervised, unsupervised, semi-supervised, and reinforcement learning tasks.

3.1.1 Multi-view learning methods (MVL)

The MVL approach has been divided into three categories [104], which are described as follows:

1. *Co-regularization style algorithms*: This approach includes the regularization terms in regression and discriminant functions. The regularization ensures a similar prediction from the distinct classifier learned from different dataset views. Recently, many algorithms have been proposed to ensure regularization. It includes multi-view twin SVM (MvTSVM) [83], SVM-2k [22], canonical correlation analysis (CCA) [35], deep canonical correlation analysis (DCCA) [71], Multi-view discriminant analysis (MvDA) [42], multi-view uncorrelated linear discriminant analysis (MULDA) [70]. The proposed algorithms perform many machine learning tasks such as multi-view supervised learning, multi-view clustering, multi-view semi-supervised learning, and multi-view dimensional reduction.
2. *Co-training style algorithm*: This algorithm style is usually used for semi-supervised learning. Iteratively, multiple classifiers are learned from the multiple dataset views to predict the test data

from each learned view. Several representative algorithms, such as co-EM [57], co-clustering [91], co-training [6, 57], and co-testing [54], have been proposed. These algorithms have been deployed for different machine learning tasks such as multi-view transfer learning and multi-view semi-supervised learning.

3. *Margin-consistency style algorithm*: This approach focuses on the characteristics of the algorithms in multiple views for the classification tasks. The methods utilized the consistency of the data to check the view's margin that have the same posteriors. Several algorithms, such as multi-view maximum entropy discrimination (MVMED) [69], soft margin consistency based multi-view maximum entropy discrimination (SMVMED) [10], and consensus and complementarity based MED (MED-2C) [11], have been proposed.

Tremendous success has been achieved by the deep learning model in various domains such as stock photography, visual search, security industry, automobile industry, and the healthcare industry. The convolutional neural network (CNN or ConvNet) has performed excellently among the deep neural networks (DNN), which follow the mechanism of a multi-layer neural network [27, 99]. The basic architecture of CNN is shown in Figure 3.2 [90]. The CNN consists of four main types of layers like

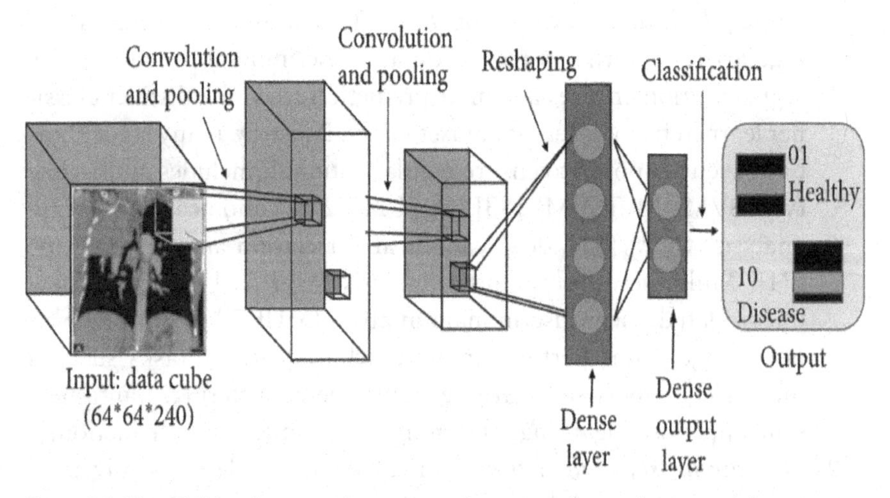

Figure 3.2 The CNN architecture having convolution, pooling reshaping and dense output layer [99].

- *Convolution layer*: It is the primary building block of CNN and has trainable filters.
- *Relu layer*: It is an activation function that reduces the overfitting of the model.
- *Pooling layers*: It provides the streamlined output by collecting the results from numerous neurons and reduces the number of factors while training the model.
- *Fully connected layer*: It is the output layer of the model. It flattens the received inputs from the previous neurons and produces the results.

Deep multi-layer neural networks have many models for the classification task such as ResNet, AlexNet, InceptionNet, Googlenet, and VGG16. Furthermore, the segmentation of images is usually performed by U-Net [99]. The more detailed description of CNN is the out-of-scope of this chapter.

Now, it is evident from the above discussion that multiple data views can provide the leverage needed to exploit the view information maximally to enhance the machine learning algorithms with suitable optimization. Moreover, deep learning models can also extract the features and learn the model effectively for the classification task. The prose of MVL and DL (called Deep MVL) opens up a new horizon of more effective and efficient learning for the classification task. Therefore, deep multi-view learning has attracted researchers to deploy this model in different domains, especially healthcare. Several diagnoses have utilized the effective performance such as Brain-related issues [80, 86], Breast cancer [14, 26, 44], seizure recognition [75, 95, 96], etc.

This chapter discusses the computation methods of deep MVL that have been successfully deployed in various diagnoses of patients in healthcare domain. Section 3.1, Introduction, includes the basic understanding of multi-view data, MVL and DL with basic architecture.The literature reviews on multi-view and deep MVL related to the healthcare domain have been described in Section 3.2. Different methodologies of deep MVL are also discussed, corresponding to their categories to understand the methods in Section 3.3. Section 3.4 describes the deep MVL computational methods for brain issue, breast cancer, and seizure detection. The research opportunity and open problems have been summarized along with their limitations in Section 3.5. At last, the conclusion of this chapter mentioned in Section 3.6.

3.2 LITERATURE REVIEW

Since the last decade, it has been seen that multi-view learning has been successfully deployed in multiple fields [19, 64, 100, 104]. However, this literature review only focuses on the healthcare applications of profound multi-view learning. Therefore, the literature review has been divided into two parts (shown in Figure 3.3):

3.2.1 Multi-view learning in healthcare domain

In Ref. [63], It considers the multi-view structure to get the relevant views, i.e., implemented using neural network architecture. This architecture has been successfully applied to classify the breast microcalcifications for two-class problems such as benign and malignant. In Ref. [59], this method considers two types of data of the patient as multi-view, i.e., magnetic resonance (MR) and ultrasound (US) image dataset. The two data views collectively extract the most significant features for dilated cardiomyopathy (DCM) patient classification. Laplacian support vector machines (MvLapSVM) and multi-view linear discriminant analysis (MLDA) are two proposed models.

In Ref. [7], A medical imaging technique (radiomics) has huge information utilized effectively because of its association with protein or

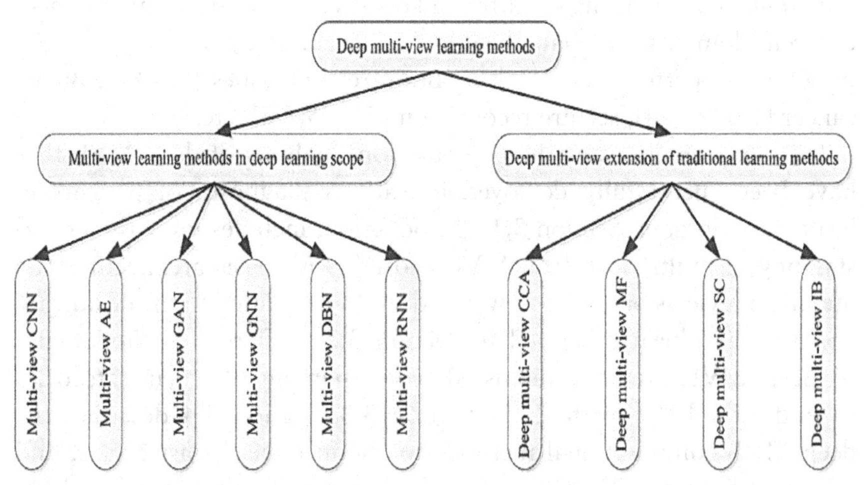

Figure 3.3 The categorization of Deep MVL methods based on MVL extension in DL and classical ML Models [90].

gene data information. The academics classification method has been proposed based on dissimilarity using multi-view learning where high dimension and low sample size. In Ref. [58], This method considered the data heterogeneity and generalized prediction and proposed a multi-view multi-task network (MuViTaNet) to predict the onset of multiple complications. MuViTaNet method has outperformed breast cancer survivors in profiling the development of cardiac complications [82]. The uncertainty-aware multi-view co-training (UMCT) is a unified framework that handles the segmentation of volumetric medical images that yield effective performance on test data. The 3D volume is permuted by the rotation of images to get multiple views.

3.2.2 Deep multi-view learning (deep MVL) in the healthcare domain

Since the last decade, deep learning has successfully processed distinct data for many machine learning tasks such as audio, video, image, text, graph, etc. However, these datasets are also previewed like a multi-view of the data that includes different perspectives of the multiple source data to enhance the learning classifiers. Therefore, many hybrid methods have recently been proposed based on DL and MVL with outstanding performance. The remarkable performance of deep MVL in many domains has recently attracted the attention of many researchers. Table 3.1 has summarized the literature based on the area of application and the proposed research's internal characteristics. Therefore, many methods have also been proposed to solve the problems in healthcare such as brain-related issues [80, 86], breast cancer [14, 26, 44], and seizure recognition [75, 95, 96].

Usually, the medical images (MR, ultrasound, and mammograms) and signals (especially EEG) are used to diagnose health-related issues using deep MVL. For the image dataset, the segmentation based on a multi-size U-net has been performed to get the different characteristics of features to perceive multiple views for the learning [9, 46, 80, 86]. In another study [75], EEG motor imagery is used to extract the feature by reducing the noise, unsteadiness, nonlinear, and time-varying characteristics. The extracted features are time-domain, frequency, spatial, time-frequency, and deep multi-view features (Deep MVF). The analysis shows that spatial domain features and time-frequency domain were the most suitable features to enhance the performance of the classifiers.

Table 3.1 List of literature related to deep multi-view learning in the healthcare domain

Area	*Dataset Name*	*Dataset type*	*Segmentation*	*DL Method(s)*	*Performance Measures*	*Reference*
Brain	The BrainWeb dataset, IBSR V2.0 dataset	MR Image	Yes	U-Net	Tissue (GM, WM, CSF), Acc	[80]
	BCI (the multi-class motor imagery EEG)	EEG signals	Yes	SVM, RBM.	Acc, Kappa	[86]
Breast Cancer	Samsung Medical Centre.	160 clinical dataset images	No	SVM, deep DCNN	Acc, AUC, ROC	[44]
	authors	264 pairs of BUS and USE images	No	SVM, DNN	Acc, ROC, AUC, Se,Sp	[26]
	Authors	Image		CNN, ResNet-50	AUC, ROC	[14]
Seizure recognition	CHB-MIT dataset	EEG signals	No	SVM, PSVM, CNN	AUC, ROC	[96]
	CHB-MIT dataset	EEG signals	No		Acc, AUC, ROC, P,R, F	[95]
	CHB MIT dataset	analyzing EEG signals	No	SVM, KNN, NB,DT, CNN	Acc, Se, Sp	[75]
Liver tumor	Malignant Breast, heart disease, fatty liver, malignant lung tumor (Lung), and a healthy control group	Image	No	KNN, SRC, CRC, VGG16, VGG19, AlexNet, ResNet	Acc, P, R, F	[105]
	Authors	ultrasound images	No	CCA, deep DCCA	Acc, sensitivity, specificity	[30] [30]

(Continued)

Table 3.1 (Continued) List of literature related to deep multi-view learning in the healthcare domain

Area	*Dataset Name*	*Dataset type*	*Segmentation*	*DL Method(s)*	*Performance Measures*	*Reference*
Others	Tommy dataset	Image (mammograms)	Yes	CNN, InceptionResNetV2	AUC, ROC	[46]
	InBreast [46] and DDSM [9].	Image (mammograms)	Yes	AlexNet	ROC	[9]
	Inbreast, DDSM and ImageNet		No CNN	ROC, AUC	[8]	
	MIMIC-III dataset	deidentified clinical records for ¿40K patients	No	SVM, SVD, Attention Autoencoder	AUC, ROC, NCDG	[14]

It has been observed that several deep learning models along with machine learning models have been applied and compared their performances. Frequently, utilized DL models are U-Net [80], DCNN [44], DNN [26], ResNet-50 [14], VGG16 [105], VGG19 [105], AlexNet, ResNet [105], DCCA [30], InceptionResNetV2 [46], etc. Many traditional machine learning algorithms are also utilized at the same time for the classification task, where the most frequent ML algorithms are SVM [86], DNN [14, 26, 75, 96], and KNN [75, 105]. The performance evaluation of deep multi-view learning has been measured with many criteria, where the most utilized criteria are Accuracy [44, 75, 80, 86, 105] , AUC [14, 44, 86, 96], and ROC [9, 14, 44, 86, 96], where others evaluation measures can be seen from Table 3.1.

Note: Some abbreviations used in Table 3.1
Acc: Accuracy
AUC: Area under the curve
ROC: Receiver operating characteristic curve
P: Precision
R: Recall
Se: Sensitivity
Sp: Specificity
F1: F1-Score

3.3 DEEP MULTI-VIEW LEARNING (DEEP MVL)

In literature, multiple MVL methods have been proposed based on DL. The deep MVL has been categorized into two categories: MVL extension in DL and Deep multi-view extension in classical learning method [90]. The further categorization of these two methods is shown in Figure 3.3. This section has a review of representative MVL methods and advancements of MVL. In the representative MVL, the following methods are discussed: the deep belief network (DBN), multi-view autoencoder (AE), and CNN. Then, the investigation of deep multi-view extensions for the classical learning approach is investigated such as deep multi-view CCA, information bottleneck (IB), matrix factorization (MF), etc. Many surveys related to MVL summarize the MVL approaches based on theories, categorization, and their real-life applications [12, 61, 68, 85, 104]. Therefore, it is important to discuss problem-specific MVL methods such as multi-model learning [61], multi-view representation learning [31, 48], multi-view clustering [12], and multi-view fusion [68, 85, 104].

3.3.1 Multi-view learning extension in deep learning

3.3.1.1 Multi-view deep belief net (DBN) [102]

The main objective of DBN is to capture the distribution of the labels and samples. The multi-view deep belief net utilizes the model of the Restricted Boltzmann Machine (RBM) that contains hidden layers and visible layers (i.e., two layers)(shown in Figure 3.4). The computation in two layers is done based on the energy function shown in eq. 3.1

$$E(X,H) = -\sum_{p} C_p X_p - \sum_{q} B_q H_q - \sum_{q}\sum_{p} H_p W_p X_q \tag{3.1}$$

where H and X indicate the hidden layers and visible unit of layers. The C_p and B_q are the variables and biases in the architecture of RBM. The hidden layers of DBN architecture may perform as shown in eq. 3.2.

$$P(X, h^1, h^2, h^3, ..., h^l) = P(X|h^1)P(h^1|h^2), ..., P(h^l) \tag{3.2}$$

where X and $P(h^l)$ indicate the input data and joint probability distribution of the top layer of DBN. Multi-view DBN model is generative model

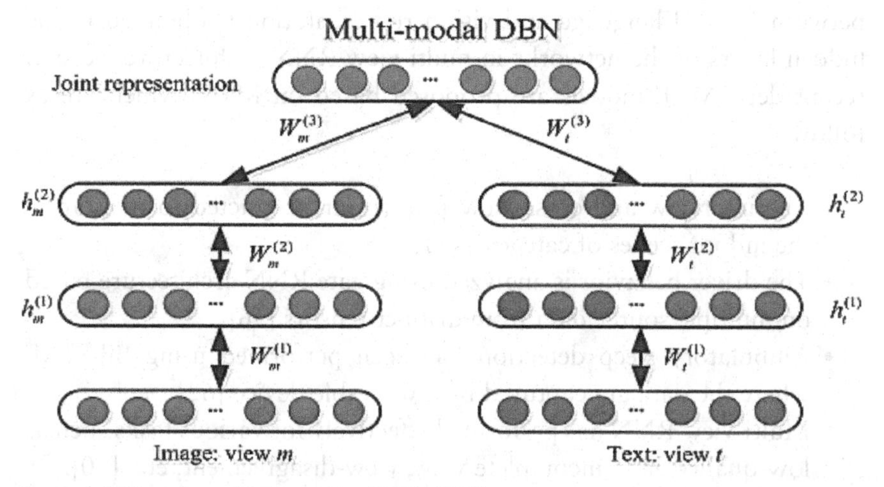

Figure 3.4 The adopted framework of DBN [102].

to fit the joint distribution of the various views of the data such as color, texture, audio, video, etc [66]. The different modalities are extracted by the model followed by the joint representation of multi-source data with a single layer of Neural network (Figure 3.4).

The multimodal deep Boltzmann machine (DBM) [74] method is applied parallel to find the importance of genes based on the expression of the genes and phenotype of the patient. To model the separate view, the multi-model correlation of DBN with RBN is also proposed [101]. The hybrid model based on conditional RBM extracts the features using inter-modality and cross-modality [3] for the sequential event. The complementary principle of multi-view learning is used for the local and deep features [2].

3.3.1.2 Multi-view recurrent neural network

The multi-view recurrent network approach has been applied over time series data for the multiple analysis with different time frames [73]. In Ref. [43], the multi-view architecture is proposed to find the relationship between textual and visual data based on a multi-view alignment model. In Ref. [53], for the visual image, three subnetworks are adopted, namely, language network, vision network, and multi-view network. The temporal dependency and task-specific representation are performed by the language network in the architecture. The vision network utilize the pre-trained deep network to extract the features of the image such as ResNet, InceptionNet, and AlexNet. Furthermore, the relationship between learned language and vision representation is obtained in the hidden layers of the networks in multi-view RNN architecture. Several recent deep MVL models are proposed based on RNN, which are as follows:

- The interview and cross-view features are extracted to reorganize the indoor scenes of categories [1].
- The driver behavior is analyzed using gate RNN architecture based on multiple source data from distinct sensors [56].
- Ambulatory sleep detection has been performed using BiLSTM, where the data are captured by a wearable device [62].
- Multi-view RNN has performed effectively for various tasks such as low-quality data, incomplete view, view-disagreement, etc. [90].

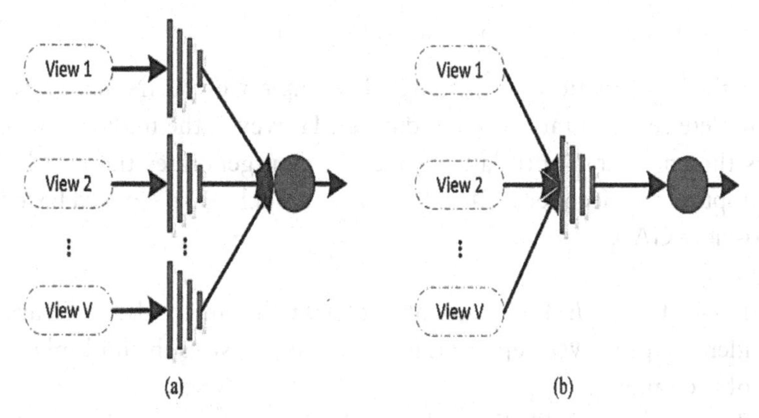

Figure 3.5 The types of the multi-view CNN fusion [17]. (a) One-view-one-network strategy and (b) multi-view-one-network strategy.

3.3.1.3 Multi-view CNN

The CNN-based architecture is superior in performance to the traditional machine learning approach for image processing because CNN extracts the high-level features by different parameter optimization [50, 60]. The multi-view CNN model incorporates the discriminative common representation of multi-views of data. Currently, multi-view CNN architecture has two types of network strategies: one-view-one-network and multi-view-one network (as shown in Figure 3.5. The one-view-one-network utilized the one CNN architecture for the multi-view of the data separately to extract the feature set for each view, then it fused subsequently [24, 45, 52, 67, 92]. In the multi-view-one-net strategy, the multi-view of the data is processed in a single network to fuse into a single representation.

3.3.1.4 Multi-view generative adversarial networks (multi-view GAN)

GAN is the unsupervised DL model and is successfully applied over multiple domains like image in painting [17] and image-to-image translation [39]. The major characteristics of adversarial training include the generative model G and discriminative model D, where G and D characterize source data distribution and find the probability distribution from training data. The main objective of the GAN is to find parameters as eq. 3.3:

$$\delta_g^* = \arg(v(\delta)_g, \delta_d) \tag{3.3}$$

where the loss function is $(v(\delta)_g, \delta_d)$. The single-view GAN may learn the incomplete representation of the dataset. However, the multi-view GAN maps the encoder E into latent space Z, then generates the novel view by adopting the decoder G. The following models are proposed based on multi-view GAN:

- *DR-GAN [77]*: The main objective of this method is to learn an identity-preserved representation that synthesizes the multiple views of the images.
- *Two-pathway* GAN *[76]*: This method collaborates and competes in sharing the parameter, enhancing the generative ability for test data. The learning embedding space is also maintained.
- *Bi-directional GAN (BiGAN) [61]*: It learns jointly by inference and generative networks, which means learning through inverse mapping by projecting into latent space. In other research [13], the multi-view extension of BiGAN has also been proposed by density estimation of distinct views of the data.
- *Multi-view embedding network based on GAN [72]*: It maintains the unique view of the network and maintains the connectivity across the different views in the GAN network.

3.3.1.5 Multi-view graph neural networks (multi-view GNN)

GNN method effectively models the graph-structured data such as knowledge graphs [33] and social networks [38]. Recently, MVL has been incorporated into GNN for multi-view graph conventional networks and multi-graph clustering. In Ref. [20], a graph autoencoder, called one2multi, has been proposed that embeds the learning node using content information with self-supervised clustering and graph autoencoder.

3.3.1.6 Multi-view autoencoder

Promising results have been seen of autoencoder (AE) in various fields such as human pose recovery [36], data retrieval [103], and disease analysis [103]. The autoencoder has two objective functions in deep learning concepts, such as encoding and decoding functions. The encoding function maps the input data, whereas decoding performs the reconstruction of the data. The square loss is utilized for the cost function of the autoencoder (shown in eq. 3.4):

$$\sum_{i=1}^{k} ||x_i - g(v_i)||_F^2 + \sum_{i=1}^{k} ||x_i - f(x_i)||_F^2 \tag{3.4}$$

where k is the volume of the data instances, $x_i \in X$ is the input data instance and $v_i \in V$ is the optimal representation.

3.3.2 Extension of deep MVL in the traditional learning models

The CCA maps two random variables into a common subspace in which correlation is maximally preserved. If views of the data are considered as a variable, then the correlation between views may be obtained precisely. An implementation of CCA for MVL can be inducted into deep networks. Therefore, much research has been proposed for deep multi-view CCA where some methods are described as given below:

- *Deep CCA*: Two neural network correlation maximization has been done using an extension of CCA in multi-layer extension [5]. A nonlinear CCA is also formulated for three feedforward networks [37].
- *Deep adversarial CCA (DACCA)*: In traditional CCA, a Deep adversarial concept has been implemented, called DACCA. It synthesizes instances of multi-view data and extracts the discriminative features [21].
- *Deep Canonical correlation autoencoders (DCCAE) [79]*: This method optimizes the reconstruction of autoencoders, where the analysis of the canonical relationship of obtained features.
- *Matrix factorization for multi-view clustering*: This method employed the deep matrix factorization method to perform clustering tasks for the multi-view data source, where Figure 3.6 shows the flow diagram of the method.
- *Deep multi-view spectral learning network*: Multi-view matrix factorization (MVMF) model is used for the final layer of the deep network. Furthermore, investigate the middle layers of the network for latent correlation. In Ref. [88], the low-rank subspace ensemble (DLRSE) has been proposed to extend the deep MVMF.

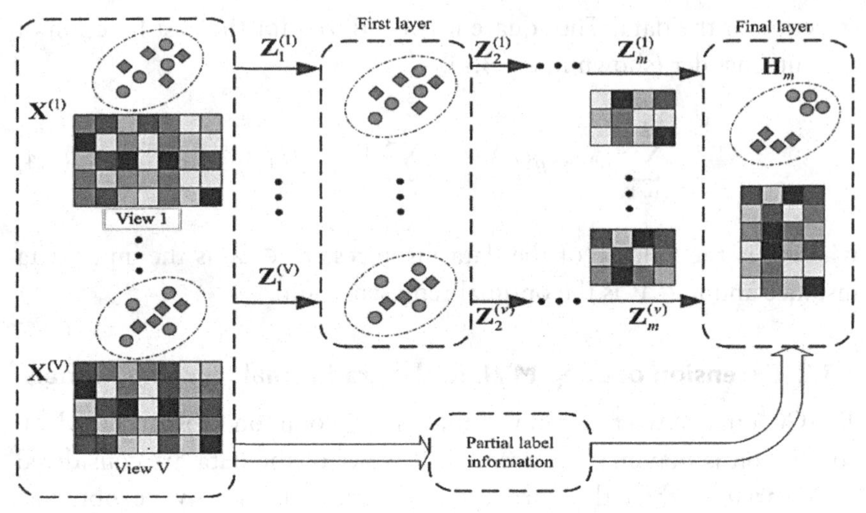

Figure 3.6 Architecture of deep MVL [84].

3.4 DEEP MVL MODELS IN HEALTHCARE DOMAIN

DL models have great success over the cross-domain, and DNN-based models have been applied in bioinformatics and health informatics, especially [23, 49, 97, 98]. It has been applied in three areas, specifically breast diagnosis [40, 44], brain issue [80, 86], and seizure recognition [95, 96]. These three areas have been discussed in this section.

3.4.1 Breast cancer diagnosis

A high morbidity and mortality rate of breast cancer is prevelent in women [40, 81]. It has been observed that the survival rate has significantly increased by identifying breast cancer at an early stage [34, 40]. This motivates the researcher to enhance the effective and efficient diagnostic power in standard clinical procedures. For decades, a breast cancer diagnosis has been performed based on histopathological image analysis. Usually, hematoxylin and eosin (H&E) are used to stain the tissues to analyze them. In the advancement of digital image processing, the manual procedure is still performed to identify the biomarkers by the pathologists using a microscope, which is very complex and time-consuming. The biomarkers are enlargement reliant on size, infiltration pattern, and invasiveness of tumors with classes color, texture, and morphology. Pathologists require efficient expertise to assess the cancer tissues. The difference in pathologist experiences causes variation and

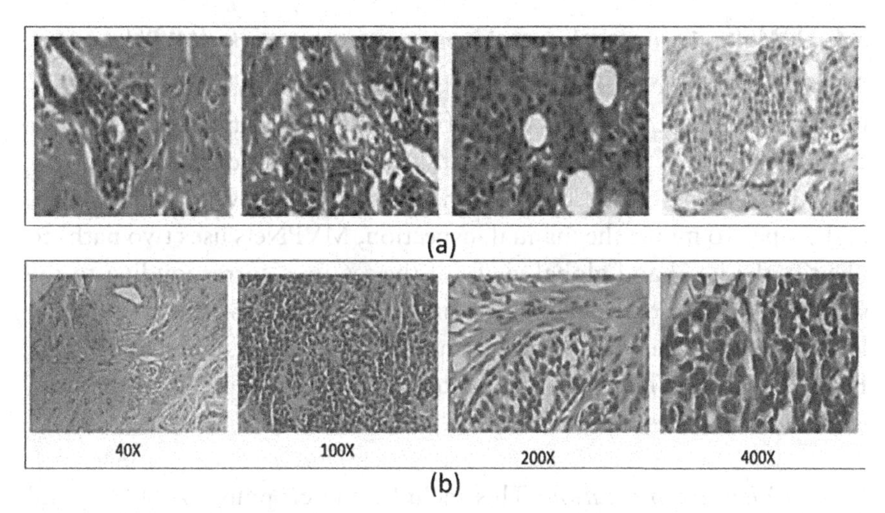

Figure 3.7 Diverse class and different magnification posing of the Breast Cancer (malignant) [40].

considerable errors in the analysis of cancer tissues. Therefore, it is required to possess an automated method to diagnose cancer irrespective of any type of magnification.

Digital breast tomosynthesis (DBT) is designed to improve to diagnose the cancer tissue overlap problem [51]. A huge number of slices of breasts (both) can be analyzed by the radiologist using DBT, which is complex. The radiologist is also considering the symmetricity of both breasts while analyzing tissue because the internal structure of both breasts is the same, which usually reduces the False Positive (FP). Now, computer-aided bilateral analysis is highly required to screen cancer tissues in the breast.

Earlier, hand-crafted features were used to analyze cancer tissues, which is a complex process to identify the suitable feature for the given problem. Now CNN has played a significant role in extracting the high-level feature to detect cancer [55, 65]. Tumor classification has been performed using CNN to identify the significance of stroma and tubules [87]. In another study, tumor segmentation has also been done successfully for the MRI images and used different kernels for CNN to locate the tumor. Breast cancer histology is highly complex and diverse because each magnification may yield a distinct feature, as shown in Figure 3.7. The different magnification posing and class diversity may be considered distinct views of the same tissue slice. Therefore, it is evident that MVL can be deployed with high-level feature extraction using CNN.

3.4.1.1 Multi-viewing path deep learning neural networks (MVPNets) [40]

This method can identify the biomarkers quantitatively in histopathology images at multiple magnifications of the tissue. Also, it can detect tumor types successfully. The biomarkers at different resolutions are as follows: size, nuclei shape, tumor location, uniformity, infiltrative growth pattern, and shape. To mimic the manual inspection, MVPNets uses two paths to identify the local and global views of the features corresponding to the small and large kernel. The smaller size of the kernel investigates the low-level features in the images, such as nuclei size, mitotic figure, and shape. Furthermore, the large size of the kernel identifies the growth pattern, tumor size, etc. description of MVPNets is as follows:

- *NuView augmentation:* This includes the cropping, zooming, and resizing of training data to get the benefit of nuclei to cluster to localize the tumor. The segmentation of images is done based on Gaussian mixture model (GMM) for the three components, where the critical component is nuclei. The clustering is performed using the expectation maximization (EM) algorithm to locate the nuclei, as shown in Figure 3.8.
- *MVPNets architecture:* The proposed architecture for magnification-invariant classification is performed based on multi-view learning where the local and global features of the tissue are used as views simultaneously. The stacked multiple convolutional layers are used as views to extract the different sets of features in parallel blocks, see

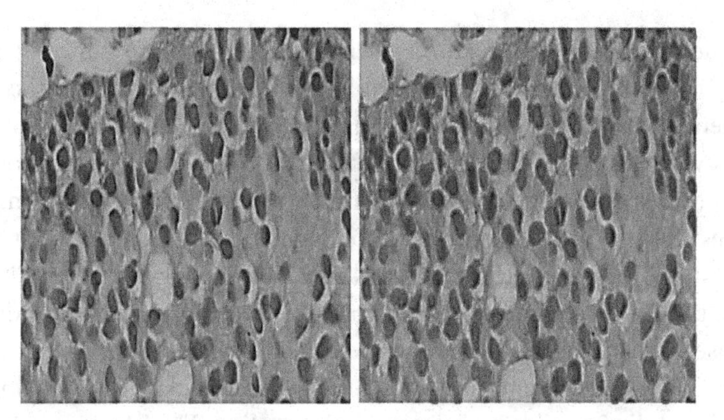

Figure 3.8 Nuclei extraction using EM based segmentation [40].

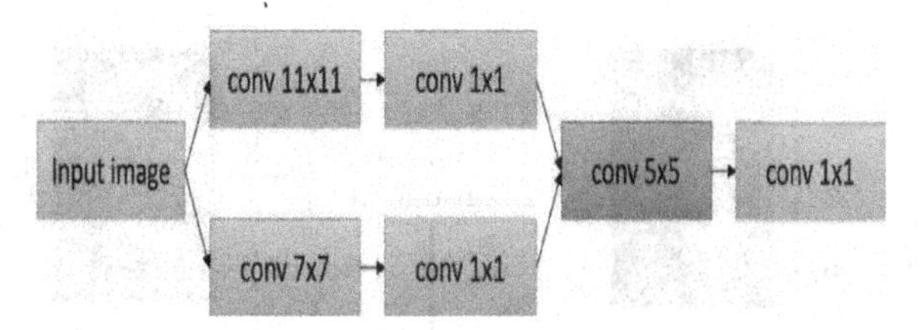

Figure 3.9 The multi-view architecture of MVPNets [40].

Figure 3.9. It utilizes different kernel size, where a large kernel size (11×11) extracts the global infiltrative growth pattern and a smaller kernel size (7×7) extracts the more regional features. MVPNets are used to train the model from scratch using Stochastic gradient descent (SGD) optimizer with an adaptive learning rate function. The models over the epoch are analyzed based on categorical cross-entropy loss performance measures.

3.4.1.2 3-D multi-view deep convolutional neural network (3D multi-view DCNN) [44]

3D multi-view DCNN is used as the bilateral feature representation in the DBT-structured volume. It utilizes self-taught learning to identify the masses based on latent bilateral feature representation. The main objective of the method is to use the data at multiple levels of abstraction for accurate models. It is expected to have symmetric masses appear in the left and right breast. However, in the case of cancer, different breast tissue structures appear that show the asymmetric volume of densities of masses. This method uses two views, called the main view (characteristics of mass volumes) and the bilateral view (corresponding volume) [44].

- *Latent bilateral feature (LBF) representation:* The LBF representation analysis process has been shown in Figure 3.10. In the analysis process, the source reconstructed volume (V_s) and target reconstructed volume (V_t) need to be calculated. The source reconstruction (R_s) and target reconstruction (R_t) can be calculated through a geometric transformation as shown in eq. 3.5.

$$R_t = \text{Trans}(R_s) \tag{3.5}$$

The VOI transformation enables the bilateral feature representation of masses as V_s and V_t.

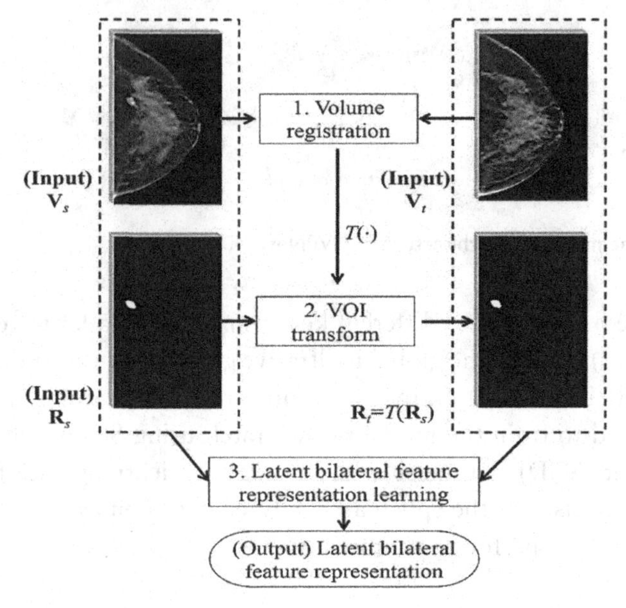

Figure 3.10 3D multi-view DCNN framework for LBF representation, where gray dots represent the normal breast tissues and mass samples [44].

- *The architecture of 3D Multi-view DCNN:* The architecture has multiple stages such as $C1$, $C1$', $C3$, and $C3$' as convolutional layer stages, where $S2$, $S2$', $S4$ & $S4'$ are the subsampling layer stages. The intensity variation in the depth direction is required to adopt 3D learnable filters for CNN, i.e., shown in eq. 3.6:

$$X_j^l = \phi\{\sum_{i=1}^{N^l} X_i^{l-1} \times w_{ij}^l + b_j^l\} \tag{3.6}$$

where $\phi\{.\}$ is the activation function. N^l and X_j^l are the numbers of feature maps and the feature map of $l-th$ layer, respectively. w_{ij}^l and b_j^l are the 3D filter and bias, respectively. The F5 hidden layer finds the high-level LBF representation of the extracted features from DBT data in the architecture. In Figure 3.10, 3D multi-view DCNN framework for LBF representation, gray dots represent the normal breast tissues and mass samples at layer F6. The last layer (F6) utilizes the softmax function to minimize the classification error, and the cross-entropy loss function is used to find the error of classification. The 160 reconstructed volumes of 40 patients' data are used to train the model, where 86 volumes have malignant mass, and 74 have normal ones. The performance of the models has been compared using ROC and AUC for the hand-crafted features and LBF .

3.4.2 Brain issue

The organs and tissues segmentation of medical images have performed successfully using DCNNs [29, 32, 41]. The segmentation and classification approaches of medical images using DCNN can be categorized into two 1) patch segmentation for the voxel classification and batch-based voxel classification. The size of the patches matters a lot for classification problems, which means large sizes of patches include multiple classes that reduce the performance. Smaller sizes have less information to learn the classifiers from the patches effectively. The performance of DCNN is not effective when each patch within images is complex. To address this issue M3Net [80] architecture has been proposed.

Electroencephalography (EEG) obtains huge information about brain nerve activity [16]. EEG analysis finds independent acts of nerves, i.e., caused by craniocerebral nerve injuries, spine injuries, and strokes. The analysis of brain activities using EEG improves the patients' communication with the outside world. Many frequencies generated by EEG show the different subject responses. Therefore, many methods have been proposed based on frequency-dependent problems of common spatial pattern (CSP) such as CSSP [47], FBCSP [4], CSSSP [18] etc. Usually, only frequency and spatial domain are used for the analysis where other domains are ignored, such as the time-frequency domain and time domain, i.e., poses the loss of information in motor imagery. Therefore, In Ref. [86], the time domain and frequency-time domain have been utilized along with the frequency and spatial domain of motor imagery and proposed MVL framework using DL for recognition systems. The details of this method have been covered in the following subsections.

3.4.2.1 Multi-model, multi-size, and multi-view deep neural network (M3Net) [80]

M3Net segments the image into the following steps, where the architecture is shown in Figure 3.11:

- *Step-1 (Pre-processing of brain MR images):* This process utilizes the CMA autoseg routine and contrast-limit adaptive histogram equalization (CLAHE) method.
- *Step-2 (Probabilistic brain atlases construction)*: This step obtains the probability of generated segmentation such as white matter, gray matter, and CSF.
- *Step-3 (Patch segmentation using multi-size U-Nets)*: The training of U-Nets with atlas patches and image patches is done then patch-by-patch segmentation is performed.
- *Step-4 (Voxel classification using multi-size BPNNs)*: The pre-trained multi-size BPNNs are utilized to classify the patch-based voxel.
- *Step-5 (Brain MR images segmentation)*: The 2D likelihood map of Multi-size U-Net and Multi-size BPNN are combined to get each view's 3D likelihood.
- *Step-6 (3D segmentation results)*: Then finally, the 3D segmentation results are obtained by combining the trans-axial, coronal, and sagittal views.

The proposed architecture has been evaluated using three BrainWeb [15], IBSR V2.0, and IBSR 20 datasets. The experimental analysis has been done based on gray matters, white matters, and CSF.

3.4.2.2 Deep multi-view feature learning for EEG signal motor imagery [12]

This method classifies the motor imagery of signals. The extracted features are frequency domain, time domain, spatial domain, and time-

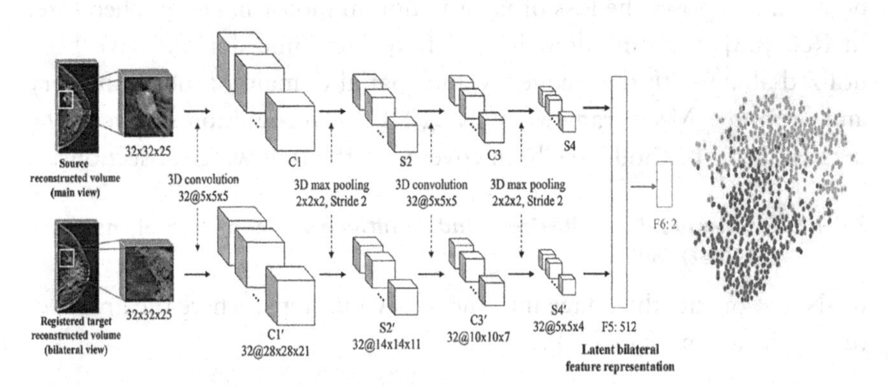

Figure 3.11 Architecture of M3Nets [80].

frequency domain, where these features are complemented and cooperated. In the process, the global characteristics have been accounted for to remove the feature redundancy that enhances the recognition by reducing the dimension of the features. Then the deep multi-view extracted features are used for classification using SVM. The proposed architecture is shown in Figure 3.12.

The traditional feature extraction is not effective in extracting the characteristics of the EEG signal because it has a low signal-to-noise ratio and is unsteady, nonlinear, and time-varying. Therefore, three feature extraction techniques are utilized to extract the distinct EEG signal characteristics to form the multi-view features, i.e., shown in the orange color (Figure 3.12). The features are described below:

- *Time-domain features:* These features are extracted by artifact removal and denoising from the original EEG signal.
- *Frequency domain feature:* The frequency bands are passed through the band-pass filter that extracts the valuable frequency band and groups them into multiple sub-bands.
- *Time-Frequency domain feature*: This feature has the frequency characteristics of EEG signals based on various periods.
- *Spatial domain feature*: These features are extracted based on different EEG signals, where the diagonalization of the matrix is used to get the optimal set of spatial filters for projection.

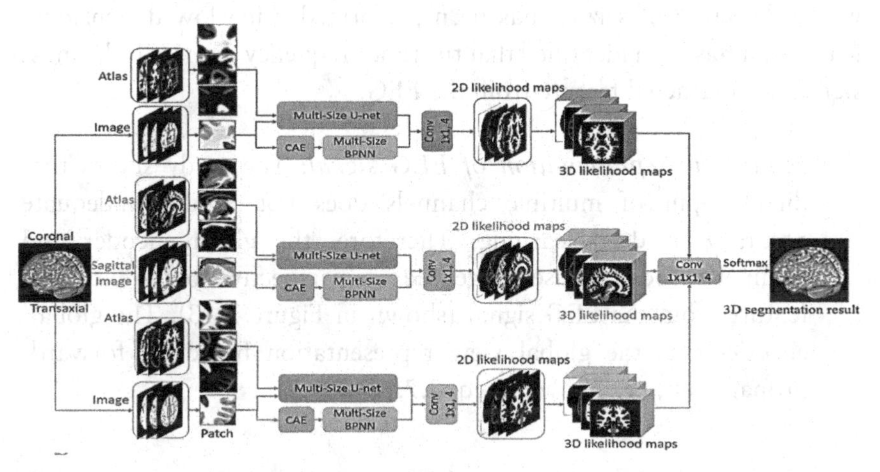

Figure 3.12 A framework of deep multi-view features learning [75].

- *Deep multi-view features*: The parametric t-SNE extracts the feature using deep network from EEG signals. It also reduces the dimension and maximizes the variance among the four types of imagery.

3.4.3 Seizure recognition

Sudden abnormal neuron discharges cause epilepsy in the brain, posing a serious neurological disorder in humans. The unpredictable epileptic seizures are chronic symptoms [25]. The study shows that EEG is utilized to detect and diagnose because of temporal resolution and affordability. The brain's electrical activities are monitored using many electrodes around the brain. Recent advancements in computing and pervasive sensing technology have empowered to analyze the EEG signals of epilepsy patients to detect and diagnose epilepsy seizures. The description of some of the methods is given in the following section.

3.4.3.1 Multi-channel EEG seizure detection using deep MVL [96]

EEG multiple channel scalp detection has been done using deep learning models [89, 94]. The EEG signal has a substantial unwanted signal (irrelevant channels) that prevents brain activity effectively. Therefore, the performance of learning methods has significantly reduced. To handle this issue, multi-channel EEG-based seizure detection has been proposed using MVL [96]. This method has proposed a novel framework, i.e., dynamic soft channel selection in multiple channels of EEG signals where detection of seizure has been performed using low dimensional features. It has been identified that the time-frequency domain is the most significant extracted feature from the EEG.

- *Multi-view representation of EEG signal*: The study shows that direct input of multiple channels does not produce adequate accuracy in deep learning. Therefore, the global-encoder and channel-encoder are used to get the two perspectives of the extracted feature from the EEG signal (shown in Figure 3.13). The global-encoder gets the global view representation based on forward-propagation, i.e., shown in eq. 3.7.

$$H_G = \phi(w_G x_{(1:c)} + b_G) \tag{3.7}$$

where w_G is weight matrix and b_G is bias vector, and the activation function is $\phi(.)$. As shown in eq, the channel-view representation can be obtained using a channel-encoder. eq. 3.7.

$$H_i = f(w_c x_i + b_c) \tag{3.8}$$

- *Channel aware attention mechanism*: The main objective of this attention mechanism is to derive the global context (relevant information of the channel). The normalized attention score is measured using the softmax function. Then, local-based and global-based attention mechanisms are used to find the channel-view representation.
- *Seizure detection:* The training of the model has been performed uniformly using S number of training samples. The final cost function of the channel attention model can be calculated using cross-entropy loss (eq. 3.9).

$$J_{CA}(W_{(g,c,e,h,s)}, b_{(g,c,e,h,s)}) \tag{3.9}$$

$$= \frac{1}{S}\sum_{i=1}^{S}\sum_{j=1}^{|\text{class}|}[y_j^{(i)}(\log(\hat{y}_j^i)) + (1 - y_j^{(i)})(\log(1 - \hat{y}_j^i))$$

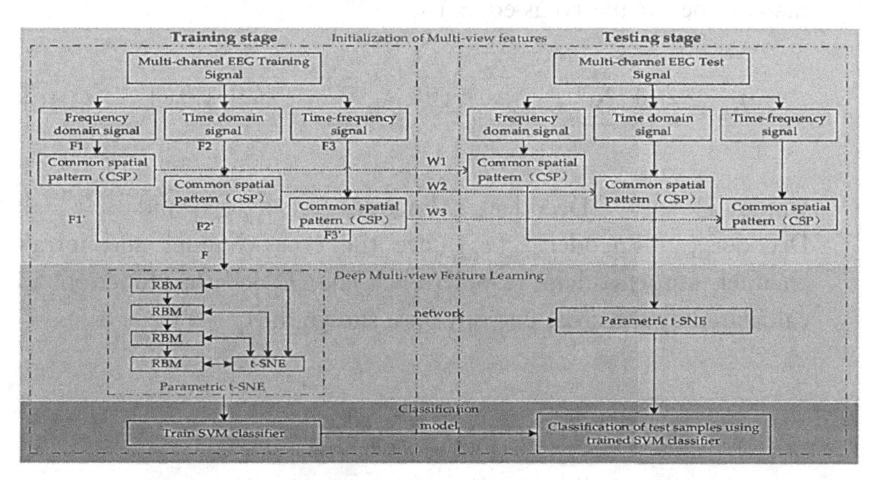

Figure 3.13 A framework of multi-view deep features learning that learns jointly from supervised seizure detection and unsupervised multi-channel EEG reconstruction [96].

3.4.3.2 *Autoencoder-based deep MVL for seizure detection [95]*

This method performs seizure classification in two-stage:

- *EEG multi-view feature learning:* The classical approach to extracting the features is to obtain the handcraft features from various aspects, which requires significant expert knowledge input. Therefore, this method uses bio-signal processing to represent the EEG spectrogram [28, 93]. The generated spectrogram transforms each segment into the time-frequency domain. Moreover, the feature extraction is performed using deep networks, where the study shows that extracted time-frequency domain is more valuable than the only time-domain feature. Moreover, autoencoders recognize the instances corresponding to the different perspective that helps the classifier learn through latent seizure characteristics [78]. The proposed feature extraction model utilized EEG channels' correlation (cross-channel and intra-cross channel). While training, the reconstruction error minimization objective function utilizes the multi-view feature extractor. A framework of multi-view deep features learning that learns jointly from supervised seizure detection and unsupervised multi-channel EEG reconstruction is shown in Figure 3.14. The multi-view autoencoder (MAE) utilizes the cost function that can be calculated as eq. 3.10.

$$J_{\text{MAE}} = \frac{1}{|S|}\sum_{i=1}^{k}[L_H(x^{(i)}, (\hat{x}_r^{(i)})) + \sum_{c=1}^{C} L_H(x_c^{(i)}, \hat{x}_c^{(i)}))] \quad (3.10)$$

where $\hat{x}_r^{(i)} = \text{Decoder}_{\text{cross}}(\text{Encoder}_{\text{cross}}(x_{(1,C)}))$ and $\hat{x}_r^{(i)} = \text{Decoder}_{\text{intra}}$ $(\text{Encoder}_{\text{intra}}(x_c))$ are the cross-channel and intra-channel autoencoders respectively. The $L_H(.)$ the function is calculated by the cross-entropy loss, shown in eq. 3.11.

$$L_H(x^{(i)}, \hat{x}_r^i) = -\sum_{j=1}^{k}[x_j^{(i)}(\log(\hat{x}_j^{(i)})) + (1 - x_j^{(i)})\log(1 - x_j^{(i)}) \quad (3.11)$$

- *Classification:* The proposed model focuses on identifying the relevant EEG signals. To achieve the same objective, an aware channel module is introduced to enhance the hidden feature learning that

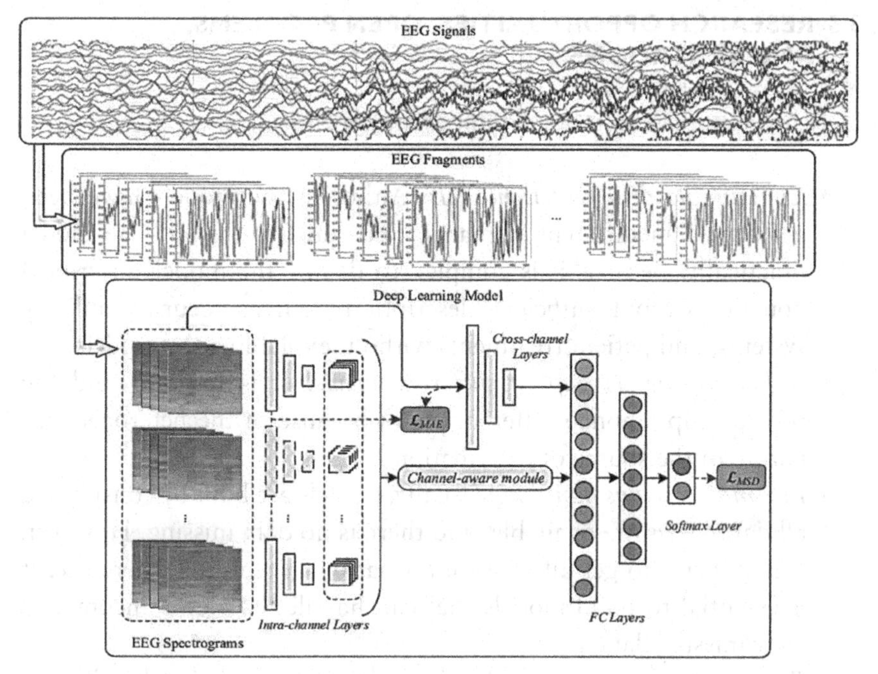

Figure 3.14 A framework of multi-view deep features learning that learns jointly from supervised seizure detection and unsupervised multi-channel EEG reconstruction [93].

incorporates the selectivity and sparsity constraints while training the model. Therefore, the training objective includes the J_{MAE} and J_{MSD} cost functions. The multi-view learning (MVL) model, including two cost functions, can be written as in eq. 3.12:

$$J_{\text{MVL}}(W_{(r,c,p,u,s)}, b_{(r,c,p,u,s)}) = \frac{1}{|S|}\sum_{i=1}^{k}[\beta_1 L_H(y^{(i)}, (\hat{y}_r^{(i)}) + \beta_2 L_H(x^{(i)}, \hat{x}_r^{(i)}) + \sum_{c=1}^{C} L_H(x_c^{(i)}, \hat{x}_c^{(i)})] \tag{3.12}$$

where β_1 and β_2 are the hyperparameters, the CHB-MIT dataset of 23 patients is used for the model's training, where each channel has 256 Hz with 16-bit resolution. The evaluation criteria of the model are used as AUC-ROC and AUC-PR.

3.5 RESEARCH OPPORTUNITIES, OPEN PROBLEMS, AND LIMITATIONS

Here are some research opportunities and open problems:

- *Explainable deep MVL models:* Although the models have been performed in different domains. It is hard to explain the model practically. Because it is complex to deploy the models in critical domain without sufficient description such as security, military systems, and patient treatments without explaining the models.
- *A heterogeneous gap of different views:* It is hard to find the relationship amonge different views because of the heterogeneous nature of the source of information.
- *Incomplete views handling:* Usually, models are built by considering all data views are available, and there is no data missing. However, it is difficult to get all views information in real life. Therefore, it is essential to build models that can handle the views' incomplete view/missing data.
- *Representation learning:* Graph feature representation handling is one of the crucial problems in multi-view graph learning. However, very few works have been done in representation learning.
- *Exploration of views relationship:* Deep multi-view learning learns through shared embedding features by fusion that explores the views relations. However, this approach is not yet effective in getting good relations among the views.

Deep MVL limitations are as follows:

- Deep MVL methods are data-hungry models. Therefore, more training data is required because deep networks learn sufficiently with massive input data [90].
- Instead of better performance of deep MVL over multiple tasks, it does explain the decision model that hinders application in critical domains [80].
- A comprehensive theoretical understanding of deep neural network learning mechanisms is not available.

3.6 CONCLUSION

Initially, multi-view learning has been described with different examples to build the basic concepts along with general categorization MVL such as co-regularization style algorithm, co-training algorithm, and margin consistency. Then, DL architecture has been elaborated based on the internal component of architecture. After this concept, the various computational method of deep MVL has been elaborated into two broad categories as a MVL method in DL and deep learning extension of traditional learning method. The main objective of this chapter is to discuss deep MVL in the healthcare domain. Therefore, deployed models of deep MVL have been described in context of three broad health issues i.e., breast diagnosis (MVPNets and 3D multi-view DCNN), brain issue (M3Net and Deep Multi-view feature learning), and seizure recognition (seizure detection suing multi-channel EEG) and Autoencoder-based deep MVL). At last, the research opportunities, open problems, and limitations have been discussed for deep MVL.

REFERENCES

[1] Abrar H Abdulnabi, Bing Shuai, Zhen Zuo, Lap-Pui Chau, and Gang Wang. Multimodal recurrent neural networks with information transfer layers for indoor scene labeling. *IEEE Transactions on Multimedia*, 20(7):1656–1671, 2017.

[2] Alaa S Al-Waisy, Rami Qahwaji, Stanley Ipson, and Shumoos Al-Fahdawi. A multimodal deep learning framework using local feature representations for face recognition. *Machine Vision and Applications*, 29(1):35–54, 2018.

[3] Mohamed R Amer, Timothy Shields, Behjat Siddiquie, Amir Tamrakar, Ajay Divakaran, and Sek Chai. Deep multimodal fusion: A hybrid approach. *International Journal of Computer Vision*, 126(2):440–456, 2018.

[4] Kai Keng Ang, Zheng Yang Chin, Haihong Zhang, and Cuntai Guan. Filter bank common spatial pattern (fbcsp) in brain-computer interface. In *2008 IEEE International Joint Conference on Neural Networks (IEEE World Congress on Computational Intelligence)*, IEEE, pp. 2390–2397, 2008.

[5] Suzanna Becker and Geoffrey E Hinton. Self-organizing neural network that discovers surfaces in random-dot stereograms. *Nature*, 355(6356):161–163, 1992.

[6] Avrim Blum and Tom Mitchell. Combining labeled and unlabeled data with co-training. In *Proceedings of the Eleventh Annual Conference on Computational Learning Theory*, pp. 92–100, 1998.

[7] Hongliu Cao, Simon Bernard, Robert Sabourin, and Laurent Heutte. Random forest dissimilarity based multi-view learning for radiomics application. *Pattern Recognition*, 88:185–197, 2019.

[8] Gustavo Carneiro, Jacinto Nascimento, and Andrew P Bradley. Automated analysis of unregistered multi-view mammograms with deep learning. *IEEE Transactions on Medical Imaging*, 36(11):2355–2365, 2017.

[9] Gustavo Carneiro, Jacinto Nascimento, and Andrew P Bradley. Deep learning models for classifying mammogram exams containing unregistered multi-view images and segmentation maps of lesions. In: S Kevin Zhou, Hayit Greenspan, and Dinggang Shen (Eds.), *Deep Learning for Medical Image Analysis*. Academic Press: Cambridge, MA, pp. 321–339, 2017.

[10] Guoqing Chao and Shiliang Sun. Alternative multiview maximum entropy discrimination. *IEEE Transactions on Neural Networks and Learning Systems*, 27(7):1445–1456, 2015.

[11] Guoqing Chao and Shiliang Sun. Consensus and complementarity based maximum entropy discrimination for multi-view classification. *Information Sciences*, 367:296–310, 2016.

[12] Guoqing Chao, Shiliang Sun, and Jinbo Bi. A survey on multi-view clustering. arXiv preprint arXiv:1712.06246, 2017.

[13] Mickaël Chen and Ludovic Denoyer. Multi-view generative adversarial networks. In *Joint European Conference on Machine Learning and Knowledge Discovery in Databases*, Springer, pp. 175–188, 2017.

[14] Shaika Chowdhury, Chenwei Zhang, Philip S Yu, and Yuan Luo. Mixed pooling multi-view attention autoencoder for representation learning in healthcare. arXiv preprint arXiv:1910.06456, 2019.

[15] D Louis Collins, Alex P Zijdenbos, Vasken Kollokian, John G Sled, Noor J Kabani, Colin J Holmes, and Alan C Evans. Design and construction of a realistic digital brain phantom. *IEEE Transactions on Medical Imaging*, 17(3):463–468, 1998.

[16] Janis J Daly and Jonathan R Wolpaw. Brain–computer interfaces in neurological rehabilitation. *The Lancet Neurology*, 7(11):1032–1043, 2008.

[17] Brian Dolhansky and Cristian Canton Ferrer. Eye in-painting with exemplar generative adversarial networks. In *Proceedings of the IEEE Conference on Computer Vision and Pattern Recognition*, pp. 7902–7911, 2018.

[18] Guido Dornhege, Benjamin Blankertz, Matthias Krauledat, Florian Losch, Gabriel Curio, and KR Muller. Combined optimization of spatial and temporal filters for improving brain-computer interfacing. *IEEE Transactions on Biomedical Engineering*, 53(11):2274–2281, 2006.

[19] Alexandrina L Dumitrescu. *Chemicals in Surgical Periodontal Therapy*. Springer: Berlin/Heidelberg, Germany, 2011.

[20] Shaohua Fan, Xiao Wang, Chuan Shi, Emiao Lu, Ken Lin, and Bai Wang. One2multi graph autoencoder for multi-view graph clustering. In *Proceedings of the Web Conference 2020*, pp. 3070–3076, 2020.

[21] Wenqi Fan, Yao Ma, Han Xu, Xiaorui Liu, Jianping Wang, Qing Li, and Jiliang Tang. Deep adversarial canonical correlation analysis. In *Proceedings of the 2020 SIAM International Conference on Data Mining*, SIAM, pp. 352–360, 2020.

[22] Jason Farquhar, David Hardoon, Hongying Meng, John Shawe-Taylor, and Sandor Szedmak. Two view learning: Svm-2k, theory and practice. In *NIPS'05: Proceedings of the 18th International Conference on Neural Information Processing Systemss*, 355–362, 2005.

[23] Xiaoyan Fei, Lu Shen, Shihui Ying, Yehua Cai, Qi Zhang, Wentao Kong, Weijun Zhou, and Jun Shi. Parameter transfer deep neural network for single-modal b-mode ultrasound-based computer-aided diagnosis. *Cognitive Computation*, 12(6):1252–1264, 2020.
[24] Yifan Feng, Zizhao Zhang, Xibin Zhao, Rongrong Ji, and Yue Gao. Gvcnn: Group-view convolutional neural networks for 3d shape recognition. In *Proceedings of the IEEE Conference on Computer Vision and Pattern Recognition*, pp. 264–272, 2018.
[25] Robert S Fisher, Walter Van Emde Boas, Warren Blume, Christian Elger, Pierre Genton, Phillip Lee, and Jerome Engel Jr. Epileptic seizures and epilepsy: definitions proposed by the international league against epilepsy (ilae) and the international bureau for epilepsy (ibe). *Epilepsia*, 46(4):470–472, 2005.
[26] Bangming Gong, Lu Shen, Cai Chang, Shichong Zhou, Weijun Zhou, Shuo Li, and Jun Shi. Bi-modal ultrasound breast cancer diagnosis via multi-view deep neural network svm. In *2020 IEEE 17th International Symposium on Biomedical Imaging (ISBI)*, IEEE, pp. 1106–1110, 2020.
[27] Ian Goodfellow, Yoshua Bengio, and Aaron Courville. *Deep Learning*. MIT Press: Cambridge, MA, 2016.
[28] J Gotman, D Flanagan, J Zhang, and B Rosenblatt. Automatic seizure detection in the newborn: methods and initial evaluation. *Electroencephalography and Clinical Neurophysiology*, 103(3):356–362, 1997.
[29] Ricardo Guerrero, Chen Qin, Ozan Oktay, Christopher Bowles, Liang Chen, Richard Joules, Robin Wolz, M del C Valdés-Hernández, David Alexander Dickie, Joanna Wardlaw, et al. White matter hyperintensity and stroke lesion segmentation and differentiation using convolutional neural networks. *NeuroImage: Clinical*, 17:918–934, 2018.
[30] Le-Hang Guo, Dan Wang, Yi-Yi Qian, Xiao Zheng, Chong-Ke Zhao, Xiao-Long Li, Xiao-Wan Bo, Wen-Wen Yue, Qi Zhang, Jun Shi, et al. A two-stage multi-view learning framework based computer-aided diagnosis of liver tumors with contrast enhanced ultrasound images. *Clinical Hemorheology and Microcirculation*, 69(3):343–354, 2018.
[31] Wenzhong Guo, Jianwen Wang, and Shiping Wang. Deep multimodal representation learning: A survey. *IEEE Access*, 7:63373–63394, 2019.
[32] Ida Häggström, C Ross Schmidtlein, Gabriele Campanella, and Thomas J Fuchs. Deeppet: A deep encoder–decoder network for directly solving the pet image reconstruction inverse problem. *Medical Image Analysis*, 54:253–262, 2019.
[33] Will Hamilton, Payal Bajaj, Marinka Zitnik, Dan Jurafsky, and Jure Leskovec. Embedding logical queries on knowledge graphs. In *32nd Conference on Neural Information Processing Systems (NeurIPS 2018)*, Montréal, Canada, 2018.
[34] Zhongyi Han, Benzheng Wei, Yuanjie Zheng, Yilong Yin, Kejian Li, and Shuo Li. Breast cancer multi-classification from histopathological images with structured deep learning model. *Scientific Reports*, 7(1):1–10, 2017.
[35] David R Hardoon, Sandor Szedmak, and John Shawe-Taylor. Canonical correlation analysis: An overview with application to learning methods. *Neural Computation*, 16(12):2639–2664, 2004.

[36] Chaoqun Hong, Jun Yu, Jian Wan, Dacheng Tao, and Meng Wang. Multimodal deep autoencoder for human pose recovery. *IEEE Transactions on Image Processing*, 24(12):5659–5670, 2015.
[37] William W Hsieh. Nonlinear canonical correlation analysis by neural networks. *Neural Networks*, 13(10):1095–1105, 2000.
[38] Wenbing Huang, Tong Zhang, Yu Rong, and Junzhou Huang. Adaptive sampling towards fast graph representation learning. *Advances in Neural Information Processing Systems*, 31, 2018.
[39] Phillip Isola, Jun-Yan Zhu, Tinghui Zhou, and Alexei A Efros. Image-to-image translation with conditional adversarial networks. In *Proceedings of the IEEE Conference on Computer Vision and Pattern Recognition*, pp. 1125–1134, 2017.
[40] Padmaja Jonnalagedda, Daniel Schmolze, and Bir Bhanu. mvpnets: Multi-viewing path deep learning neural networks for magnification invariant diagnosis in breast cancer. In *2018 IEEE 18th International Conference on Bioinformatics and Bioengineering (BIBE)*, IEEE, pp. 189–194, 2018.
[41] Konstantinos Kamnitsas, Christian Ledig, Virginia FJ Newcombe, Joanna P Simpson, Andrew D Kane, David K Menon, Daniel Rueckert, and Ben Glocker. Efficient multi-scale 3d cnn with fully connected crf for accurate brain lesion segmentation. *Medical Image Analysis*, 36:61–78, 2017.
[42] Meina Kan, Shiguang Shan, Haihong Zhang, Shihong Lao, and Xilin Chen. Multi-view discriminant analysis. *IEEE Transactions on Pattern Analysis and Machine Intelligence*, 38(1):188–194, 2015.
[43] Andrej Karpathy and Li Fei-Fei. Deep visual-semantic alignments for generating image descriptions. In *Proceedings of the IEEE Conference on Computer Vision and Pattern Recognition*, pp. 3128–3137, 2015.
[44] Dae Hoe Kim, Seong Tae Kim, and Yong Man Ro. Latent feature representation with 3-d multi-view deep convolutional neural network for bilateral analysis in digital breast tomosynthesis. In *2016 IEEE International Conference on Acoustics, Speech and Signal Processing (ICASSP)*, IEEE, pp. 927–931, 2016.
[45] Roman Klokov and Victor Lempitsky. Escape from cells: Deep kd-networks for the recognition of 3d point cloud models. In *Proceedings of the IEEE International Conference on Computer Vision*, pp. 863–872, 2017.
[46] Trent Kyono, Fiona J Gilbert, and Mihaela Van Der Schaar. Triage of 2d mammographic images using multi-view multi-task convolutional neural networks. *ACM Transactions on Computing for Healthcare*, 2(3):1–24, 2021.
[47] Steven Lemm, Benjamin Blankertz, Gabriel Curio, and K-R Muller. Spatio-spectral filters for improving the classification of single trial eeg. *IEEE Transactions on Biomedical Engineering*, 52(9):1541–1548, 2005.
[48] Yingming Li, Ming Yang, and Zhongfei Zhang. A survey of multi-view representation learning. *IEEE Transactions on Knowledge and Data Engineering*, 31(10):1863–1883, 2018.
[49] Weibo Liu, Zidong Wang, Xiaohui Liu, Nianyin Zeng, and David Bell. A novel particle swarm optimization approach for patient clustering from emergency departments. *IEEE Transactions on Evolutionary Computation*, 23(4):632–644, 2018.
[50] Weibo Liu, Zidong Wang, Yuan Yuan, Nianyin Zeng, Kate Hone, and Xiaohui Liu. A novel sigmoid-function-based adaptive weighted particle swarm optimizer. *IEEE Transactions on Cybernetics*, 51(2):1085–1093, 2019.

[51] C Loukas, Spiros Kostopoulos, Anna Tanoglidi, Dimitris Glotsos, C Sfikas, and Dionisis Cavouras. Breast cancer characterization based on image classification of tissue sections visualized under low magnification. *Computational and Mathematical Methods in Medicine*, 2013, 2013.

[52] Ravikiran Mane, Neethu Robinson, A Prasad Vinod, Seong-Whan Lee, and Cuntai Guan. A multi-view cnn with novel variance layer for motor imagery brain computer interface. In *2020 42nd Annual International Conference of the IEEE Engineering in Medicine & Biology Society (EMBC)*, IEEE, pp. 2950–2953, 2020.

[53] Junhua Mao, Wei Xu, Yi Yang, Jiang Wang, Zhiheng Huang, and Alan Yuille. Deep captioning with multimodal recurrent neural networks (m-rnn). arXiv preprint arXiv:1412.6632, 2014.

[54] Ion Muslea, Steven Minton, and Craig A Knoblock. Active learning with multiple views. *Journal of Artificial Intelligence Research*, 27:203–233, 2006.

[55] Vinod Nair and Geoffrey E Hinton. Rectified linear units improve restricted boltzmann machines. In *Icml*, 2010.

[56] Athma Narayanan, Avinash Siravuru, and Behzad Dariush. Sensor fusion: Gated recurrent fusion to learn driving behavior from temporal multimodal data. arXiv preprint arXiv:1910.00628, 2019.

[57] Kamal Nigam and Rayid Ghani. Analyzing the effectiveness and applicability of co-training. In *Proceedings of the Ninth International Conference on Information and Knowledge Management*, pp. 86–93, 2000.

[58] Thai-Hoang Pham, Changchang Yin, Laxmi Mehta, Xueru Zhang, and Ping Zhang. Cardiac complication risk profiling for cancer survivors via multi-view multi-task learning. In *2021 IEEE International Conference on Data Mining (ICDM)*, IEEE, pp. 499–508, 2021.

[59] Esther Puyol-Antón, Bram Ruijsink, Bernhard Gerber, Mihaela Silvia Amzulescu, Helene Langet, Mathieu De Craene, Julia A Schnabel, Paolo Piro, and Andrew P King. Regional multi-view learning for cardiac motion analysis: application to identification of dilated cardiomyopathy patients. *IEEE Transactions on Biomedical Engineering*, 66(4):956–966, 2018.

[60] Izaz Ur Rahman, Zidong Wang, Weibo Liu, Baoliu Ye, Muhammad Zakarya, and Xiaohui Liu. An n-state markovian jumping particle swarm optimization algorithm. *IEEE Transactions on Systems, Man, and Cybernetics: Systems*, 51(11):6626–6638, 2020.

[61] Dhanesh Ramachandram and Graham W Taylor. Deep multimodal learning: A survey on recent advances and trends. *IEEE Signal Processing Magazine*, 34(6):96–108, 2017.

[62] Akane Sano, Weixuan Chen, Daniel Lopez-Martinez, Sara Taylor, and Rosalind W Picard. Multimodal ambulatory sleep detection using lstm recurrent neural networks. *IEEE Journal of Biomedical and Health Informatics*, 23(4):1607–1617, 2018.

[63] Yaniv Shachor, Hayit Greenspan, and Jacob Goldberger. A mixture of views network with applications to multi-view medical imaging. *Neurocomputing*, 374:1–9, 2020.

[64] Ming Shao and Yun Fu. Deeply self-taught multi-view video analytics machine for situation awareness. In *AFA Cyber Workshop. White Paper*, 2015.

[65] Nitish Srivastava, Geoffrey Hinton, Alex Krizhevsky, Ilya Sutskever, and Ruslan Salakhutdinov. Dropout: A simple way to prevent neural networks

from overfitting. *The Journal of Machine Learning Research*, 15(1):1929–1958, 2014.

[66] Nitish Srivastava and Russ R Salakhutdinov. Multimodal learning with deep boltzmann machines. In *Advances in Neural Information Processing Systems (NIPS 2012)*, 25, 2012.

[67] Hang Su, Subhransu Maji, Evangelos Kalogerakis, and Erik Learned-Miller. Multi-view convolutional neural networks for 3d shape recognition. In *Proceedings of the IEEE International Conference on Computer Vision*, pp. 945–953, 2015.

[68] Shiliang Sun. A survey of multi-view machine learning. *Neural Computing and Applications*, 23(7):2031–2038, 2013.

[69] Shiliang Sun and Guoqing Chao. Multi-view maximum entropy discrimination. In *Twenty-Third International Joint Conference on Artificial Intelligence*, 2013.

[70] Shiliang Sun, Xijiong Xie, and Mo Yang. Multiview uncorrelated discriminant analysis. *IEEE Transactions on Cybernetics*, 46(12):3272–3284, 2015.

[71] Tingkai Sun, Songcan Chen, Jingyu Yang, and Pengfei Shi. A novel method of combined feature extraction for recognition. In *2008 Eighth IEEE International Conference on Data Mining*, IEEE, pp. 1043–1048, 2008.

[72] Yiwei Sun, Suhang Wang, Tsung-Yu Hsieh, Xianfeng Tang, and Vasant Honavar. Megan: A generative adversarial network for multi-view network embedding. arXiv preprint arXiv:1909.01084, 2019.

[73] Ilya Sutskever, James Martens, and Geoffrey E Hinton. Generating text with recurrent neural networks. In *ICML*, 2011.

[74] Arida Ferti Syafiandini, Ito Wasito, Setiadi Yazid, Aries Fitriawan, and Mukhlis Amien. Multimodal deep boltzmann machines for feature selection on gene expression data. In *2016 International Conference on Advanced Computer Science and Information Systems (ICACSIS)*, IEEE, pp. 407–412, 2016.

[75] Xiaobin Tian, Zhaohong Deng, Wenhao Ying, Kup-Sze Choi, Dongrui Wu, Bin Qin, Jun Wang, Hongbin Shen, and Shitong Wang. Deep multi-view feature learning for eeg-based epileptic seizure detection. *IEEE Transactions on Neural Systems and Rehabilitation Engineering*, 27(10):1962–1972, 2019.

[76] Yu Tian, Xi Peng, Long Zhao, Shaoting Zhang, and Dimitris N Metaxas. Cr-gan: Learning complete representations for multi-view generation. arXiv preprint arXiv:1806.11191, 2018.

[77] Luan Tran, Xi Yin, and Xiaoming Liu. Disentangled representation learning gan for pose-invariant face recognition. In *Proceedings of the IEEE Conference on Computer Vision and Pattern Recognition*, pp. 1415–1424, 2017.

[78] Pascal Vincent, Hugo Larochelle, Yoshua Bengio, and Pierre-Antoine Manzagol. Extracting and composing robust features with denoising autoencoders. In *Proceedings of the 25th International Conference on Machine Learning*, pp. 1096–1103, 2008.

[79] Weiran Wang, Raman Arora, Karen Livescu, and Jeff Bilmes. On deep multi-view representation learning. In *International Conference on Machine Learning*, PMLR, pp. 1083–1092, 2015.

[80] Jie Wei, Yong Xia, and Yanning Zhang. M3net: A multi-model, multi-size, and multi-view deep neural network for brain magnetic resonance image segmentation. *Pattern Recognition*, 91:366–378, 2019.

[81] Elisabete Weiderpass and Bernard W Stewart. *World Cancer Report*. WHO Regional Office for the Western Pacific: Manila, PH, 2020

[82] Yingda Xia, Dong Yang, Zhiding Yu, Fengze Liu, Jinzheng Cai, Lequan Yu, Zhuotun Zhu, Daguang Xu, Alan Yuille, and Holger Roth. Uncertainty-aware multi-view co-training for semi-supervised medical image segmentation and domain adaptation. *Medical Image Analysis*, 65:101766, 2020.

[83] Xijiong Xie and Shiliang Sun. Multi-view twin support vector machines. *Intelligent Data Analysis*, 19(4):701–712, 2015.

[84] Cai Xu, Ziyu Guan, Wei Zhao, Yunfei Niu, Quan Wang, and Zhiheng Wang. Deep multi-view concept learning. In *IJCAI*, Stockholm, pp. 2898–2904, 2018.

[85] Chang Xu, Dacheng Tao, and Chao Xu. A survey on multi-view learning. arXiv preprint arXiv:1304.5634, 2013.

[86] Jiacan Xu, Hao Zheng, Jianhui Wang, Donglin Li, and Xiaoke Fang. Recognition of eeg signal motor imagery intention based on deep multi-view feature learning. *Sensors*, 20(12):3496, 2020.

[87] Jun Xu, Xiaofei Luo, Guanhao Wang, Hannah Gilmore, and Anant Madabhushi. A deep convolutional neural network for segmenting and classifying epithelial and stromal regions in histopathological images. *Neurocomputing*, 191:214–223, 2016.

[88] Zhe Xue, Junping Du, Dawei Du, and Siwei Lyu. Deep low-rank subspace ensemble for multi-view clustering. *Information Sciences*, 482:210–227, 2019.

[89] Guangxu Xun, Xiaowei Jia, and Aidong Zhang. Detecting epileptic seizures with electroencephalogram via a context-learning model. *BMC Medical Informatics and Decision Making*, 16(2):97–109, 2016.

[90] Xiaoqiang Yan, Shizhe Hu, Yiqiao Mao, Yangdong Ye, and Hui Yu. Deep multi-view learning methods: A review. *Neurocomputing*, 448:106–129, 2021.

[91] Pei Yang and Wei Gao. Information-theoretic multi-view domain adaptation: A theoretical and empirical study. *Journal of Artificial Intelligence Research*, 49:501–525, 2014.

[92] Tan Yu, Jingjing Meng, and Junsong Yuan. Multi-view harmonized bilinear network for 3d object recognition. In *Proceedings of the IEEE Conference on Computer Vision and Pattern Recognition*, pp. 186–194, 2018.

[93] Ye Yuan, Guangxu Xun, Kebin Jia, and Aidong Zhang. A multi-view deep learning method for epileptic seizure detection using short-time fourier transform. In *Proceedings of the 8th ACM International Conference on Bioinformatics, Computational Biology, and Health Informatics*, pp. 213–222, 2017.

[94] Ye Yuan, Guangxu Xun, Kebin Jia, and Aidong Zhang. A novel wavelet-based model for eeg epileptic seizure detection using multi-context learning. In *2017 IEEE International Conference on Bioinformatics and Biomedicine (BIBM)*, IEEE, pp. 694–699, 2017.

[95] Ye Yuan, Guangxu Xun, Kebin Jia, and Aidong Zhang. A multi-view deep learning framework for eeg seizure detection. *IEEE Journal of Biomedical and Health Informatics*, 23(1):83–94, 2018.

[96] Ye Yuan, Guangxu Xun, Fenglong Ma, Qiuling Suo, Hongfei Xue, Kebin Jia, and Aidong Zhang. A novel channel-aware attention framework for multi-channel eeg seizure detection via multi-view deep learning. In *2018 IEEE EMBS International Conference on Biomedical & Health Informatics (BHI)*, IEEE, pp. 206–209, 2018.

[97] Wenbin Yue, Zidong Wang, Weibo Liu, Bo Tian, Stanislao Lauria, and Xiaohui Liu. An optimally weighted user-and item-based collaborative filtering approach to predicting baseline data for friedreich's ataxia patients. *Neurocomputing*, 419:287–294, 2021.

[98] Nianyin Zeng, Han Li, Zidong Wang, Weibo Liu, Songming Liu, Fuad E Alsaadi, and Xiaohui Liu. Deep-reinforcement-learning-based images segmentation for quantitative analysis of gold immunochromatographic strip. *Neurocomputing*, 425:173–180, 2021.

[99] Aston Zhang, Zachary C Lipton, Mu Li, and Alexander J Smola. Dive into deep learning. arXiv preprint arXiv:2106.11342, 2021.

[100] Haotian Zhang, Gaoang Wang, Zhichao Lei, and Jenq-Neng Hwang. Eye in the sky: Drone-based object tracking and 3d localization. In *Proceedings of the 27th ACM International Conference on Multimedia*, pp. 899–907, 2019.

[101] Nan Zhang, Shifei Ding, Hongmei Liao, and Weikuan Jia. Multimodal correlation deep belief networks for multi-view classification. *Applied Intelligence*, 49(5):1925–1936, 2019.

[102] Nan Zhang, Shifei Ding, Jian Zhang, and Yu Xue. An overview on restricted boltzmann machines. *Neurocomputing*, 275:1186–1199, 2018.

[103] Zheng Zhang, Qi Zhu, Guo-Sen Xie, Yi Chen, Zhengming Li, and Shuihua Wang. Discriminative margin-sensitive autoencoder for collective multi-view disease analysis. *Neural Networks*, 123:94–107, 2020.

[104] Jing Zhao, Xijiong Xie, Xin Xu, and Shiliang Sun. Multi-view learning overview: Recent progress and new challenges. *Information Fusion*, 38:43–54, 2017.

[105] Jianhang Zhou, Qi Zhang, and Bob Zhang. An automatic multi-view disease detection system via collective deep region-based feature representation. *Future Generation Computer Systems*, 115:59–75, 2021.

Chapter 4

Precision healthcare in the era of IoT and big data

Monitoring of self-care activities

Sujit Bebortta and Dilip Senapati
Ravenshaw University

CONTENTS

4.1 INTRODUCTION

In recent years, the emergence of wireless sensor networks (WSNs) has led to large-scale growth in data acquisition, interfacing, interoperability among devices, and scalability [12, 15, 17]. These sensory devices have played a pivotal role in strengthening the foundation of Internet of Things (IoT). From the time of its inception, the IoT has been encompassed as

DOI: 10.1201/9781003368342-4

a heterogeneous collection of sensory devices connected to the Internet, thus giving rise to a network of self-organized, identifiable, and remotely manageable smart devices [8, 15]. Following, cutting-edge advancements in computational capabilities of the smart devices connected to an IoT network, there has been tremendous innovation in intelligent applications [1, 3, 15, 18, 23, 59]. These include diverse applications such as smart industry, smart transportation, smart cities, smart medical support systems, and smart agriculture [6, 8, 9, 12, 13, 28]. To this end, the role of statistical models has remained significant in modeling and analyzing the fluctuations in the captured signals generated from different IoT devices [46, 47, 56]. In Figure 4.1, the deployment scenario for different smart IoT devices in a cloud-based environment is presented. The model comprises a tripartite architecture, where the IoT device layer represents the IoT end-users, mobile users, and IoT devices connected from several application areas such as industry, healthcare, and smart homes. The second layer constitutes the Random Access Network (RAN), through

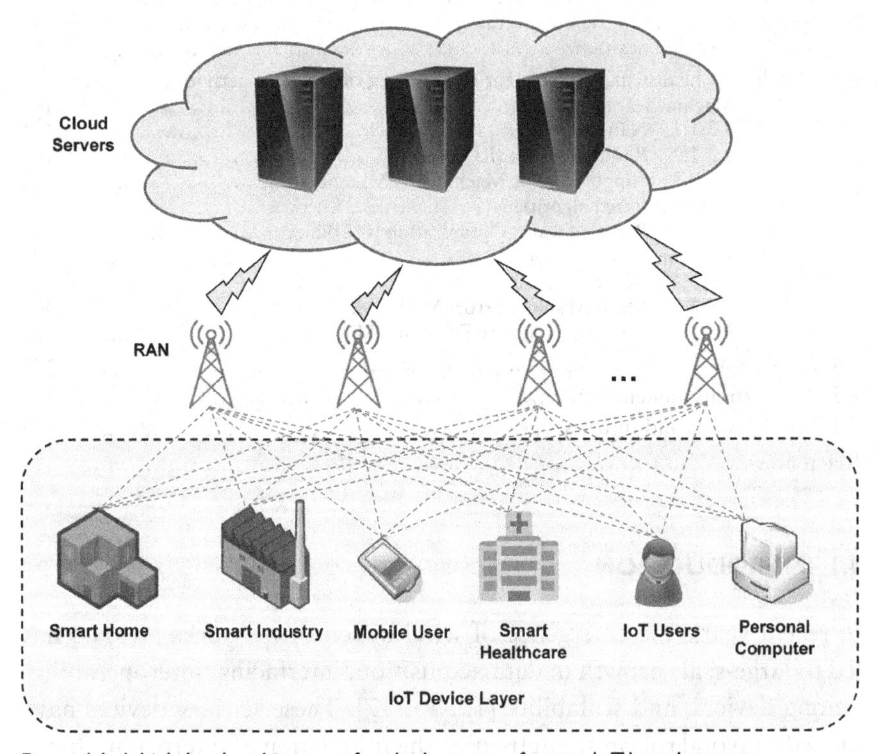

Figure 4.1 A high-level architecture for deployment of smart IoT-based systems.

which the captured data packets are forwarded to the cloud computing platform for further operations over the IoT data [18].

Several studies have depicted the successful deployment of such intelligent and innovative IoT applications in numerous fields of research including healthcare systems, smart geospatial applications, and wireless channel modeling [10, 19, 42–44]. With the continual increase in the number of interconnected devices associated with IoT several challenges such as energy efficiency, big data issues, security vulnerabilities, and Quality of Service (QoS) have surfaced [1, 2, 13, 14, 16]. There has been a substantial amount of research directed toward this field which addresses the issues of big data in IoT [1, 13]. A major goal toward this end remains in achieving low complexity execution of tasks and better provisioning of resources to overcome the issues of big data [1, 13, 14]. The issues pertaining to big data arise as a consequence of the massive amount of data being continually generated from interconnected IoT devices and IoT-based applications. Recently, there has been a phenomenal growth in research directed toward analysis and management of big data. In this direction, big data generated from healthcare sector has attracted much interest [5]. Thus, it becomes challenging to handle the massive amount of data generated as a consequence of digital transformation in healthcare sector. In remote health monitoring applications, big data mostly involves data acquired from various wearable sensory devices mounted on the patients or deployed in their surroundings. The data is usually encompassed within electronic health records (EHRs), which provide a summary of the patients' medical history [7]. EHRs play a crucial role in managing patients' medical statistics along with obtaining the hospital's performance.

The advancements in precision healthcare have witnessed enormous growth with the inception of intelligent healthcare systems and progress in big data research. This has resolved most of the complex computational tasks encountered by conventional healthcare systems. To this end, Wireless Body Area Networks (WBANs) have proved to be a major breakthrough in addressing the requirements for remote health monitoring and capturing daily life activities in developing medical Decision Support Systems (m-DSS). With the recent advent of Healthcare 4.0, the fourth revolution in healthcare industry was marked [7, 28, 29]. This not only provided a faster and cheaper alternative to traditional electronic health (e-Health) systems but also added intelligence toward remote management of EHRs, with optimized bandwidth, computing costs, and predictive analysis of patient records.

This chapter provides a framework for monitoring of self-care activities in children with physical and motor disabilities. Considering the flexibility and adaptability of nature-inspired learning models, this study considers the Particle Swarm Optimization (PSO)-based learning framework to predict different classes of disabilities. The proposed framework is tested with three different learning classifiers, namely, Naïve Bayes (NB), Random Forest (RF), and Support Vector Machine (SVM). The efficacy of the proposed PSO-based approach was compared with the baseline models and was observed to provide better prediction accuracy. Further, the optimized models in convergence with baseline models were tested for error statistics corresponding to Mean Absolute Error (MAE) and the Root Mean Square Error (RMSE). It was observed that the proposed approach provided comparatively lower error values corresponding to different number of generations over the considered dataset.

4.1.1 Motivations

At present, e-health systems have witnessed tremendous transformation with the emergence of wearable technology and intelligent remote health monitoring systems. To this end, machine learning models have served as a backbone for enhancing the performance of such systems by facilitating accurate and on-time diagnosis of clinical conditions. Considering the risk of cardiovascular diseases, a wearable cardiovascular activity monitoring scheme was proposed [2]. Their proposed system was claimed to provide continuous monitoring of risks associated with patients suffering from cardiovascular diseases through biosignals generated from the wearable sensory devices. The work in Ref. [30] proposed an intelligent machine-learning-driven model toward ambient assisted living for patients with blood-pressure disorder. The efficacy in timely diagnosis and real-time prediction of clinical conditions has largely benefitted from the conjecture of big data and machine learning frameworks [5]. To deliver healthcare services to the elderly, several studies focused on devising intelligent AI-based models which involved data acquired for different health parameters [38, 39]. However, in case of children with disabilities delivering remote healthcare is crucial as it requires specialized set of EHRs and patient history acquired from clinical trials. The studies in Refs. [11, 22, 58, 62], classified various categories of disability in children with compliance to International Classification of Functioning, disability and health: Children and Youth (ICF-CY). In favor of designing healthcare system for exceptional children, the authors in Ref. ([62], presented an Artificial Neural Network (ANN) model for characterizing self-care activities in children. Their proposed framework could assist in training AI-based models for specific set of self-care activities in the expert system domain. Considering the above studies, the present work focuses on developing prediction models for classifying different self-care activities using the PSO algorithm. The outcomes obtained for different error statistics and prediction accuracy were provided over the considered dataset. It was observed that the proposed approach outperformed the baseline models. Further, the convergence of different optimized classification models was also provided where the PSO-based NB classifier was observed to provide promising results. It can be inferred from the above discussions that the selection of an optimal classification framework is inevitable for developing intelligent healthcare system toward attaining precision healthcare.

4.1.2 Contributions

The contributions of the present study can be summarized as follows:

i. Provide a precise background on state-of-the-art precision healthcare systems and the role of IoT toward delivering real-time health monitoring services.
ii. Analysis of classification models for characterizing different self-care activities in exceptional children.
iii. Optimizing the learning classifiers over the considered dataset using PSO algorithm.
iv. Presenting a novel PSO-based algorithm for classifying self-care activities.
v. Providing experimental outcomes for prediction accuracy and error statistics of proposed PSO-based approach with baseline learning models.
vi. Discussions on challenges and limitations of existing literature.
vii. Providing relevant future scopes for research in extending the efficacy of learning models in the precision healthcare domain.

4.1.3 Organization

The rest of this chapter is organized as follows: In Section 4.2, a comprehensive background regarding the role of IoT, cloud computing, and machine learning in healthcare. Section 4.3, provides an overview of the intelligent healthcare system for monitoring of self-care activities in children. The results and observations pertaining to the study are illustrated in Section 4.4. The limitations of the present study and possible challenges for extending IoT-based healthcare systems are provided in Section 4.5. Finally, in Section 4.6, the conclusions drawn from this chapter and the possible future directions to extend research in the direction of smart healthcare and remote monitoring are provided.

4.2 BACKGROUND

Remote health monitoring systems have gained enormous popularity with the advent of precision healthcare paradigms to facilitate real-time monitoring of patients' clinical parameters and keeping track of daily life activities. To this end machine learning models have induced clinicians and healthcare organizations to obtain routine monitoring and comprehensive analysis of the patients' ailments and past medical history. These technologies are most commonly driven by wearable sensory devices which capture the physiological conditions of the patients and transmit them through biosignals over numerous connected devices belonging to patients' healthcare providers or family members. Further, the health parameters are recorded to perform advanced analytics in deciding the line of treatment for the patients. In this view, the present section deals with the major driving forces behind the success of precision healthcare systems.

4.2.1 IoT-based healthcare (IoTH) systems

With the growth in IoT-enabled healthcare systems, the proficiency in remote monitoring and exchange of health reports through EHRs over multiple healthcare units has become more accessible. To obtain a precise account of a patient's health parameters and the surrounding environment, a smart health monitoring system was proposed [32]. An early epidemic detection framework using semantic rule-based complex event processing (CEP) was proposed for identifying symptoms in activities of daily living (ADL) [63]. The IoTH paradigm was observed to witness disruptive innovations at the time of COVID-19 [33]. To understand the technological capabilities of such systems, an extensive literature-driven study is required to guide clinicians and caregivers to devise better solutions in overcoming the severance induced by such pandemics [33]. In sophisticated IoTH systems, multimedia data plays a crucial role in capturing data from diverse sources through texts, images, audio signals, and video frames being generated from different smart objects in IoT [53]. Thus, a blockchain framework was deployed to facilitate secure and low-cost solution toward allocation of medical resources to patients in user-centric systems [53]. Considering the low security architecture of WSNs in IoTH, privacy preserving framework based on homomorphic encryption for secure exchange of data was proposed [29]. In view of safeguarding both security and efficacy of e-Health systems, a Physical Unclonable Function (PUF) authentication scheme was proposed to secure health monitoring devices against physical attacks [27]. Further, considering secure and on-time delivery/retrieval requirements of healthcare information in IoTH for inter and intra-care facilities across diverse remotely distributed platforms, a secure blockchain-based solution was proposed for promoting traceability and ubiquity in futuristic IoTH systems [7].

4.2.2 Cloud-healthcare architecture

The healthcare industry has largely benefitted with the conglomeration of cloud computing infrastructure to facilitate better processing of healthcare data and information storage [57]. This has also provided the consolidation of tasks and secure maintenance of EHRs over desired period of time. However, the explosive growth witnessed in IoTH systems has posed certain limitations over conventional cloud-based computing infrastructures. The major challenges being those of latency, optimal utilization of bandwidth, processing costs, and centralized service architecture [14, 18]. To overcome the above challenges, a fog computing-based healthcare framework was proposed which extends the capabilities of cloud infrastructure closer to the sources of healthcare data [40]. To better access the mobility information of the patients during emergency events, an edge-fog-cloud-based collaborative network was proposed to capture users' precise location and provide persistent and time-sensitive health information [41]. Considering the criticality and time-sensitivity of healthcare data acquisition and transmission, an IoT-based fog computing approach was proposed for mobility aware scheduling of tasks and their allocation in the healthcare domain [1]. For addressing the requirements of near real-time healthcare applications in Internet of Medical Things (IoMT), solutions based on AI and fog/edge computing paradigms were proposed to intelligently and efficiently process healthcare data [28]. To augment the reliability and failure-tolerance of IoMT systems, an integrated physical infrastructure comprising Cloud-Fog-Edge computing paradigms was proposed [49]. An integrated healthcare solution with IoT and Cyber-Physical Systems (CPS) based on fog computing for developing e-Health gateways was presented [51]. Further, health monitoring through early warning scores was analyzed in realistic IoT-based scenarios. A non-intrusive IoT-cloud-based self-care system for monitoring patients with diabetes was proposed by exploring SVM-based intelligent model on cloud platform along with an integration to android-based application [31]. The android-based application facilitated generating notifications and alerts to the patients and their associated healthcare providers to monitor vital health parameters.

4.2.3 Precision healthcare

Precision healthcare involves extensive study of a patient's health records including daily lifestyle habits, treatment history, and genetic profiles to predict a precise line of treatment [50]. To this end query processing and document ranking plays a vital role in health information retrieval over online healthcare systems for facilitating precision medicine [50]. Thus, in the design of clinical DSS, such challenges of retrieving healthcare information from disparate sources and cross platform exchange of health information through information gateways network remains crucial [45]. This could however, be achieved by designing smart healthcare tools that leverage healthcare providers and clinicians to collaboratively curate, analyze, and store the patient's health parameters over a common analytics portal like the one presented in HINGE (Healthcare INformation Gateway and Exchange) framework [45]. Considering the complexity associated with acquiring precision medicine information for predicting accurate treatment regimens, AI plays a pivotal role in facilitating early drug discovery by taking into account the role of biomarkers [20]. For the diagnosis of serious diseases such as brain tumor, early diagnosis and adoption of appropriate treatment have been the key toward better survival rate and quality of life. In this perspective, partial tree (PART) unsupervised learning model, which considers dependency among data to generate decision rules to train the learning algorithm has been observed to supersede conventional learning models for classifying different stages of progression for the tumor [35].

4.3 INTELLIGENT HEALTHCARE SYSTEMS FOR MONITORING OF SELF-CARE ACTIVITIES

This section presents the strategies adopted in this chapter to analyze and classify the self-care activities in children belonging to different age groups with physical and motor disorders [62]. The dataset was categorized as per the guidelines of ICF-CY to determine the degree of various disabilities and hence could better assist the caregivers in classifying the amount of care required for each individual patient [61]. For our analysis, three different classification algorithms, namely, NB, RF, and SVM were considered to train the intelligent system with the supplied self-care activity dataset. The learning models were further optimized by employing PSO algorithm to extract the significant features from the featureset toward improving prediction accuracy. Further, different performance evaluation strategies such as prediction accuracy and error statistics viz., MAE and RMSE were adopted to depict the convergence of the proposed PSO-based intelligent system. The above performance metrics lead to appropriate recommendations for classifying the type of disability and required care to be delivered to each individual based on their degree of disability. Figure 4.2 presents an overview of the intelligent healthcare system.

An architecture for managing and processing healthcare big data for IoT-based systems toward monitoring self-care activities is provided in Figure 4.3. Initially data regarding health parameters and different self-care activities of the patients is acquired. These data are stored in a local database from where it is channelized over access routers for processing over big data platforms [5]. The processed healthcare data is further analyzed for useful patterns using intelligent learning techniques. Finally, the prediction outcomes after performing the above analytics are produced as log files to the respective users or care givers over their mobile phones or PCs.

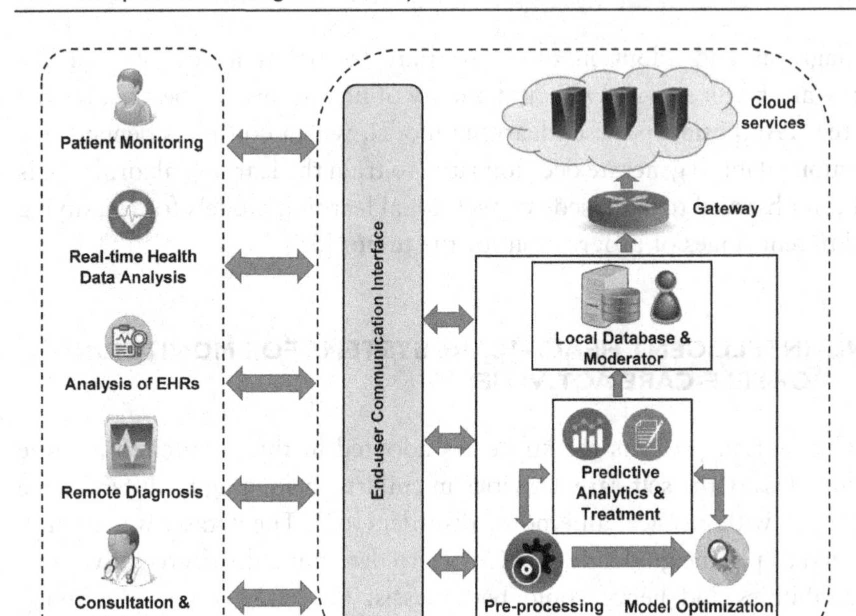

Figure 4.2 Overview of an intelligent healthcare system.

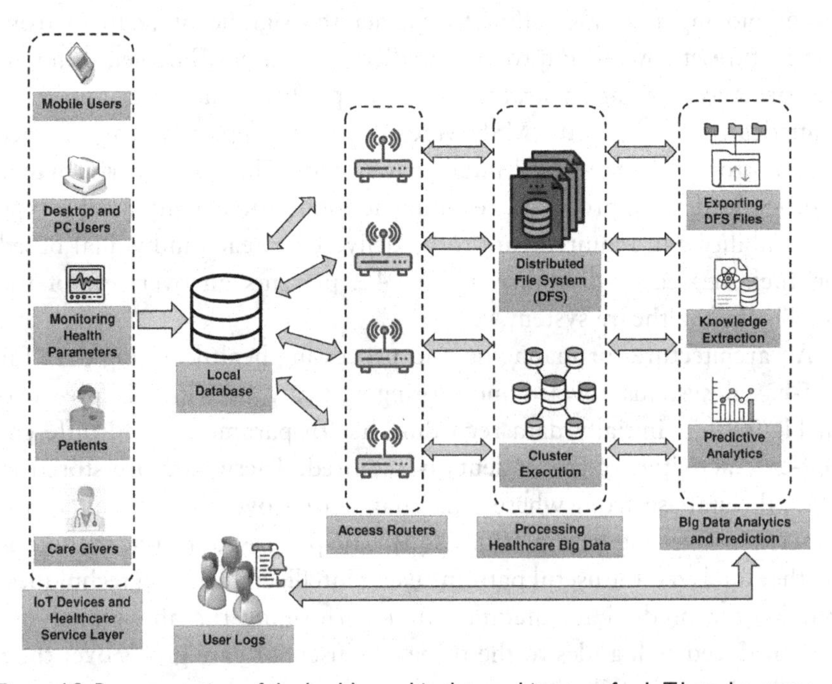

Figure 4.3 Representation of the healthcare big data architecture for IoT-based systems.

4.3.1 Machine learning models

In this section, three different machine learning models considered for our analysis have been discussed. The following classification models have been used considering their robustness and efficacy toward designing intelligent healthcare systems.

4.3.1.1 Naïve Bayes (NB) model

The NB model is a popularly used probabilistic learning approach which is based on Bayes' theory for determining the probability corresponding to some specific feature given some prior knowledge [54]. It is experimentally observed that the NB model can provide high prediction accuracy for featuresets subject to the existence of dependencies among the features [54]. Therefore, it can be stated that the performance of the NB model would be optimal if the degree of dependency between respective features is high. This has further harnessed the popularity of NB model across several cross-disciplinary fields, to be well-suited as a statistical tool for achieving high prediction accuracy. Thus, from Bayes' theorem considering X to be some dataset consisting of C_i classes, the conditional probability pertaining to NB can be obtained as follows:

$$F(C_i|X) = \frac{F(C_i)F(X|C_i)}{F(X)}, \tag{4.1}$$

where $F(X|C_i)$ provides the likelihood of considered dataset X upon C_i classes.

Now, the joint probability can be obtained as,

$$F(X|C_i) = F(x_1|C_i) \times F(x_2|C_i) \times F(x_3|C_i) \times \cdots \times F(x_n|C_i). \tag{4.2}$$

$$F(X|C_i) = \prod_j F(x_j|C_i). \tag{4.3}$$

Considering $F(X)$ as constant for all classes C_i, the joint probability $F(X|C_i)$ requires to be maximized to maximize the probability $F(C_i|X)$. Therefore, in our case for any disability belonging to class C_i, we can maximize the posterior probability $F(C_i|X)$ as,

$$\hat{f} = \arg\max_i \prod_j F(x_j|C_i), \tag{4.4}$$

where $j = 1, 2, \ldots, n$, such that $x_j \in X$.

4.3.1.2 Random Forest (RF) model

In the RF classification model, a collection of independent decision trees which are generated randomly through the input vector are employed in facilitating classification of the considered dataset [21]. Here, the independent decision trees generated within the model are capable of making decision based on voting [21]. It further enables the individual trees to select the most popular class to make appropriate prediction based on the input dataset. This represents the efficacy of RF models toward handling complex real-world problems and further depicts its suitability toward classifying multi-class datasets [21]. In this view, a crucial aspect remains toward developing strategies for selection of attributes in a dataset. To accomplish this, the RF model employs Gini Index which builds the model based on impurity measure with respect to classes in the supplied dataset. This further assists in computing the probability of misclassified class variables and hence it is popularly used with decision trees. Thus, for any given dataset X, the Gini Index pertaining to selection of some random feature belonging to class C may be given as,

$$\text{Gini Index} = \prod \sum_{i} \frac{f\left(C_i, X\right)}{|X|} \sum_{j} \frac{f\left(C_j, X\right)}{|X|}, \tag{4.5}$$

where $f(C_i, X)$ shows that the selected attribute belongs to some class C_i such that $i \neq j$.

4.3.1.3 Support Vector Machine (SVM) model

The SVM model has managed to find its application in plethora of fields and has been extensively employed to model complex processes [4, 37]. Its efficacy to handle both classification and regression problems in real-world intelligent machine learning applications has further contributed toward its popularity [37]. Further, the SVM leverages the users for appropriate kernel selection strategies to build the learning model results in efficient classifiers with comparably low variance and bias. Some major application areas where the use of SVM has been observed to be most befitting include forecasting weather statistics, modeling environmental phenomena, financial market trend prediction, and toward prediction in m-DSS [11]. This work considers the SVM model for facilitating classification of multi-class self-care activities using the Gaussian kernel function for generating the decision rules in our system. Thus, the kernel-generating function can be defined as,

$$\text{Kern}(x, x_i) = \exp\left(-\lambda |x - x_i|^2\right), \tag{4.6}$$

where x,x_i denotes two vectors, λ provides the risk parameter, and the function $Kern(x, x_i)$ is dependent of distance between vectors $|x-x_i|$. Using eq. (4.6), decision rules for SVM model can be given as follows:

$$s(x) = \text{sign}\left(\sum_i \text{Kern}(x, x_i) \times \alpha_i - \beta\right), \tag{4.7}$$

where α_i and β represent coefficients of model such that $i = 1, 2, \ldots, n$ which provides number of support vectors involved in the learning model.

4.3.2 Nature inspired algorithms

Nature inspired optimization has found tremendous applications for solving complex optimization problems to facilitate fast convergence to an optimal solution. The fundamental inception behind these algorithms has traced back from natural processes and social behavior of creatures in their natural living habitat. These algorithms hold a well-established background of reducing computational complexity, time, and costs for multi-dimensional problems having large search spaces. In this perspective, nature-inspired optimization algorithms play a crucial role toward feature selection in minimizing the data acquisition costs associated with medical datasets. These datasets are highly correlated in nature and entail an extensive collection of features to assist the clinicians and care givers a precise account of the patients' underlying health condition. Thus, several heuristic search techniques and bio-inspired schemes have been adopted by different researchers toward achieving optimality in prediction models.

Several industries including healthcare have extensively employed nature-inspired optimization techniques for reducing computational complexity associated with big data issues. In view of facilitating accurate diagnosis and predicting treatment regimens nature-inspired algorithms in conjunction with machine intelligence and data mining have analogously played an imperative role in the healthcare sector [48]. To address the issues of big data in healthcare, the firefly algorithm has been observed to be suitable in solving combinatorial problems and hence eliminates possibility of untimely convergence and local optima for the optimization problem [52]. For managing healthcare data flows and improving request/response mechanism in AI-based healthcare services, Ant Colony Optimization (ACO) plays an important role in handling flow concentration of healthcare data, thus preventing outages and improving processing time [3]. To address the issues of low response time associated with resource-constrained cloud health systems deployed for monitoring patients with heart disorders, the efficacy of ACO model was realized for efficient allocation of Virtual Machines (VM) over conventional First Come First Serve (FCFS) approach [36]. In home healthcare applications, dynamic vehicle routing has been of interest toward delivering concurrent specialized healthcare services. However, to facilitate minimum travel time and optimize number of patient visits, the Mutated Cuckoo Search Algorithm (MCSA) was employed [55]. Considering widespread applicability of EHRs and big data, a major utilization remains toward early detection and management of high mortality diseases such as cancer [36]. Following the drawbacks of conventional Gabor filter technique which was extensively used by radiologists for extracting features from mammography, the Cuckoo search was used for selecting the optimal filters for extracting highly descriptive features [36]. For IoT-based e-Health systems operating over cloud computing environment, an energy-efficient PSO approach was employed for optimal data forwarding and reducing transmission overheads [19].

4.3.2.1 Particle Swarm Optimization (PSO) model

The PSO was primarily proposed by Kennedy and Eberhart [34] and was modeled on the social behavior of birds, fish, and some insects by mimicking their swarming behavior. The fundamental objective behind this algorithm was to optimize space and time complexities associated with complex computations. The social creatures are generically referred to as particles which appear in an apparently disorganized group capable of moving in random direction with a certain velocity [34]. The PSO has found extensive applications in several real-world problems toward developing mathematical optimization frameworks [60]. This work adopts the PSO model toward selecting an optimal number of features from the supplied self-care activity dataset. Here, the PSO model assists in finding an optimal solution for efficient prediction of self-care activities in children with physical and motor disorders through the swarming agents which are otherwise known as particles. The particle's underlying trajectory is modeled through stochastic and deterministic techniques. Hence, the position update equation for the particles is defined as follows:

$$x_i^{k+1} = x_i^k + \varphi_i^{k+1}, \tag{4.8}$$

where, $x_i = (x_{i1}, x_{i2}, \dots, x_{in})$, with $i = 1, 2, \dots, m$ and φ_i^{k+1} denotes velocity for i^{th} particles with inertia weight k. Thus, the above expression depicts position for i^{th} particles in an n-dimensional search space. The particles while being positioned on a search space are uniformly distributed as,

$$x_i^k \sim U\left(x_{\min}, x_{\max}\right), k = 0. \tag{4.9}$$

where $U(.)$ denotes the uniform distribution function, and $x_{\min}$ and $x_{\max}$ represent minimum and maximum particles characterized within the search space at some instance $k = 0$.

Now, the velocity vector for the ith particles can be given as below,

$$\varphi_i^{k+1} = \omega \times \varphi_i^k + a_1 \times \ell_1 \left(p_{\text{best}_i} - x_i^k\right) + a_2 \times \ell_2 \left(g_{\text{best}_i} - x_i^k\right), \tag{4.10}$$

where:

p_{best_i} = denotes best position for some i^{th} particle.

g_{best_i} = depicts global best position corresponding to some i^{th} particle in the swarm.

a_1 = represents the confidence factor for intelligence of particle corresponding to p_{best_i}.

a_2 = represents confidence factor for collaboration of particle corresponding to g_{best_i} within the swarm.

ℓ_1, ℓ_2 = depict uniformly distributed random numbers between $[0, 1]$.

Thus, the primary objective behind considering PSO model for healthcare sector above other nature-inspired optimization models lies in its simplicity of implementation, efficient computation of optimal solution and robustness toward defining control parameters.

4.3.3 Performance evaluation

To understand the efficacy of PSO-based approach for predicting different classes of self-care activities, we need to observe its convergence in comparison with baseline approaches. This assists in appropriate decision-making for classifying between different categories of disabilities and hence leads to an efficient design of intelligent healthcare systems. This study depicts the efficacy of the PSO-based approach over metrics such as prediction accuracy along with error statistics like MAE and RMSE. A precise discussion of the performance metrics is provided below:

4.3.3.1 Accuracy

The prediction accuracy for any learning model can be defined by considering the ratio between the sum of T_{p_i} and T_{n_i} to the sum of $T_{p_i} + F_{p_i} + T_{n_i} + F_{n_i}$ and is defined as follows:

$$\text{Accuracy} = \frac{\sum_i \left(T_{p_i} + T_{n_i}\right)}{\sum_i \left(T_{p_i} + F_{p_i} + T_{n_i} + F_{n_i}\right)}, \tag{4.11}$$

where:

T_{p_i} = represents true positives.
T_{n_i} = shows the true negatives.
F_{p_i} = denotes the false positives.
F_{n_i} = illustrates the false negatives.

4.3.3.2 Mean Absolute Error (MAE)

The MAE is a popularly used error statistic for obtaining the performance error for learning models over some specific variable of interest within the supplied dataset. This method produces an absolute value $|\hat{x}_i - x_i|$ corresponding to the prediction error incurred between predicted and actual values respectively. Therefore, the MAE pertaining to N^{th} observations in the considered dataset can be given as follows:

$$\text{MAE} = \frac{\sum_i |\hat{x}_i - x_i|}{N}. \tag{4.12}$$

4.3.3.3 Root Mean Square Error (RMSE)

The RMSE is a crucial error statistic for analyzing how better a model fits to the predicted values. It is illustrated by a measure of standard deviation of the Nth sample in the supplied dataset with the errors incurred in the prediction model. The RMSE for a model can be computed as follows:

$$\text{RMSE} = \sqrt{\frac{\sum_{i} (\hat{x}_i - x_i)^2}{N}}. \tag{4.13}$$

4.4 RESULTS AND OBSERVATIONS

This section deals with the results corresponding to the proposed PSO-based approach for classification of self-care activities in children [62]. The considered dataset initially constituted of records acquired from 70 individuals for portraying various classes of physical and motor disabilities. These classifications to signify different degrees of disability are made in compliance with WHO's ICF-CY guidelines [61]. The dataset provides an explicitly distinctive account of self-care problems encountered while performing daily life activities in children with motor disorders. A detailed study on different categorizations of such disorders can be found in Ref. [62]. In this study, we consider the inertia weight for PSO algorithm as $k = 0.33$, the random state was considered as 52, and number of particles was specified as, $i = 20$. The number of generations for which the performance metrics viz., accuracy, MAE, and RMSE are considered is set to 50. We initially present the performance of PSO-based approach with baseline models, and further depict the convergence of PSO-based models to provide an inter-model analysis for the selection of the best learning model for the suggested healthcare scenario. Table 4.1 provides the performance metrics for PSO-NB model with corresponding prediction accuracy, MAE, and RMSE values where the most optimal values are highlighted in bold text. In Table 4.2, the performance metrics obtained for PSO-RF model is summarized. The performance of PSO-SVM model can be visualized in Table 4.3. Further,

Table 4.1 Performance metrics for PSO-NB

	Generations					
	0	10	20	30	40	50
Accuracy	0.790428	0.871143	0.876429	**0.883428**	0.878430	0.877572
MAE	0.065525	0.037899	0.034159	0.032950	0.032804	**0.032803**
RMSE	0.228843	0.186575	0.18048	0.180447	**0.176442**	0.177356

Table 4.2 Performance metrics for PSO-RF

	Generations					
	0	10	20	30	40	50
Accuracy	0.795715	0.846429	0.850715	0.853999	0.856856	**0.857717**
MAE	0.088382	0.064467	0.060378	0.056218	0.053586	**0.053086**
RMSE	0.209159	0.188450	0.186806	0.183260	0.180422	**0.179391**

Table 4.3 Performance metrics for PSO-SVM

	Generations					
	0	10	20	30	40	50
Accuracy	0.715428	0.758427	0.776858	0.778556	0.778857	**0.788428**
MAE	0.081307	0.069022	0.063754	0.062899	0.062428	**0.062186**
RMSE	0.283282	0.260168	0.255759	0.251806	0.226179	**0.217529**

Table 4.4 Performance metrics for NB model

	Generations					
	0	10	20	30	40	50
Accuracy	0.770412	0.855121	0.857812	0.861201	0.860121	**0.866124**
MAE	0.079921	0.056711	0.053119	0.051111	0.050112	**0.050001**
RMSE	0.446123	0.318657	0.318044	0.318001	0.301762	**0.300018**

Table 4.5 Performance metrics for RF model

	Generations					
	0	10	20	30	40	50
Accuracy	0.777465	0.812890	0.828010	0.821361	0.836120	**0.839918**
MAE	0.098112	0.076123	0.076412	0.069013	0.066218	**0.060113**
RMSE	0.331286	0.290129	0.281001	0.280011	0.271810	**0.261891**

the performance for baseline models viz., NB, RF, and SVM are provided in Tables 4.4–4.6 respectively.

In Figure 4.4, the accuracy obtained for the PSO-based approach and baseline learning models over the considered dataset is provided. The PSO-based approach entails learners viz., PSO-NB, PSO-RF, and PSO-SVM. It was observed that the PSO-NB provided the best prediction accuracy of 0.883428 pertaining to different generations. A detailed account of this can be observed from Table 4.1. Figure 4.5 provides

Table 4.6 Performance metrics for SVM model

	Generations					
	0	10	20	30	40	50
Accuracy	0.687120	0.718101	0.731051	0.739901	0.740001	**0.741270**
MAE	0.089012	0.071028	0.070010	0.069910	0.065010	**0.064012**
RMSE	0.441320	0.421080	0.417060	0.401891	0.400010	**0.399071**

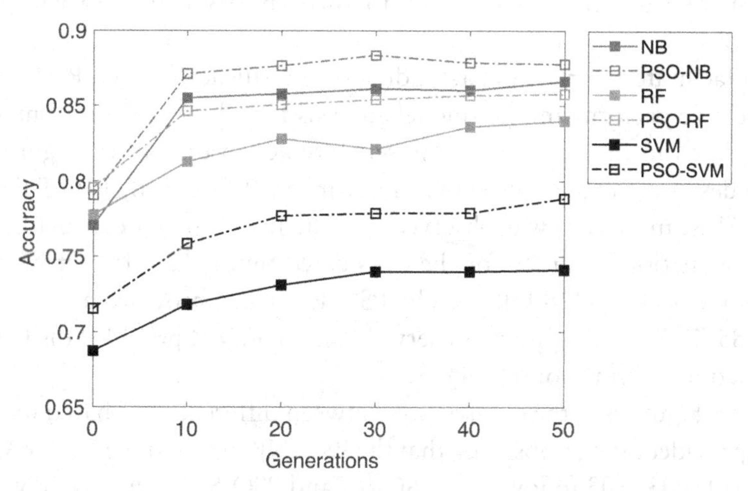

Figure 4.4 Comparison of accuracy for PSO-based models (viz., PSO-NB, PSO-RF, and PSO-SVM) with baseline learning models (viz., NB, RF, and SVM).

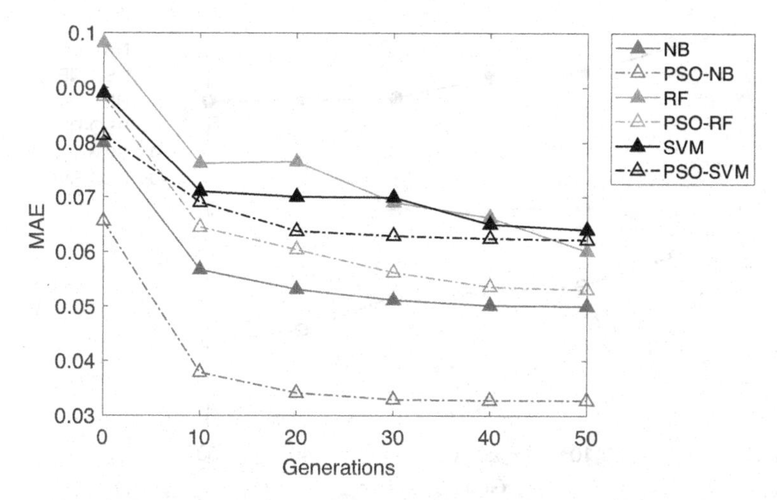

Figure 4.5 Comparison of MAE values for PSO-based models (viz., PSO-NB, PSO-RF, and PSO-SVM) with baseline learning models (viz., NB, RF, and SVM).

the MAE for different learning models. It was observed that the MAE for PSO-NB was the minimum with MAE $=$ 0.032803 for the 50th generation as observed from Table 4.1. Further, the next lowest MAE was obtained for the NB model with MAE $=$ 0.050001 as observed from Table 4.4. The comparative analysis between the RMSE values of the PSO-based models and baseline models was provided in Figure 4.6. It is worthwhile to note that the PSO-NB model provided minimum RMSE vale of RMSE $=$ 176,442 followed by PSO-RF with RMSE $=$ 0.179391.

To facilitate a better understanding of the efficacy of each PSO-based model, we perform an inter-model analysis for all the three PSO-models considered in this study over the self-care activities dataset. Figure 4.7 provides the comparison between accuracy of PSO-NB, PSO-RF, and PSO-SVM models. It was observed that the PSO-NB model provides the best prediction accuracy for the considered multi-class dataset with an accuracy of 0,883428 followed by PSO-RF which provided an accuracy of 0.857717. Further, it was observed that PSO-SVM provided the lowest prediction accuracy of 0.788428.

From Figure 4.8, the comparison between different PSO-based models was provided. It was observed that the PSO-NB incurred the lowest MAE value of 0.032803 followed by PSO-RF and PSO-SVM with MAE values

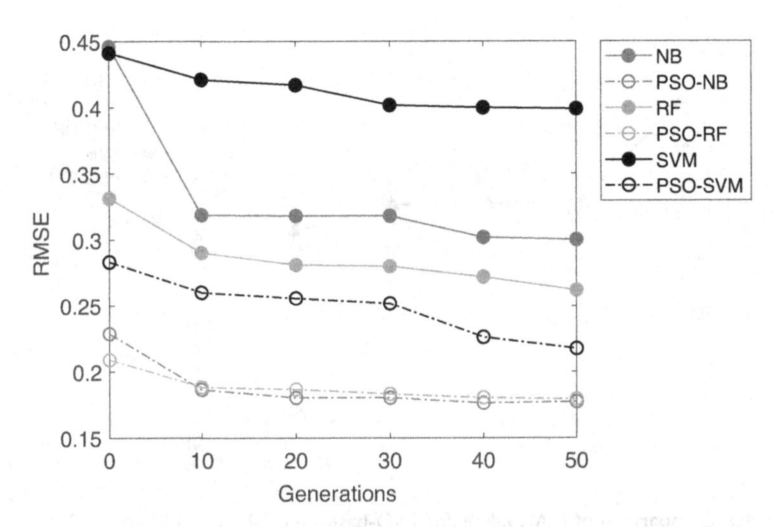

Figure 4.6 Comparison of RMSE values for PSO-based models (viz., PSO-NB, PSO-RF, and PSO-SVM) with baseline learning models (viz., NB, RF, and SVM).

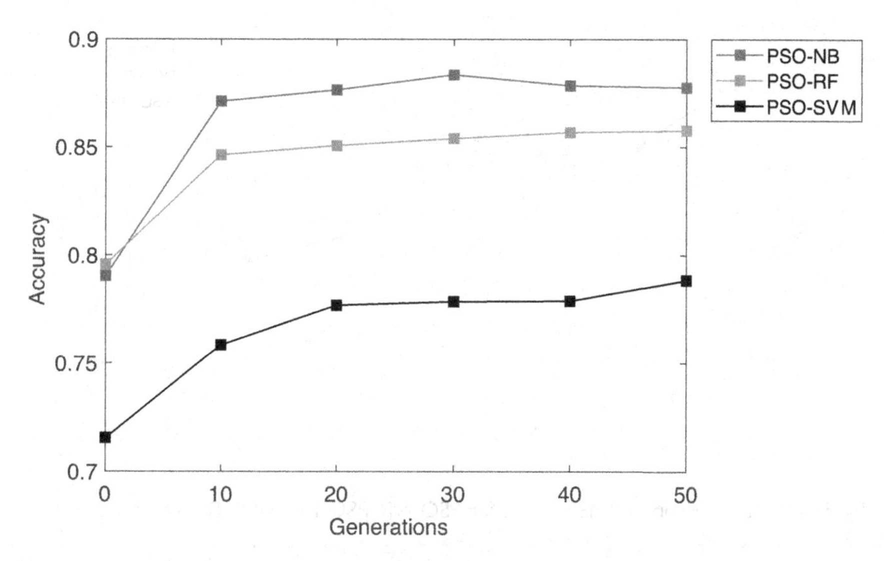

Figure 4.7 Comparison of accuracy for PSO-NB, PSO-RF, and PSO-SVM models.

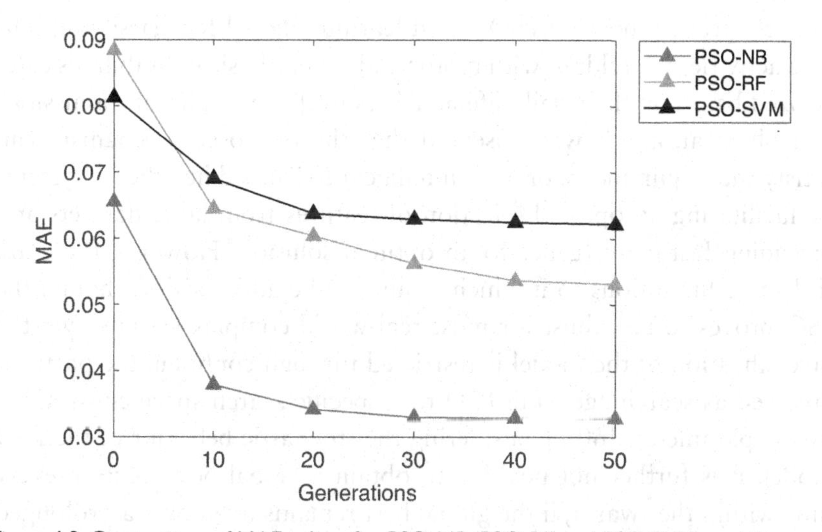

Figure 4.8 Comparison of MAE values for PSO-NB, PSO-RF, and PSO-SVM models.

of 0.053086 and 0.062186 respectively. In Figure 4.9, the RMSE values for PSO-NB, PSO-RF, and PSO-SVM were compared, where PSO-NB provided the lowest RMSE value of 0.176442 followed by RMSE value of PSO-RF at 0.179391. The RMSE value for PSO-SVM was observed to be the highest among all three learning models at 0.217529.

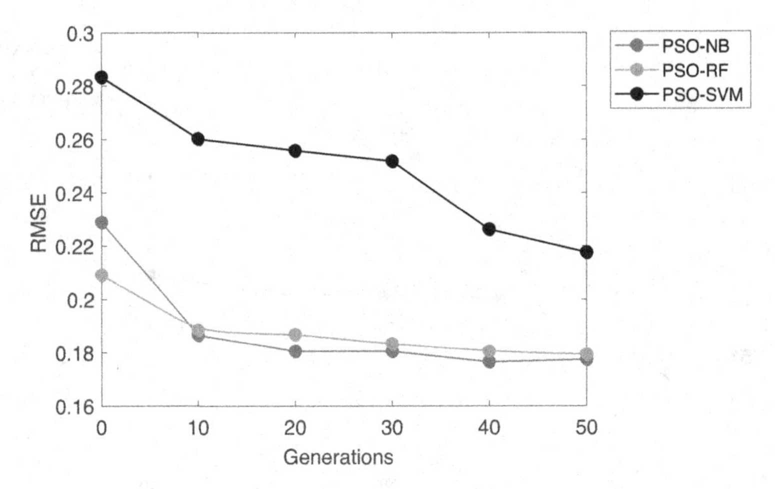

Figure 4.9 Comparison of RMSE values for PSO-NB, PSO-RF, and PSO-SVM models.

4.5 LIMITATIONS AND CHALLENGES

This chapter proposed a PSO-based learning model for classifying self-care activities in children with motor and other physical disabilities categorized based on their daily life activities [62]. Through our discussions and observations, it was observed that the proposed mechanism can satisfy the requirements of most intelligent IoT-based healthcare systems by facilitating an optimal selection of features from large datasets and providing fast convergence to an optimal solution. However, there are still some limitations to it which require to be addressed. Although the PSO proves to be robust for most real-world complex systems, yet the diversification of the model is restricted through confining the particles involved as search agents in PSO to a specific search space constrained by the parameters [60]. Considering the stochastic behavior of the PSO model, it is further not possible to obtain a global best solution every time within the swarm, if the global best remains fixed over a prolonged duration [60]. Thus, in that case, the model may provide a local optimal solution. Further, as the healthcare data generated incurs an exceptionally high degree of dimensionality with the exponential growth in size, the present model may encounter intractable computational demands [25].

Considering the challenges of large featuresets associated with complex big datasets, requirement for reduction in attributes, and premature convergence associated with PSO is crucial. Several studies have attempted to extend the PSO for achieving better performance [24, 25].

Some studies have also suggested the combination of co-evolutionary techniques and quantum computing models in convergence with PSO for attaining better computational performance for big datasets with reduced complexity [24]. Further, when it comes to cloud-based IoTH systems, the management of resources, energy efficiency, security, and ubiquity may be somewhat compromised through conventional nature-inspired algorithms [26]. To this end, the adoption of some recently emerging paradigms such as Quantum Computing as a Service (QCaaS), Deep Learning as a Service (DLaaS), and Blockchain as a Service (BaaS) can prove to increase security, sustainability, energy efficiency, and scalability of futuristic healthcare systems [7, 26].

4.6 CONCLUSIONS AND FUTURE SCOPE

In this chapter, a framework toward monitoring self-care activities in children with physical and motor disabilities based on their daily life activities was provided. In view of the flexibility and adaptability furnished by nature-inspired learning models, this work exploited the PSO model to predict different classes of disabilities for the considered multi-class dataset. The proposed framework was tested for PSO-NB, PSO-RF, and PSO-SVM models in convergence with baseline models for different performance metrics. It was observed through the experimental results that the PSO-NB model outperformed all other learning models in terms of prediction accuracy and error statistics viz., MAE and RMSE. The PSO-NB model incurred an accuracy of 0.883428 (or, 88.3428%) along with MAE and RMSE values of 0.032803 and 0.176442 respectively. Hence, the PSO-NB model successfully minimized the error statistics and provided satisfying prediction accuracy for classifying different categories of disabilities in children for the proposed intelligent healthcare system.

Although the proposed PSO-NB model can satisfy most of the requirements of emerging healthcare systems and can facilitate optimal selection of features, yet some issues such as managing extensively large datasets over cloud-based platforms in perspective of Cloud-Healthcare Systems remain a crucial task. In this view, several factors such as offloading the massive healthcare data, sustainability, scalability, resource utilization and management, security, and overall computational complexity are to be considered while designing cloud-based IoTH systems.

REFERENCES

[1] Abdelmoneem, R. M., Benslimane, A., & Shaaban, E. (2020). Mobility-aware task scheduling in cloud-Fog IoT-based healthcare architectures. *Computer Networks*, 179, 107348.

[2] Akbulut, F. P., & Akan, A. (2018). A smart wearable system for short-term cardiovascular risk assessment with emotional dynamics. *Measurement*, 128, 237–246.

[3] Alarifi, A., & Alwadain, A. (2021). Relative traffic management scheme for robot-assisted healthcare applications. *Swarm and Evolutionary Computation*, 64, 100887.

[4] Amari, S. I., & Wu, S. (1999). Improving support vector machine classifiers by modifying kernel functions. *Neural Networks*, 12(6), 783–789.

[5] Amirian, P., van Loggerenberg, F., Lang, T., Thomas, A., Peeling, R., Basiri, A., & Goodman, S. N. (2017). Using big data analytics to extract disease surveillance information from point of care diagnostic machines. *Pervasive and Mobile Computing*, 42, 470–486.

[6] Bebortta, S., & Das, S. K. (2020). Assessing the Impact of Network Performance on Popular E-Learning Applications. In *2020 Sixth International Conference on e-Learning (econf)* (pp. 61–65). IEEE.

[7] Bebortta, S., & Senapati, D. (2021). A secure blockchain-based solution for harnessing the future of smart healthcare. In: S. K. Singh, R. S. Singh, A. K. Pandey, S. S Udmale, & A. Chaudhary (Eds.), *IoT-Based Data Analytics for the Healthcare Industry* (pp. 167–191). Academic Press: Cambridge, MA.

[8] Bebortta, S., & Senapati, D. (2021). Empirical characterization of network traffic for reliable communication in IoT devices. In: A. I. Awad, S. Furnell, M. Paprzycki, & S. K. Sharma (Eds.), *Security in Cyber-Physical Systems: Foundations and Applications* (pp. 67–90). Springer Nature: London.

[9] Bebortta, S., & Singh, S. K. (2021). An Adaptive Machine Learning-based Threat Detection Framework for Industrial Communication Networks. In *2021 10th IEEE International Conference on Communication Systems and Network Technologies (CSNT)* (pp. 527–532). IEEE.

[10] Bebortta, S., Das, S. K., Kandpal, M., Barik, R. K., & Dubey, H. (2020). Geospatial serverless computing: Architectures, tools and future directions. *ISPRS International Journal of Geo-Information*, 9(5), 311.

[11] Bebortta, S., Panda, M., & Panda, S. (2020). Classification of pathological disorders in children using random forest algorithm. In *2020 International Conference on Emerging Trends in Information Technology and Engineering (ic-ETITE)* (pp. 1–6). IEEE.

[12] Bebortta, S., Rajput, N. K., Pati, B., & Senapati, D. (2020). A real-time smart waste management based on cognitive IoT framework. In: T. Sengodan, M. Murugappan, & S. Misra (Eds.), *Advances in Electrical and Computer Technologies* (pp. 407–414). Springer: Singapore.

[13] Bebortta, S., Senapati, D., Panigrahi, C. R., & Pati, B. (2021). Adaptive performance modeling framework for QoS-aware offloading in MEC-based IIoT systems. *IEEE Internet of Things Journal*, 9(12), 10162–10171.

[14] Bebortta, S., Senapati, D., Panigrahi, C. R., & Pati, B. (2021). An Adaptive Modeling and Performance Evaluation Framework for Edge-enabled Green IoT Systems. *IEEE Transactions on Green Communications and Networking*.

[15] Bebortta, S., Senapati, D., Rajput, N. K., Singh, A. K., Rathi, V. K., Pandey, H. M., ... & Tiwari, P. (2020). Evidence of power-law behavior in cognitive IoT applications. *Neural Computing and Applications*, 32(20), 16043–16055.
[16] Bebortta, S., Singh, A. K., & Senapati, D. (2022). Performance analysis of multi-access edge computing networks for heterogeneous IoT systems. *Materials Today: Proceedings*.
[17] Bebortta, S., Singh, A. K., Mohanty, S., & Senapati, D. (2020). Characterization of range for smart home sensors using tsallis entropy framework. In: C. R. Panigrahi, B. Pati, B. K. Pattanayak, S. Amic, & K.-C. Li (Eds.), *Advanced Computing and Intelligent Engineering* (pp. 265–276). Springer Nature: Singapore.
[18] Bebortta, S., Singh, A. K., Pati, B., & Senapati, D. (2021). A robust energy optimization and data reduction scheme for iot based indoor environments using local processing framework. *Journal of Network and Systems Management*, 29(1), 1–28.
[19] Bharathi, R., Abirami, T., Dhanasekaran, S., Gupta, D., Khanna, A., Elhoseny, M., & Shankar, K. (2020). Energy efficient clustering with disease diagnosis model for IoT based sustainable healthcare systems. *Sustainable Computing: Informatics and Systems*, 28, 100453.
[20] Boniolo, F., Dorigatti, E., Ohnmacht, A. J., Saur, D., Schubert, B., & Menden, M. P. (2021). Artificial intelligence in early drug discovery enabling precision medicine. *Expert Opinion on Drug Discovery*, 16(9), 991–1007.
[21] Breiman, L. (2001). Random forests. *Machine Learning*, 45(1), 5–32.
[22] Bushehri, S. F., & Zarchi, M. S. (2019). An expert model for self-care problems classification using probabilistic neural network and feature selection approach. *Applied Soft Computing*, 82, 105545.
[23] Das, S. K., & Bebortta, S. (2021). Heralding the Future of Federated Learning Framework: Architecture, Tools and Future Directions. In *2021 11th International Conference on Cloud Computing, Data Science & Engineering (Confluence)* (pp. 698–703). IEEE.
[24] Ding, W., Lin, C. T., Chen, S., Zhang, X., & Hu, B. (2018). Multiagent-consensus-MapReduce-based attribute reduction using co-evolutionary quantum PSO for big data applications. *Neurocomputing*, 272, 136–153.
[25] Fong, S., Wong, R., & Vasilakos, A. V. (2015). Accelerated PSO swarm search feature selection for data stream mining big data. *IEEE Transactions on Services Computing*, 9(1), 33–45.
[26] Gill, S. S., & Buyya, R. (2019). Bio-inspired algorithms for big data analytics: a survey, taxonomy, and open challenges. In: N. Dey, H. Das, B. Naik, & H. S. Behera (Eds.), *Big Data Analytics for Intelligent Healthcare Management* (pp. 1–17). Academic Press: Cambridge, MA.
[27] Gope, P., Gheraibia, Y., Kabir, S., & Sikdar, B. (2020). A secure IoT-based modern healthcare system with fault-tolerant decision making process. *IEEE Journal of Biomedical and Health Informatics*, 25(3), 862–873.
[28] Greco, L., Percannella, G., Ritrovato, P., Tortorella, F., & Vento, M. (2020). Trends in IoT based solutions for health care: Moving AI to the edge. *Pattern Recognition Letters*, 135, 346–353.
[29] Guo, X., Lin, H., Wu, Y., & Peng, M. (2020). A new data clustering strategy for enhancing mutual privacy in healthcare IoT systems. *Future Generation Computer Systems*, 113, 407–417.

[30] Hassan, M. K., El Desouky, A. I., Elghamrawy, S. M., & Sarhan, A. M. (2018). Intelligent hybrid remote patient-monitoring model with cloud-based framework for knowledge discovery. *Computers & Electrical Engineering*, 70, 1034–1048.

[31] Hebbale, A., Vinay, G. H. R., Krishna, B. V., & Shah, J. (2021). IoT and Machine Learning based Self Care System for Diabetes Monitoring and Prediction. In *2021 2nd Global Conference for Advancement in Technology (GCAT)* (pp. 1–7). IEEE.

[32] Islam, M. M., Rahaman, A., & Islam, M. R. (2020). Development of smart healthcare monitoring system in IoT environment. *SN Computer Science*, 1, 1–11.

[33] Javaid, M., & Khan, I. H. (2021). Internet of Things (IoT) enabled healthcare helps to take the challenges of COVID-19 Pandemic. *Journal of Oral Biology and Craniofacial Research*, 11(2), 209–214.

[34] Kennedy, J., & Eberhart, R. (1995). Particle swarm optimization. *Proceedings of ICNN'95-International Conference on Neural Networks*, Vol. 4. IEEE, 1995.

[35] Khan, S. R., Sikandar, M., Almogren, A., Din, I. U., Guerrieri, A., & Fortino, G. (2020). IoMT-based computational approach for detecting brain tumor. *Future Generation Computer Systems*, 109, 360–367.

[36] Khan, S., Khan, A., Maqsood, M., Aadil, F., & Ghazanfar, M. A. (2019). Optimized gabor feature extraction for mass classification using cuckoo search for big data e-healthcare. *Journal of Grid Computing*, 17(2), 239–254.

[37] Kwok, J. Y. (1999). Moderating the outputs of support vector machine classifiers. *IEEE Transactions on Neural Networks*, 10(5), 1018–1031.

[38] Lousado, J. P., Pires, I. M., Zdravevski, E., & Antunes, S. (2021). Monitoring the Health and Residence Conditions of Elderly People, Using LoRa and the Things Network. *Electronics*, 10(14), 1729.

[39] Luna-Perejón, F., Muñoz-Saavedra, L., Castellano-Domínguez, J. M., & Domínguez-Morales, M. (2021). IoT garment for remote elderly care network. *Biomedical Signal Processing and Control*, 69, 102848.

[40] Mahmud, R., Koch, F. L., & Buyya, R. (2018). Cloud-fog interoperability in IoT-enabled healthcare solutions. In *Proceedings of the 19th International Conference on Distributed Computing and Networking* (pp. 1–10).

[41] Mukherjee, A., Ghosh, S., Behere, A., Ghosh, S. K., & Buyya, R. (2021). Internet of health things (IoHT) for personalized health care using integrated edge-fog-cloud network. *Journal of Ambient Intelligence and Humanized Computing*, 12, 943–959.

[42] Mukherjee, T., Nayak, G., & Senapati, D. (2021). Evaluation of symbol error probability using a new tight Gaussian Q approximation. *International Journal of Systems, Control and Communications*, 12(1), 60–71.

[43] Mukherjee, T., Pati, B., & Senapati, D. (2021). Performance evaluation of composite fading channels using q-weibull distribution. In: C. R. Panigrahi, B. Pati, B. K. Pattanayak, S. Amic, & K.-C. Li (Eds.), *Progress in Advanced Computing and Intelligent Engineering* (pp. 317–324). Springer: Singapore.

[44] Mukherjee, T., Singh, A. K., & Senapati, D. (2019). Performance evaluation of wireless communication systems over Weibull/q-lognormal shadowed fading using Tsallis' entropy framework. *Wireless Personal Communications*, 106(2), 789–803.

[45] Nalluri, J. J., Syed, K., Rana, P., Hudgins, P., Ramadan, I., Nieporte, W., ... & Ghosh, P. (2018). A smart healthcare portal for clinical decision making and precision medicine. In *Proceedings of the Workshop Program of the 19th International Conference on Distributed Computing and Networking* (pp. 1–6).

[46] Nayak, G., Singh, A. K., & Senapati, D. (2021). Computational modeling of non-gaussian option price using non-extensive Tsallis' entropy framework. *Computational Economics*, 57(4), 1353–1371.

[47] Nayak, G., Singh, A. K., Bhattacharjee, S., & Senapati, D. (2021). A new tight approximation towards the computation of option price. *International Journal of Information Technology*, 14(3), 1295–1303.

[48] Nayar, N., Ahuja, S., & Jain, S. (2019). Swarm intelligence and data mining: A review of literature and applications in healthcare. In *Proceedings of the Third International Conference on Advanced Informatics for Computing Research* (pp. 1–7).

[49] Nguyen, T. A., Min, D., Choi, E., & Lee, J. W. (2021). Dependability and Security Quantification of an Internet of Medical Things Infrastructure based on Cloud-Fog-Edge Continuum for Healthcare Monitoring using Hierarchical Models. *IEEE Internet of Things Journal.*

[50] Nguyen, V., Karimi, S., & Jin, B. (2019). An experimentation platform for precision medicine. In *Proceedings of the 42Nd International ACM SIGIR Conference on Research and Development in Information Retrieval* (pp. 1357–1360).

[51] Rahmani, A. M., Gia, T. N., Negash, B., Anzanpour, A., Azimi, I., Jiang, M., & Liljeberg, P. (2018). Exploiting smart e-Health gateways at the edge of healthcare Internet-of-Things: A fog computing approach. *Future Generation Computer Systems*, 78, 641–658.

[52] Rahul, K., & Banyal, R. K. (2021). Firefly algorithm: an optimization solution in big data processing for the healthcare and engineering sector. *International Journal of Speech Technology*, 24(3), 581–592.

[53] Rathee, G., Sharma, A., Saini, H., Kumar, R., & Iqbal, R. (2020). A hybrid framework for multimedia data processing in IoT-healthcare using blockchain technology. *Multimedia Tools and Applications*, 79(15), 9711–9733.

[54] Rish, I. (2001). An empirical study of the naive Bayes classifier. In *IJCAI 2001 Workshop on Empirical Methods in Artificial Intelligence* (Vol. 3, No. 22, pp. 41–46).

[55] Sangeetha, R. V., & Srinivasan, A. G. (2021). Mutated cuckoo search algorithm for dynamic vehicle routing problem and synchronization occurs within the time slots in home healthcare. *International Journal of System Assurance Engineering and Management*, 1–17.

[56] Senapati, D., & Karmeshu. (2016). Generation of cubic power-law for high frequency intra-day returns: Maximum Tsallis entropy framework. *Digital Signal Processing*, 48, 276–284.

[57] Sharma, D. K., Chakravarthi, D. S., Shaikh, A. A., Ahmed, A. A. A., Jaiswal, S., & Naved, M. (2021). The aspect of vast data management problem in healthcare sector and implementation of cloud computing technique. *Materials Today: Proceedings.*

[58] Sharma, M. (2022). Categorization of self care problem for children with disabilities using partial swarm optimization approach. *International Journal of Information Technology*, 14, 1835–1843.

[59] Singh, A. K., Senapati, D., Bebortta, S., & Rajput, N. K. (2021). A non-stationary analysis of erlang loss model. In: C. R. Panigrahi, B. Pati, B. K. Pattanayak, S. Amic, & K.-C. Li (Eds.), *Progress in Advanced Computing and Intelligent Engineering* (pp. 286–294). Springer: Singapore.
[60] Usman, M. J., Ismail, A. S., Abdul-Salaam, G., Chizari, H., Kaiwartya, O., Gital, A. Y., ... & Dishing, S. I. (2019). Energy-efficient Nature-Inspired techniques in Cloud computing datacenters. *Telecommunication Systems*, 71(2), 275–302.
[61] World Health Organization. (2007). *International Classification of Functioning, Disability, and Health: Children & Youth Version: ICF-CY*. World Health Organization: Geneva, Switzerland.
[62] Zarchi, M. S., Bushehri, S. F., & Dehghanizadeh, M. (2018). SCADI: A standard dataset for self-care problems classification of children with physical and motor disability. *International Journal of Medical Informatics*, 114, 81–87.
[63] Zgheib, R., Kristiansen, S., Conchon, E., Plageman, T., Goebel, V., & Bastide, R. (2020). A scalable semantic framework for IoT healthcare applications. *Journal of Ambient Intelligence and Humanized Computing*, 1–19.

Chapter 5

Machine learning approach for classification of stroke patients using clinical data

Rafiqul Islam and Bharti Rana
University of Delhi

CONTENTS

5.1 INTRODUCTION

A brain stroke is a major worldwide health problem and the second leading cause of death globally. Approximately 5.87 million people died globally due to brain stroke, and there has been a 26% increase in world stroke deaths during the past 20 years (Global Burden of Diseases (GBD) study [1]). In India, the incidence of brain strokes is 130 persons out of one lakh population [2]. Indian Stroke Association (ISA) [3] reported that about 17 million people are affected by stroke every year, out of which 6.2 million die and 5 million suffer handicaps.

Brain stroke occurs when there is bleeding in the brain due to a sudden break or burst of a blood vessel. It may also occur when something obstructs the supply of blood to a portion of the brain. The unexpected obstruction in blood supply and oxygen to the brain's tissues causes brain stroke. The symptoms are [4]: sudden weakness of your face, arm, leg,

DOI: 10.1201/9781003368342-5

and one side of the body; sudden confusion; problems in dialogue or understanding; loss of balance or coordination; problem in walking; and eye blindness. The risk factors for strokes [5] are diabetes, hypertension, and external factors such as smoking, alcohol, and heart-related diseases. A stroke can cause permanent death of the brain, handicap, or even death [4]. The early diagnosis of stroke and its treatment are essential to save the lives of patients, although they are challenging tasks for clinicians.

In the literature [6–10], the researchers have proposed supervised machine learning approaches to classify patients with stroke and healthy controls using clinical data. In the research work [6], classification of stroke is proposed on the heart disease dataset (from UCI Machine learning repository websites[1]). The research group explored the performance of three supervised machine learning algorithms, namely, support vector machine (SVM), Naïve Bayes, and deep learning. The missing values present in the dataset were removed. For training SVM, the constraint of the regularization parameter was set to 0.1, and ten-fold cross-validation (CV) was used. A forward multilayer artificial neural network with a backpropagation algorithm was employed in the deep learning approach. They reported that the deep learning model resulted in a Mean Square Error (MSE) of 0.2596 and achieved the best results while the MSE for Naïve Bayes and SVM were 0.49 ± 0.038 and 0.4778 ± 0.1106, respectively.

Monteiro et al. [7] used machine learning algorithms to forecast the functional outcome of ischemic stroke patients. A dataset of 541 patients was recorded for 3 months in the hospital of Santa Maria, Lisbon, Portugal. The acute stroke patients had undergone the Safe Implementation of Treatments in Stroke. The modified Rankin Scale (mRS) for three months was recorded for 425 patients. The features with missing values were deleted and one-hot encoding was applied to categorical variables. After cleaning the data, there were 425 patients and 152 features. The authors categorized the features into five sets based on time of collection: (i) baseline features collected at admission time; (ii) features collected 2 hours after admission; (iii) 24 hours after admission; (iv) 7 days after admission; and (v) features collected at discharge. Based on the mRS score, the problem is classified into binary classifiers as a good outcome when mRS ≤ 2 and a poor outcome when mRS > 2.

[1] https://archive.ics.uci.edu/ml/datasets/heart+disease.

They applied five classifiers, namely, L1 regularized Logistic regression (LR), Decision tree (DT), SVM, Random machine, and XGBoost. The dataset was imbalanced, so they used area under the curve (AUC) to capture the performance of the decision model. The ten-fold CV approach was used for training the model and recording the performance of the model.

Saleh et al. [8] attempted to compare the performance of different distributed machine learning algorithms, namely, LR, Random Forest (RF), DT, and SVM for the classification of stroke patients and healthy controls. They used the Healthcare Dataset Stroke for training and testing. The dataset is imbalanced, so they handled imbalanced data using random resampling techniques. They used a ten-fold CV process for training and testing. They evaluated the performance in accuracy, precision, recall, and f-measure. The RF classifier resulted in the highest classification accuracy, followed by DT, SVM, and LR.

Heo et al. [9] applied three machine learning models, namely, deep neural network (DNN), RF, and LR to analyze long-term results in ischemic stroke patients. They used a dataset consisting of 38 features, including clinical data, demographic details of patients' past diseases, medication history, some laboratory test results, and modified Rankin Scale (mRS) scores at 3 months. They have used three hidden layers and 15 artificial neural network units for deep neural networks. They have used 300 decision trees for the RF. The research group used six variables for calculating the Acute Stroke Registry and Analysis of Lausanne (ASTRAL) score. They used 67% of the data for training and the remaining data for testing. The DNN model accuracy is better than the ASTRAL score. In addition, the DNN model was the best among all the tested models.

Emon et al. [10] also emphasized the use of machine learning approaches for the early prediction of stroke. To prepare the dataset, they used clinical features like hypertension, BMI, heart disease, previous stroke, smoking status, and age. Data were pre-processed to handle missing values and duplicate values. They investigated ten supervised machine learning algorithms, namely LR, SGD, DT, AdaBoost, Multi-Layer Perceptron (MLP), Gaussian, Quadratic Discriminant Analysis (QDC), *K*-nearest Neighbors, Gradient Boosting Classifier (GBC), and XGBoost (XGB). Also, a weighted voting classification approach was proposed to attain the highest accuracy. Confusion matrix was computed for every algorithm to evaluate precision, recall, F1-score, the AUC, False Positive Rate, and False Negative Rate. It was observed that improved classification results were observed using the weighted voting classifier for predicting Stroke.

Working in the same direction, the present study aims to explore the existing machine learning algorithms for classifying stroke patients and healthy controls using clinical data. Also, a comparative investigation of the machine learning algorithms' performance is conducted for the same. Further, different datasets were created to understand the relevance of clinical features.

5.2 METHODOLOGY

5.2.1 Dataset preprocessing

The "Stroke Prediction dataset" provided by WHO, SPAIN, and MADRID was used for experiments. It is available on the Kaggle platform.[2] In the dataset, there are 5,110 data samples. Out of 5,110 samples, only 249 samples belonged to stroke patients, which means the dataset is highly imbalanced. The gender-wise details of the dataset are shown in Table 5.1. Also, in the dataset, there were several missing values.

Thus, the following steps were carried out for preprocessing of the dataset:

Table 5.1 Basic details of the Stroke Prediction dataset

Class/label (total samples)	*Gender*	*Number of samples*	*Age range (in years) (min–max)*
Healthy (4,861)	Male	2,007	0.08–82.0
	Female	2,853	0.08–82.0
	others	1	26.0–26.0
Stroke (249)	Male	108	42.0–82.0
	Female	141	1.32–82.0

[2] https://www.kaggle.com/fedesoriano/stroke-prediction-dataset.

a. An attribute named ID was removed since ID is a unique identifier for each sample, and it does not correlate with the prediction of the stroke.
b. *Removal of samples*: The following samples were removed from the datasets:
   i. The samples with missing values
   ii. The samples of children and those who never worked.
   iii. The samples with attribute gender are mentioned as 'other'.
c. *Level encoding*: A few attributes, such as gender, work type, and marital status, were nominal data represented in the strings. Thus, nominal data is converted to numeric values using level encoding for training and testing the decision model.

5.2.2 Dataset preparation

After preprocessing the dataset, the dataset was still highly unbalanced and may result in biased classification results. Thus, a balanced dataset is required to compare the performance of the decision models. Also, age is a significant factor that may affect the clinical scores. Thus, an age-matched balanced dataset called "*Balanced*" was created and utilized.

Further, to study the impact of stroke on gender, two datasets referred to as "*Male*" and "*Female,*" were created and used for the experiments.

Also, a person's work type (Government employees, employees of private institutes, or self-employed) may bring job security, work pressure, or hope for a better life. Hence, it may be a reason for being healthy or suffering from a stroke. Thus, three more datasets referred to as "*Govt*", "*private*", and "*self-emp*" corresponding to data of those working in Government institutes, private institutes, and self-employed, respectively, were created.

The details of all the utilized datasets are shown in Table 5.2.

5.2.3 Classifiers used

In this work, the performance of the following five classifiers is evaluated and compared: LR, DT, RF, SVM, and *K*-nearest Neighbors (KNN).

LR works on sigmoid function with an S-shaped curve. It gives a probability of belongingness to a class. For a two-class classification problem with labels 0 and 1, when the value of the sigmoid function

Table 5.2 The details of the prepared datasets

Name of the dataset	*Class/label*	*Samples*	*Age range (in years) (min–max)*	*Number of features*
Balanced	Healthy	188 (87M, 101F)	(44–82)	10
	Stroke	188 (87M, 101F)	(44–82)	
Male	Healthy	87 (87M, 0F)	(44–82)	9
	Stroke	87 (87M, 0F)	(44–82)	
Female	Healthy	101 (0M, 101F)	(53–82)	9
	Stroke	101 (0M, 101F)	(53–82)	
Govt	Healthy	37 (16M, 21F)	(44–76)	9
	Stroke	27 (9M,18F)	(61–81)	
Private	Healthy	104 (58M, 46F)	(43–82)	9
	Stroke	113 (59M, 54F)	(45–82)	
Self–emp	Healthy	46 (13M, 33F)	(45–82)	9
	Stroke	49 (20M, 29F)	(43–81)	

is <0.5, then the sample belongs to class 0; otherwise, it belongs to class 1.

A *Decision tree* (DT), a robust machine learning algorithm, is used for classification and regression problems. It generates a tree-like structure with a root node, intermediate or internal nodes, leaf nodes, and branches. The internal nodes of the tree are features, and the leaf node corresponds to the class of the samples like stroke or healthy. A feature with the most discriminative tendency or a feature that gives maximum information about the class label is present at the root node.

RF, a well-known and popularly used algorithm, comprises *k*-numbers of the DTs. It creates multiple DTs based on the training data and combines the results of each decision tree. It is assumed to be more robust than DT.

SVM is well-known and a powerful machine learning algorithm. It can be applied to both linear and nonlinearly separable data. It learns a hyperplane with the help of support vectors to separate the two classes. A hyperplane is chosen such that it maximizes the distance between two classes.

K-nearest Neighbor (k-NN) is the simplest but lazy classification algorithm. In this algorithm, distance from the training dataset is computed for a test sample, and the class label is predicted based on the top *k*-nearest samples.

5.2.4 Performance measures

The performance of each decision model is calculated in terms of average classification accuracy, recall, precision, and F1-score.

Classification accuracy measures the number or fraction of accurately classified samples. *Recall* measures the fraction of correctly classified samples belonging to stroke class out of the total samples of stroke class (test samples) inputted to the decision model. *Precision* is the fraction of correctly classified stroke samples out of those classified as stroke. *F1-score* measures harmonic mean of recall and precision.

A high value of precision, recall, classification accuracy, and F1-score are desired for adapting any decision model in real-life.

5.2.5 Overview of the decision model

A flowchart of the building decision model is shown in Figure 5.1. The flow comprises the following four steps:

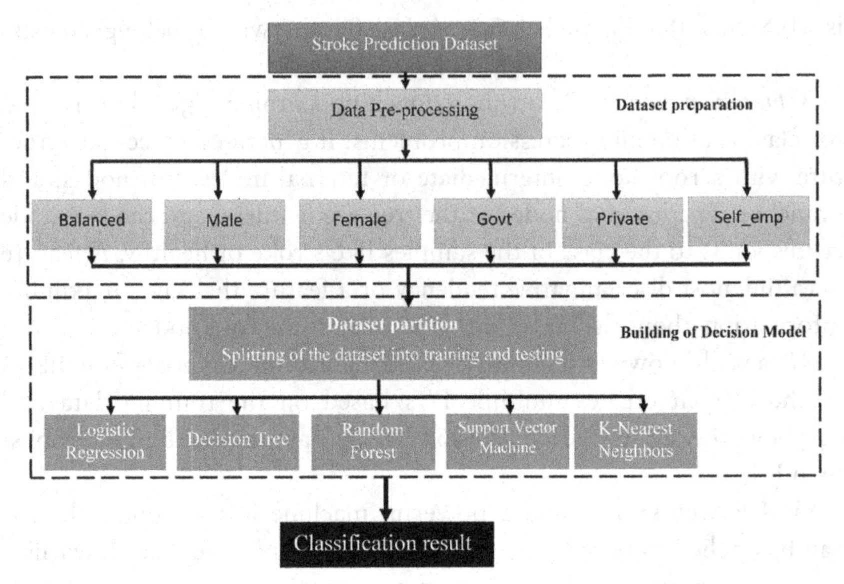

Figure 5.1 A flowchart of the building decision model.

a. Data preparation, as mentioned in the above section
b. *Partitioning of the dataset*: For training and testing of the decision models, the dataset was partitioned using ten-fold CV, where ten-folds of datasets were prepared randomly. Each fold is taken as testing exactly once, and the rest nine-folds were used to train the model.
c. *The following five classifiers were trained*: LR, DT, RF, SVM, and KNN. The hyperparameter(s) of the classifiers was(were) tuned.
d. Finally, the performance of a decision model was calculated using average classification accuracy, recall, precision, and F1-score.

5.3 RESULTS AND DISCUSSION

5.3.1 Classification results

The experiments were conducted with six datasets, namely *Balanced, Male, Female, Govt, Private,* and *Self-emp*. The performance of five machine learning algorithms, DT, LR, KNN, RF, and SVM, was compared using ten-fold CV. Tables 5.3–5.8 show the classification results of five algorithms on *Balanced, Male, Female, Govt, Private,* and *Self-emp*, respectively. The average value and the standard deviation of each

Table 5.3 The classification results for the Balanced dataset

Classifier	*Average classification accuracy*	*Precision*	*Recall*	*F1-score*
LR	0.6509 ± 0.0579	0.6543 ± 0.0866	0.6400 ± 0.1191	0.6411 ± 0.0798
DT	0.5980 ± 0.0990	0.5888 ± 0.1406	0.6012 ± 0.1665	0.5885 ± 0.1372
RF	0.6346 ± 0.04906	0.6234 ± 0.0793	0.6589 ± 0.0695	0.6386 ± 0.0643
SVM	**0.6876** ± **0.0837**	**0.6834** ± **0.1029**	**0.6752** ± **0.1337**	**0.6762** ± **0.1084**
KNN	0.6267 ± 0.0703	0.6111 ± 0.0908	0.6651 ± 0.1172	0.6340 ± 0.0928

Table 5.4 The classification results for the Male dataset

Classifier	*Average classification accuracy*	*Precision*	*Recall*	*F1-score*
LR	0.6647 ± 0.1321	0.6529 ± 0.1876	0.6650 ± 0.1337	0.6523 ± 0.1539
DT	0.6250 ± 0.096	0.5865 ± 0.1229	0.5919 ± 0.1578	0.5745 ± 0.1075
RF	0.5846 ± 0.1006	0.6929 ± 0.1119	0.6923 ± 0.0972	0.6867 ± 0.0713
SVM	**0.7104** ± **0.0732**	**0.6994** ± **0.0964**	**0.7169** ± **0.1165**	**0.7022** ± **0.0908**
KNN	0.6519 ± 0.1203	0.6313 ± 0.1692	0.6666 ± 0.1954	0.6374 ± 0.1557

Table 5.5 The classification results for the Female dataset

Classifier	*Average classification accuracy*	*Precision*	*Recall*	*F1-score*
LR	**0.6597 ± 0.1393**	**0.6679 ± 0.1977**	0.6262 ± 0.2014	**0.6348 ± 0.1732**
DT	0.5890 ± 0.0960	0.5934 ± 0.0934	0.5494 ± 0.1380	0.5656 ± 0.1046
RF	0.6347 ± 0.1467	0.6361 ± 0.1962	**0.6412 ± 0.1702**	0.6309 ± 0.1664
SVM	0.6197 ± 0.1345	0.6324 ± 0.2047	0.5897 ± 0.2031	0.5920 ± 0.1789
KNN	0.6138 ± 0.1093	0.6303 ± 0.1569	0.6165 ± 0.1670	0.6055 ± 0.1292

Table 5.6 The classification results for the Govt dataset

Classifier	*Average classification accuracy*	*Precision*	*Recall*	*F1-score*
LR	0.7142 ± 0.188	0.7012 ± 0.0045	0.7154 ± 0.0002	0.7212 ± 0.0080
DT	0.7714 ± 0.180	0.7521 ± 0.0135	0.7712 ± 0.0043	0.7600 ± 0.0012
RF	0.6421 ± 0.163	0.6312 ± 0.00309	0.6451 ± 0.0100	0.6700 ± 0.01000
SVM	0.7124 ± 0.062	0.7321 ± 0.0050	0.715 ± 0.00509	0.7123 ± 0.0052
KNN	**0.8550 ± 0.182**	**0.8500 ± 0.01500**	**0.8500 ± 0.0089**	**0.8500 ± 0.0139**

Table 5.7 The classification results for the Private dataset

Classifier	*Average classification accuracy*	*Precision*	*Recall*	*F1-score*
LR	0.7142 ± 0.109	0.7012 ± 0.0105	0.7200 ± 0.01994	0.7142 ± 0.0070
DT	0.79999 ± 1418	0.7985 ± 0.0367	0.7890 ± 0.0299	0.7900 ± 0.0324
RF	0.7245 ± 0.112	0.7251 ± 0.0025	0.7232 ± 0.0009	0.7245 ± 0.00045
SVM	0.7142 ± 0.087	0.7102 ± 0.0074	0.7010 ± 0.0119	0.7175 ± 0.037
KNN	**0.8571 ± 0.112**	**0.8200 ± 0.0344**	**0.8500 ± 0.0150**	**0.8552 ± 0.0025**

Table 5.8 The classification results for the Self-emp dataset

Classifier	*Average classification accuracy*	*Precision*	*Recall*	*F1-score*
LR	0.6232 ± 0.116	0.6140 ± 0.006	0.6200 ± 0.0030	0.6232 ± 0.0045
DT	0.6500 ± 0.128	0.6400 ± 0.0084	0.6500 ± 0.005	0.6510 ± 0.0055
RF	0.7200 ± 0.138	0.7150 ± 0.0070	0.7012 ± 0.0068	0.7120 ± 0.0053
SVM	**0.7730 ± 0.094**	**0.7545 ± 0.0212**	**0.7323 ± 0.0110**	**0.7412 ± 0.0066**
KNN	0.5990 ± 0.122	0.5890 ± 0.00109	0.5985 ± 0.00475	0.5975 ± 0.00425

performance measure over a ten-fold CV are reported. The bold values represent the maximum classification accuracy.

Further, to compare the efficacy of the classifiers, ranking of classifiers is carried out based on classification accuracy. The best classifier is ranked one, and the worst classifier is ranked five. Then, the average rank of each classifier is obtained, and the final ranking is done on average ranking. The ranks are shown in Table 5.9. Further, a summary of the utilized datasets, dataset partitioning approach, classifiers employed, and performance metrics used in the related literature is presented in Table 5.10. The following can be observed from Tables 5.3 to 5.9:

- The best classification results of 68.76% were achieved for *Balanced* dataset with SVM classifier, 71.04% achieved for *Male* dataset with SVM classifier, 65.97% for *Female* dataset with LR classifier, 85.50% for *Govt* dataset with KNN classifier, 85.71% for *Private* dataset with KNN classifier, and 77.30% for *Self-emp* dataset with SVM classifier.
- From Table 5.9, the overall rank of SVM is one which means it is working well for all the datasets, followed by LR, whose overall ranking is two. On the other hand, the rank of DT is five, which represents that DT is not able to correctly classify the samples.
- Overall, the performance of the classifiers is dataset dependent, *i.e.*, no classifier is observed to be robust.

5.3.2 T-test analysis

The relevance of each feature is calculated with the help of a two-sample t-test. The t-test values of each feature for *Balanced, Male, Female, Govt, Private,* and *Self-emp* datasets are shown in Figures 5.2–5.7, respectively. The bars with light grey color represent a significant feature. From the two-sample t-test analysis (Figures 5.2 to 5.7), the following is observed:

- The features, namely *age, heart_disease, hypertension,* and *avg_glucose_level,* were statistically significant for *Balanced* and *Male* datasets.
- For the *Female* dataset, the features, namely *age, hypertension,* and *smoking_status* were statistically significant.
- For the *Govt* dataset, the feature *age*, while for *Private* dataset, the features namely, *age, heart_disease, hypertension, avg_glucose_level,*

Table 5.9 The overall ranks of the classifiers.

Datasets	*Balanced*	*Male*	*Female*	*Govt*	*Private*	*Self-emp*	*Average_ranks*	*Overall_ranks*
Classifier ↓								
LR	2	2	1	3.5	4.5	4	2.83	2
DT	5	4	5	2	2	3	3.5	5
RF	3	5	2	5	3	2	3.33	4
SVM	1	1	3	3.5	4.5	1	2.33	1
KNN	4	3	4	1	1	5	3	3

Table 5.10 A summary of used datasets, classifiers used, and performance metrics in the related literature and the current work.

Research work	*Dataset source*	*Number of samples*	*Number of features*	*Dataset partitioning approach*	*Used classifiers*	*Performance measure(s)*
Monteiro et al. [7]	Collected at Hospital of Santa Maria, in Lisbon, Portugal	425	152	Ten-fold CV	L1 regularized LR, DT, SVM, Random machine, and XGBoost	Mean Square Error and Standard Deviation and AUC
Heo et al. [9]	Available with authors	2,604	38	67% of the data for training and the remaining 33% data for testing	Deep neural network, RF, and LR	Accuracy, ASTRAL score
Saleh et al. [8]	Stroke Prediction Dataset (from Kaggle)	5,110	10	Ten-fold CV	LR, RF, DT, and SVM	Precision Recall F1-score
Emon et al. [10]	Data was collected from the hospitals of Bangladesh	5,110	10	Training = 3,554; testing = 1,556	LR, SGD, DT, AdaBoost, Gaussian, QDC, MLP, KNN GBC, and XGB	Accuracy, Precision Recall, F1-score, AUC, FP rate and FN rate
Present research work	Balanced	376	10	Ten-fold CV	DT, LR, KNN, RF, and SVM	Average classification accuracy, Precision, Recall, F1-score
	Male	174	9			
	Female	202	9			
	Govt	64	9			
	Private	217	9			
	Self-emp	95	9			

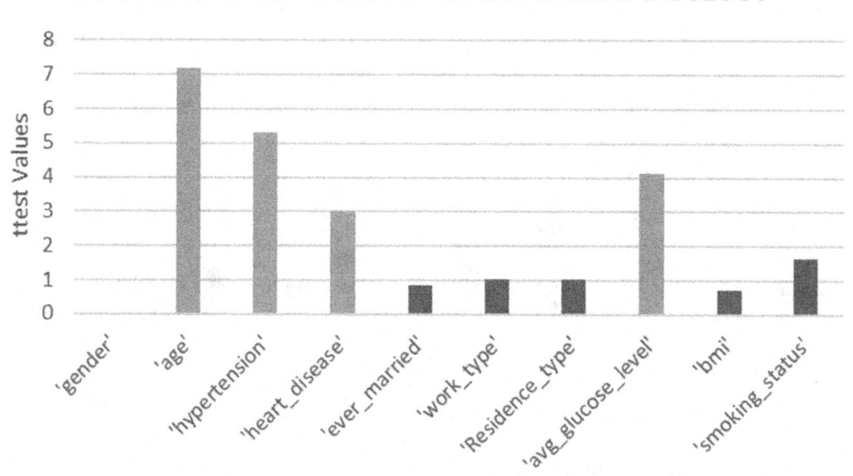

Figure 5.2 T-test results for Balanced dataset. The bars with light grey color represent a significant feature.

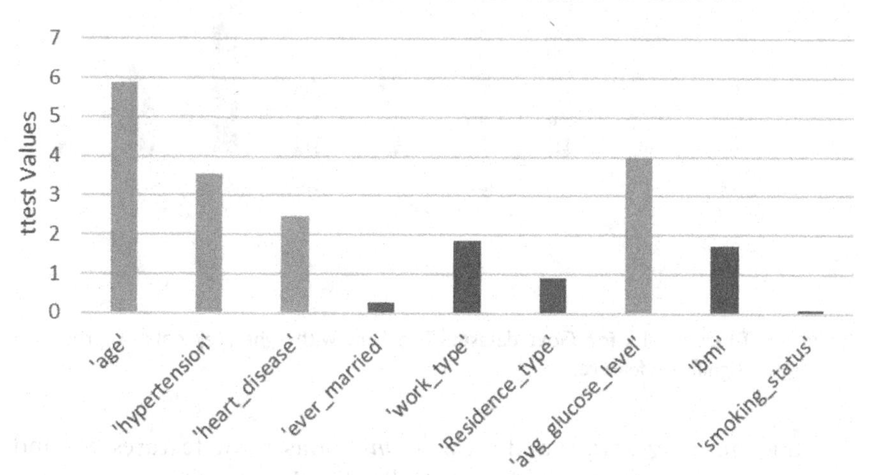

Figure 5.3 T-test results for Male dataset. The bars with light grey color represent a significant feature.

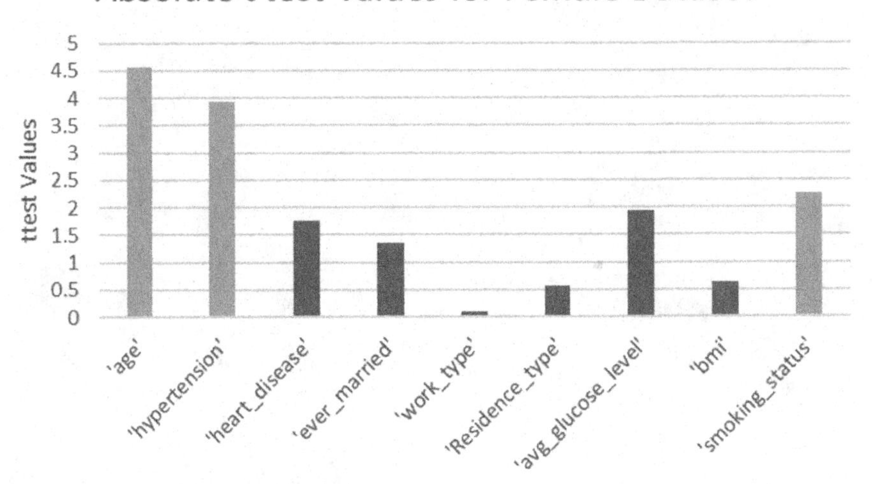

Figure 5.4 T-test results for Female dataset. The bars with light grey color represent a significant feature.

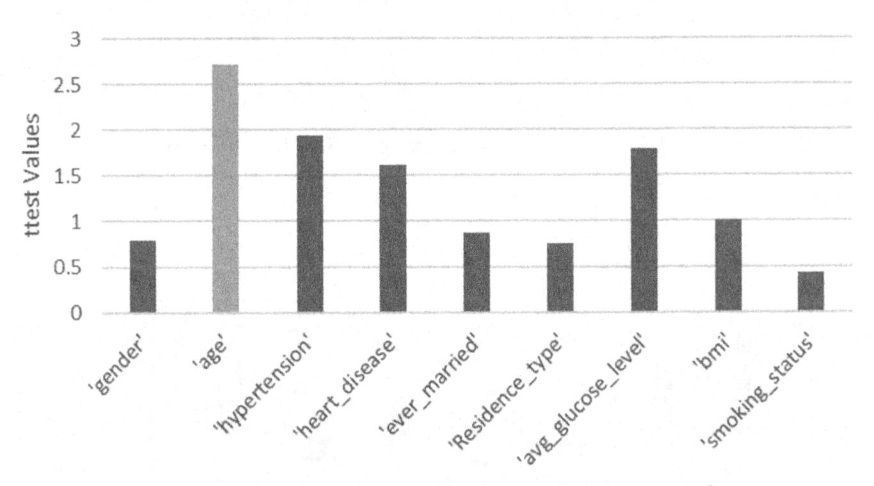

Figure 5.5 T-test results for Govt dataset. The bars with light grey color represent a significant feature.

and *smoking_status;* and for *Self-emp* dataset, the features *age* and *hypertension* were found statistically significant.

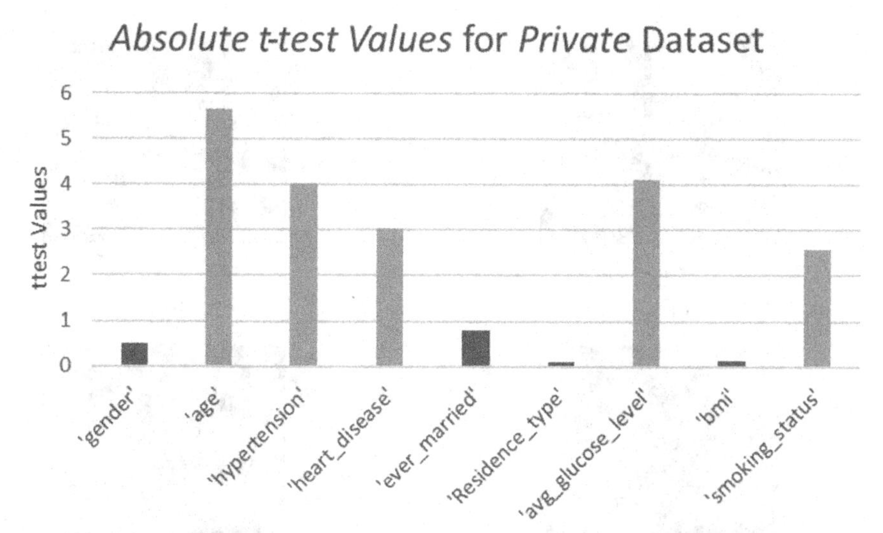

Figure 5.6 T-test results for Private dataset. The bars with light grey color represent a significant feature.

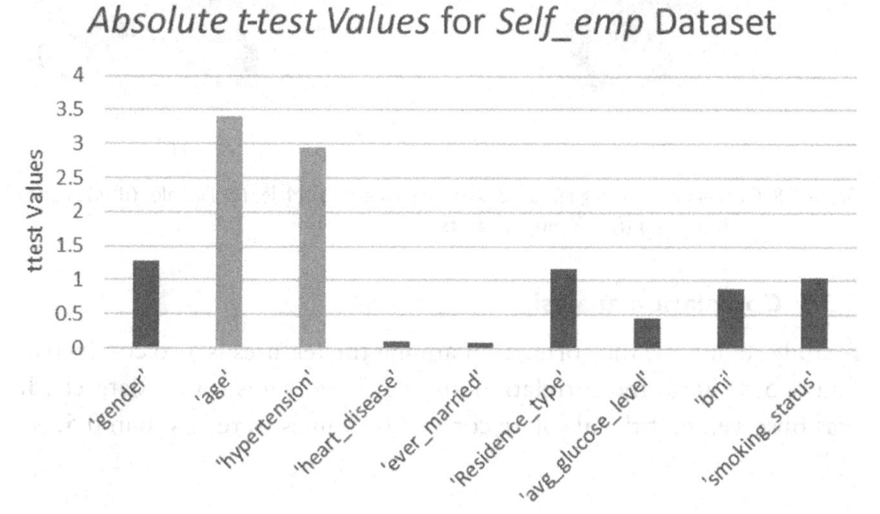

Figure 5.7 T-test results for Self-emp dataset. The bars with light grey color represent a significant feature.

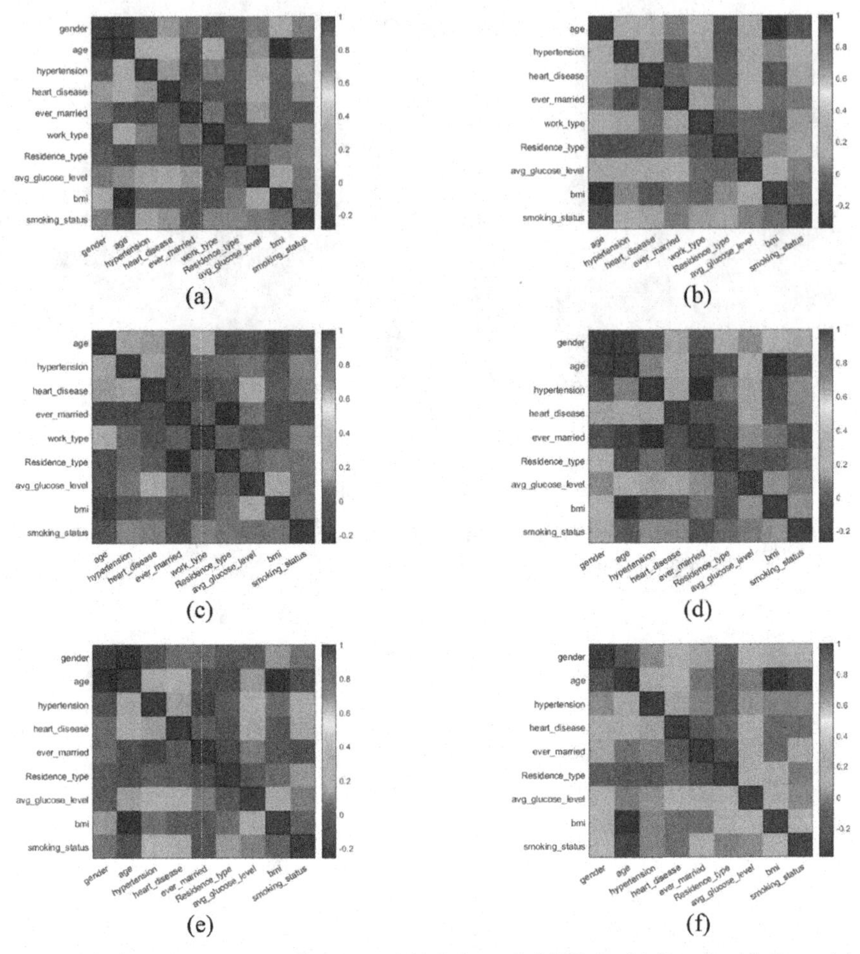

Figure 5.8 Correlation among features of (a) Balanced, (b) Male, (c) Female, (d) Govt, (e) Private, and (f) Self-emp datasets.

5.3.3 Correlation analysis

A study to analyse the correlation among the features is also conducted. Figure 5.8 shows the correlation among the features for all datasets. It was observed that the absolute correlation values were less than 0.5.

5.4 CONCLUSION AND FUTURE WORK

In the present work, a machine learning approach for classifying stroke patients and healthy controls is conducted using clinical data. A total of six datasets, namely, *Balanced, Male, Female, Govt, Private,* and *Self-emp*, were created from the publically available dataset and were utilized. A comparison of five classifiers, DT, LR, KNN, RF, and SVM, is conducted for the classification of stroke and healthy controls. Further, *age* and *hypertension* were the two main significant features for all the datasets except *Govt*. The correlation study revealed that there does not exist high correlation among the features.

In the future, a dataset with more clinical features may be prepared and utilized to predict stroke.

REFERENCES

[1] Kamalakannan, S., Gudlavalleti, A. S., Gudlavalleti, V. S. M., Goenka, S., & Kuper, H. (2017). Incidence & prevalence of stroke in India: A systematic review. *The Indian Journal of Medical Research*, 146(2), 175.

[2] Pandian, J. D., & Sudhan, P. (2013). Stroke epidemiology and stroke care services in India. *Journal of Stroke*, 15(3), 128.

[3] Sehgal, V. (2021). *The Indian Express*, 2 February, 2021, https://indianexpress.com/article/lifestyle/health/stroke-recovery-home-tipscaregivers-7171008/.

[4] CDC, https://www.cdc.gov/stroke/types_of_stroke.htm.

[5] Johns Hopkins Medicine. Risk factors for stroke, https://www.hopkinsmedicine.org/health/conditions-and-diseases/stroke/risk-factors-for-stroke.

[6] Chantamit-o-pas, P., & Goyal, M. (2017, November). Prediction of stroke using deep learning model. In *International Conference on Neural Information Processing* (pp. 774–781). Springer, Cham.

[7] Monteiro, M., Fonseca, A. C., Freitas, A. T., e Melo, T. P., Francisco, A. P., Ferro, J. M., & Oliveira, A. L. (2018). Using machine learning to improve the prediction of functional outcome in ischemic stroke patients. *IEEE/ACM Transactions on Computational Biology and Bioinformatics*, 15(6), 1953–1959.

[8] Saleh H. A., Abd-el ghany, S. F., Younis, E., Omran, N., & Ali, A. A. (2019). Stroke prediction using distributed machine learning based on apache spark. *Stroke*, 28(15), 89–97.

[9] Heo, J., Yoon, J. G., Park, H., Kim, Y. D., Nam, H. S., & Heo, J. H. (2019). Machine learning–based model for prediction of outcomes in acute stroke. *Stroke*, 50(5), 1263–1265.

[10] Emon, M. U., Keya, M. S., Meghla, T. I., Rahman, M. M., Al Mamun, M. S., & Kaiser, M. S. (2020, November). Performance analysis of machine learning approaches in stroke prediction. In *2020 4th International Conference on Electronics, Communication and Aerospace Technology (ICECA)*, Coimbatore, Tamil Nadu, India, (pp. 1464–1469). IEEE.

of six datasets, namely, Bu[illegible], [illegible] Schizophrenia [illegible] were [illegible] tested [illegible] the [illegible] dataset and were analyzed. A comparison of [illegible] classifiers [illegible] KNN, NB, [illegible] and SVM were conducted [illegible] the [illegible] datasets except [illegible] that there does not exist [illegible]

In the future, a dataset with more clinical features must be prepared and utilized to predict stroke.

REFERENCES

[1] [illegible] 2018 [illegible]

[2] [illegible]

[3] [illegible]

[4] [illegible]

[5] [illegible]

[6] [illegible]

[7] [illegible]

[8] [illegible]

Chapter 6

A comparative analysis of noise robust Fuzzy Clustering algorithms for medical image segmentation

Inder Khatri, Dhirendra Kumar, and Aaryan Gupta
Delhi Technological University

CONTENTS

6.1 INTRODUCTION

Clustering is an unsupervised learning technique used to group data points without a label on the basis of some similarity measures. This technique is generally used to find out the meaningful patterns and further any associated relationship between various data points. Clustering has recently gained a lot of popularity due to its immense applicability in the areas of data mining [4, 18], image segmentation [6] , document classification [21], data compression [28], bio-informatics [20, 27], and other research domains. Clustering is of various types: connectivity-based clustering (hierarchical clustering), density-based clustering (model-based methods), distribution-based clustering, and centroid-based clustering [32]. Among these, the centroid-based clustering is one of the simplest and effective ways which gives compact clusters by obtaining prototype of different groups present in dataset [34]. Depending on the way these

DOI: 10.1201/9781003368342-6

clusters are computed, the centroid-based clustering can be of two kinds, namely, hard clustering and soft clustering.

Hard clustering is a clustering technique in which each data point either belongs to a cluster completely or not. It assigns each data point to clusters by computing membership values, i.e. '0,1' 0 for not being a member of the respective cluster and 1 for being the member of the respective cluster. The hard clustering doesn't leave much room to consider other possibilities due to its rigidness on assigning the data to clusters. This leads to loss of important structural information; therefore, to tackle this problem, the concept of soft clustering was formulated. In soft clustering, instead of putting each data point into a separate cluster, the likelihood of a data point to be present in these various clusters is computed.

J.C. Dunn in 1973 introduced a fuzzy set theory-based soft clustering method termed as fuzzy c-means (FCM) [13]. FCM is one of the widely used soft clustering techniques on a variety of real world problems. The concept of FCM revolves around assigning a separate quantified value of belongingness to each data point for each cluster. It assigns membership values to a data point on the basis of its proximity to the center of the respective clusters. The membership value generally lies in the range of [0,1] and also for a given data point sum of all the membership values is 1.

In today's world, medical imaging has turned out to be a very helpful tool for the diagnosis, monitoring, and treatment of medical conditions. Since medical imaging provides an accurate representation of what's happening inside the patient's body, it significantly affects the decision of doctors and makes it a lot more accurate. The problems don't end here as with a large number of medical images being generated each day; it becomes difficult to manually analyze each and every image with high precision. Also the limited number of skilled radiologists in healthcare system makes the situation even more cumbersome to handle. Therefore, computer-aided Medical Image Analysis (MIA) has turned out to be a real boon for today's medical science [8, 24, 26].

Medical image segmentation(MIS) is one of the subsidiaries of MIA [30]. It helps us in identifying anomalies and abnormalities present in medical images, which is a crucial and time-taking task in diagnosis of various diseases such as brain injuries, cancer, strokes, development irregularities, etc. Hence, MIS reduces the diagnosis time and saves energy of doctors, which leads to a more efficient healthcare system. With constant research being done in this field, MIA techniques are emerging to be more reliable with each passing day. Therefore, with passing time, MIA would turn out to be one of the most convenient tools for healthcare services.

X-ray radiography, computed tomography (CT) scan, medical resonance imaging (MRI), endoscopy, positron emission tomography (PET), nuclear medical image functioning, and ultrasound are some of the modern medical imaging modalities [14]. Among these medical image modalities, MRI is considered to be one of the most productive and safest options of medical imaging. It provides better contrast in imaging of soft tissues, better differentiation between fat, water, muscle, and other soft tissues in comparison to other medical imaging modalities. It doesn't use harmful ionizing radiation, whereas some of the other modalities do utilize them for imaging. The ionizing radiations have a bad impact on the patient's body; therefore, it makes MRI a very safe option. Due to these advantages, MRI imaging technology is found to be very effective for delineating the brain soft tissues such as white matter(WM), gray matter(GM), and cerebrospinal fluid(CSF) for quantization.

The MR images are often found corrupted by various imaging artifacts such as noise, intensity in-homogeneity, and partial volume effect. These artifacts arise during the image acquisition due to human errors, technical inconsistency, and uneven radio frequencies, which ultimately result in making manual medical image segmentation inconsistent. These artifacts induce out-of-distribution like cases while analysis and deviate the decision-making of image segmentation. The most common artifact affecting the MR images is noise, which adds some additive deviation in the original signal[2, 29]. To handle the noise, several modified FCM versions have been proposed in the literature. Most of these works focus on integrating neighbor pixel's information in the cost function which tries to solve the problem by incorporating available neighborhood spatial information instead of just concentrating on a single central pixel.

A lot of methods have been proposed to tackle the noise associated with image segmentation. These methods are effective against several types of corruption which have been authenticated on the basis of different performance metrics. The fact that these methods aren't authenticated on a single parameter and have different areas of action creates a sense of uncertainty while making a choice. To our knowledge, there have been no recent works that particularly compare noise robust fuzzy clustering algorithms for MR image segmentation. Therefore, in this chapter, we present an analytical comparison between different noise segmentation methods. We compared and checked their performances, particularly against Rician Noise on a standard MR dataset.

The rest of this chapter is organized as follows. Section 6.2 describes the preliminaries and related work. The proposed method is described in Section 6.3. The experimental results on various synthetic and real data are presented in Section 6.4. Finally, Section 6.5 includes the conclusion.

6.2 PRELIMINARIES AND NOTATIONS

The description of notations used in this work and related definition is described here in this section.

Definition 6.1 *Fuzzy set: A fuzzy set is a set in which each member element will have the fractional membership through a membership function $\mu_A : X \rightarrow [0, 1]$ which gives the degree of belongingness [41]. If A is a fuzzy set defined over a set X, it can be represented as:*

$$A = \{(x, \mu_A(x)) : x \in X\}$$

Definition 6.2 *Intuitionistic fuzzy set (IFS): A intuitionistic fuzzy set B, is an extension of fuzzy set over set X, which is represented as [3]:*

$$B = \{(x, \mu_B(x), \nu_B(x)) : x \in X \text{ and } 0 \leq \mu_B(x) + \nu_B(x) \leq 1\} \quad (6.1)$$

Where $\mu_B : X \rightarrow [0, 1]$ and $\nu_B : X \rightarrow [0, 1]$ are membership and non-membership functions of an element x in the IFS B, respectively. The IFS B is reduced to FS B when $\mu_B(x) + \nu_B(x) = 1$ for all x in X.

Definition 6.3 *Picture fuzzy set (PFS): A picture fuzzy set B, is an extension of fuzzy set over X which is represented as [11]:*

$$B = \{(x, \mu_B(x), \eta_B(x), \gamma_B(x)) : x \in X \text{ and } 0 \leq \mu_B(x) + \eta_B(x) + \gamma_B(x) \leq 1\}$$

where $\mu_B : X \rightarrow [0, 1]$, $\eta_B : X \rightarrow [0, 1]$, $\gamma_B : X \rightarrow [0, 1]$ are positive membership value, neutral and negative membership functions of an element x in the set B.

The refusal degree $\xi_B(x)$ of an element x in the set B is represented as $\xi_B(x) = 1 - (\mu_B(x) + \eta_B(x) + \gamma_B(x))$. In case $\xi_B(x) = 0$, the PFS B reduces to IFS B and when $\eta_B(x) = 0; \xi_B(x) = 0$ then the PFS B is reduced to FS B for all x in B.

6.3 RELATED WORKS

One of the major problems associated with medical image segmentation is the non-robust performance in the presence of noise corruption in images. The noise corruptions are additive disturbances, which deviates the real pixel intensities and makes the segmentation inconsistent. To solve this problem, several methods have been proposed in the literature, which rely upon the neighborhood spatial information. These methods focus over the improvements in objective function, distance metrics and fuzzy sets to solve different noise-related problems associated with image segmentation algorithms using neighborhood information. This section presents an overview of these methods.

Ahmad et al. [1] proposed a modified Fuzzy C-means namely FCM_S to suppress the outliers. They assumed that the intensity distribution of a noise free image would be homogeneous in a pixel's neighborhood and hence, included an additional term in the optimization problem consisting of the immediate neighbor pixels distance from the centroid intensities. The neighborhood information acts like a regularizer and facilitates the optimization toward piece wise homogeneous labeling of pixels. This method is found to be highly dependent on the input spatial parameter alpha, which is responsible for controlling the extent of neighbor influence. Optimization of alpha usually takes a lot of time as it involves grid-search for finding optimal value. Furthermore, the computational efficiency per iteration was also poor since the neighbor information, over the given local window was incorporated in each optimization step. Chen and Zheng [7] proposed FCM_S1 and FCM_S2 where a statistical approximation of mean and median over the neighbors was used respectively, in order to reduce the time complexity. Although it achieved a better time complexity, yet the methods were not found to be effective as their performance was not up to the mark for a lot of noises especially for salt and pepper and mix noise.

The above methods used the Euclidean distance to measure the distance between pixel intensity values. The noise induced in an image usually act like an irregularity and the Euclidean distance become incapable of recognizing patterns behind these irregularities as they turn more complex. Therefore, an alternative to Eucledian distance i.e. kernel distance metric was employed in KFCM_S [7], which was found to be more efficient in handling noises in comparison to Euclidean distance. Szilgayi et al. [33] proposed Enhanced Fuzzy C-means (ENFCM), which proved to be a major breakout in making the segmentation faster. The method proposed two novelties, i.e. first the spatial information was incorporated with the original image in advance by adding the weighted sum of the immediate neighbor pixels intensity and second the whole image was represented by the gray-level histogram on the basis of which clustering was done to get the final segmentation.

One major drawback associated with the FCM_S, FCM_S1, FCM_S2, and EnFCM was the use of the same value of the spatial parameter alpha throughout the whole image. The different regions of image were often found to be affected by different noise levels, and therefore, the performance was not found to be consistent. To overcome this problem, Cai et al. [5] proposed FGFCM algorithm containing an adaptive varying spatial parameter alpha, which depended on the local statistics in a given window. This adaptive parameter alpha was calculated by using the differences between the spatial and gray level of the pixels lying in a local window. The computation of adaptive varying spatial parameter depends on two input parameter i.e. λ_s and λ_g. Similar to FGFCM, Guo et al. [38] also proposed a Noise detecting Fuzzy C-means (NDFCM) focusing on the problem of in-homogeneous noise distribution. NDFCM is able to efficiently suppress the noise and also preserve the sharp image details. Compared to FGFCM, it contained less input parameters and hence was time-efficient.

Most of the above methods are dependent upon some input parameters, which are required to be fine tuned for getting the optimal results. Krindis et al. [22] proposed a parameter free method named as Fuzzy Local Information C-means Algorithm (FLICM), which consisted of a spatial distance weighted neighborhood information term. FLICM gave good segmentation results along with preserved shapes. Gong et al. [16] further introduced kernel metric in FLICM instead of Euclidean distance along with weighted fuzzy tradeoff factor, which was proficient in capturing the irregularities due to the noise. However, both FLICM and KWFLICM were not found to be stable during optimization as the objective function was not found to be converging. Kang et al. [19] proposed Fuzzy C-means with Spatially weighted Information (FCM-SWI). The method is parameter free and tackled the problem of varying noise distribution throughout the image. The weight coefficients in FCMSWI are calculated using the neighbor pixels intensity. Lin et al. [44] introduced a novel membership constraint in FCM clustering, named as Generalized Fuzzy Clustering with improved partition, which helped in the rapid convergence. To improve robustness against noise, Zhao et al.[43] extended the GIFP to kernelized version with spatial information, i.e. KGFCM .

Recently, Lei et al.[25] proposed a fast and robust fuzzy C-means algorithm (FRFCM), which gave impressive results with considerably low time complexity. The method employed a morphological reconstruction operation as a pre-processing step, which made it more robust to a variety of noises. To avoid the heavy computation which calculating distance between the neighbor pixels and centroids, the method used membership filtering as a post-processing step. Although the method was robust to a variety of noises, it was not able to perform well on high noise samples. When encountered with high noise samples, FRFCM was not able to preserve the sharp edges and shapes. Another research work [42], termed as DSFCM_N, modeled the deviation between the original pixel values and measured noisy pixels value as residual and used this value in optimization function. They considered the residual term to be sparse matrix and used the l1 norm measure in objective function as a constraint over residuals. However, DSFCM_N did not show reliable performances when tested with higher noise samples. Further, Wang et. al. proposed Weighted Residual Fuzzy C-means (WRFCM) which used weighted l2-norm fidelity for making the residual estimation more reliable and showed better results compared to the previous works [37].

In real life data, there is always some uncertainty associated with the data due to imprecise measurement and noise, hence relying only on the membership value makes clustering a bit imprecise. To handle the vagueness associated in data Atanassov [3] proposed the Intuitionistic Fuzzy Set Theory(IFS). IFS consisted of one additional factor namely hesitancy degree, which helped in better representation of data which further resulted in a better decision-making. In recent years, some authors have incorporated several advancements with IFS theory to handle the noisy image segmentation. Verma et al.[35] proposed an Improved

Intuitionistic Fuzzy C-means (IIFCM), which incorporated the spatial and gray scale information over the local window. The algorithm is effective for dealing with a wide variety of noises, but was found to be inefficient w.r.t. to time. Kumar et al. [23] proposed Intuitionistic Fuzzy C-means with Spatial Neighborhood Information (IFCMSNI). IFCMSNI consisted of a membership weighted neighbor's deviation from centroids in the objective function. The method was insensitive to the varying noise distribution in image and hence was able to preserve sharp edges and other details.

Further an extension on IFS was presented by Cuong et al. [11] namely PFS consisting of additional refusal and neutrality degree to make the decision-making more realistic. PFS's application in Image Segmentation have shown to be effective compared to previous Fuzzy counterparts. Another work proposed Improved Picture Fuzzy Clustering Algorithm (IPFCM) [40] which considered the spatial information in the framework of Picture Fuzzy Clustering. IPFCM was dependent on the input spatial weighting parameter and was sensitive to the strength of noise, hence the parameter had to be fine tuned for getting the results which further extended the processing time. Further Wu et al. [39] proposed Adaptive Improved Picture Fuzzy Clustering Algorithm (AIPFCM), which resolved the problem of fine-tuning the parameter and also worked upon updating the parameter adaptively while optimizing the weighing parameter.

Research work also proposed an Adaptive entropy weighted weighted Picture Fuzzy Clustering Algorithm with spatial Information (APFCMS), which included a novel spatial information function that modified the membership degree using the neighbors membership values resulting in robustness to noise and outliers.

6.4 EXPERIMENTAL SETUP AND RESULTS

To check the effectiveness of the different proposed method on practical grounds experiments have been performed on a publicly available Brain MR dataset. We do evaluation for the 18 methods namely FCM_S, FCM_S1, FCM_S2, KFCM_S, EnFCM, FGFCM, NDFCM, FLICM, KWFLICM, FCMSWI, KGFCM, FRFCM, DSFCMN, WRFCM, IIFCM, IFCMSNI, IPFCM, AIPFCM, and APFCMS. The performance measures that we use for comparison are average segmentation accuracy (ASA) and

Dice score (DS) [9, 31, 36], which are shown as below:

$$\text{ASA} = \sum_{i=1}^{c} \frac{|X_i \cap Y_i|}{\sum_{j=1}^{c} |X_j|} \tag{6.1}$$

$$\text{DS} = \frac{2|X_i \cap Y_i|}{|X_i| + |Y_i|} \tag{6.2}$$

where c is the number of cluster, N is the total number of datapoints, μ_{ij} is the membership of jth datapoint in i^{th} cluster, m is the fuzzifier factor, X_i denote the pixels belonging to the manual segmented image (ground truth), Y_i denote the pixels belonging to the experimental segmented image and $|X_i|$ denotes the cardinality of X_i. The optimal values of parameters involve for each of the methods are obtained using grid search.

6.4.1 Datasets

BrainWeb simulated MRI brain volumes, a publicly available dataset[1] from the McConnell Brain Imaging Center of the Montreal Neurological Institute, McGill University [10] consist of several simulated T1-weighted brain volume data with different intensity inhomogeneity (0%, 20%, and 40%) and noise (1%, 3%, 5%, 7%, and 9%) of resolution $1 \times 1 \times 1$ mm with $181 \times 217 \times 181$ dimension.

For all the MRI images, scull striping is done using the brain extraction tool[2].

6.4.2 Results on simulated MRI dataset

To check the effectiveness of different methods against noise, we evaluate them on Brainweb Images with (5%, 7%, and 9%) noise levels. The experimental results on the BrainWeb dataset would be evident to validate the efficiency of the works proposed till now in segmentation of brain MR images into GM, WM, and CSF. The enlisted methods did score well in the metrics of average segmentation accuracy and dice score.

It could be observed that with the increase in the noise in MR images, the performance of almost every method decreased. It was observed that

[1] BrainWeb [online], available: http://www.brainweb.bic.mni.mcgill.ca/brainweb.
[2] Brain Extraction Tool (BET) [online], available: http://www.fmrib.ox.ac.uk/fsl/.

FCM_S1 and FCM_S2 showed an improved performance in comparison to FCM_S, which validated the effectiveness of mean and median filters used. Further KFCM_S also gave superior performance to FCM_S which showed the superiority of kernel metric distance. EnFCM performed better in comparison to FCM_S indicating that the prior aggregation of the neighbors pixel intensity is more helpful than the distance-based aggregation of the neighbors. FGFCM and NDFCM being adaptive to the in-homogeneous noise distribution did not work well on the brainweb dataset, possibly due to a uniform noise throughout the images and hence reported the worst results. FLICM showed comparable performance to EnFCM, FCM_S, and other related variants and KWFLICM couldn't validate itself as the improved version of FLICM as it didn't show much improvement in performance and was somewhat similar to FLICM. For the less noisy MR Images, FCMSWI showed some decent performance, but it showed a drastic drop in performance on increasing the noise showing its inefficiency for higher noises. In our analysis, we found that KGFCM showed above average performance over the other fuzzy-based segmentation methods; however, when compared to KFCM_S, its performance was slightly lower. IFS-based IIFCM and IFCMSNI performed relatively better than fuzzy sets-based methods, validating the advanced intuitionistic fuzzy sets. Further, IFCMSNI showed best results in experimentation among all the 16 methods. On the other hand, picture fuzzy sets-based method, i.e. IPFCM, AIPFCM, and APFCMS did not show much improvements and were similar to Fuzzy sets-based methods. IPFCM showed the best performance among the PFS-based methods.

In the metric of Dice score, somewhat similar trend to that of ASA was observed. IFCMSNI performed distinguishably better in most of the cases of white and gray matter, i.e. best in seven out nine cases in white matter and six out of nine cases in gray matter. Although FCMSWI and IIFCM did perform best in case of CSF, yet IFCMSNI performed reasonably good with similar results in comparison to the best scores. KFCM_S also performed better in one case of white matter, three cases of gray matter and two cases of CSF though it performed well in most of the other cases as well. It is an improvement of FCM_S which is evident from the obtained results since KFCM_S performed better than FCM_S in all the cases (Tables 6.1–6.5).

Experimental results over synthetic simulated brain MRI data can be seen as in 6.4. On comparing with ground truth, it can be seen that

Table 6.1 List of methods

Method	*Year*	*Main points*	*Input hyperparameters*
FCM_S	2002	Added neigbor's information term containing neighbors distance from the centroids	m, α
FCM_S1	2004	Replaced the average neighbors distance from centroid by the distance of mean over the neighor pixel from centroid	m, α
FCM_S2	2004	Replaced mean in FCM_S1 by median over the neighbor pixels.	m, α
KFCM_S	2004	Improvement over FCM_S by using Kernel Metric instead of Euclidean Distance	m, α, σ
EnFCM	2003	Clustering done over image histogram and neighbor pixels information was added to center pixel in prior	m, α
FGFCM	2006	Improvement over EnFCM. Instead of giving equal weight to all pixel in neighbor, pixels were weighted adaptively on the basis of spatial and grayscale distance	m, λ_s, λ_g
NDFCM	2015	Improved over EnFCM by removing parameter alpha and making it parameter free	m, $\lambda_a, \lambda_s, \lambda_g$
FLICM	2010	Added a parameter free novel neighbor information term weighted by spatial distance	m
KWFLICM	2013	Improved FLICM by using Kernel Distance and Fuzzy weighted tradeoff	m
KGFCM	2012	Added a membership constraint for faster convergence and used kernel metric	m, α, β
FCMSWI	2014	Proposed a noise adaptive parameter free neighborhood information	m
FRFCM	2018	Used morphological reconstruction as pre-processing step and membership filtering as post-processing step	m

(Continued)

Table 6.1 (Continued) List of methods

Method	*Year*	*Main points*	*Input hyperparameters*
DSFCMN	2019	Considered the residual to be sparse and used l_1 norm as constraint over residual	m, λ
WRFCM	2020	Improved DSFCMN by introducing a weight term for residuals and used l_2 norm fidelity	m, β, ζ
IIFCM	2015	Used IFS Clustering with neighborhood information dependent on the spatial and grayscale distance of neighbor pixels	m, λ
IFCMSNI	2019	Proposed a novel Spatial Neighborhood Information term in IFS clustering	m, α, β
IPFCM	2017	Extended FCM_S to the Picture Fuzzy Sets Framework with a symmetric picture fuzzy regulaizing term	m, α, β
AIPFCM	2019	Improved IPFCM by adding adaptive weights to Neigborhood information optimized with algorithm	m, λ, β
APFCMS	2019	Further improved AIPFCM by making the membership value neighbrhood weighted in cost function	m, λ, β, p, q

most of the methods couldn't identify different parts to full extent. As it can be seen in column 1 or CSF, most methods couldn't segment it properly except EnFCM, FGFCM, IPFCM, APFCMS, and KWFLICM. In the case of second column or gray matter, most of the methods couldn't preserve the shape of the part except FCM_S, KWFLICM, KFCPFSKLD, and IFCMSNI. Noise was well handled by most of the methods except IPFCM, IFCMSNI, and EnFCM. In column 3 or white matter, shape was preserved by most of the methods except FLICM, FCM_S, IPFCM, and FGFCM, whereas noise wasn't handled properly by FCM_S, IPFCM, and IFCMSNI (Figures 6.1–6.4).

Following are some key observations based on the experimental results:

1. Methods such as FCM_S, ENFCM, FGFCM, NDFCM, and IPFCM considering the local spatial information into account for denoising were not able to preserve finer details resulting in edge blurring.

Table 6.2 Average segmentation accuracy for BrainWeb dataset

Methods images	*Noise level 5*			*Noise level 7*			*Noise level 9*		
	INU 0	INU 20	INU 40	INU 0	INU 20	INU 40	INU 0	INU 20	INU 40
FCM_S	0.9478	0.9312	0.9093	0.9387	0.9347	0.9030	0.9321	0.9196	0.8957
FCM_S1	0.9509	0.9482	0.9280	0.9390	0.9327	0.9123	0.9287	0.9219	0.9028
FCM_S2	0.9564	0.9514	0.9326	0.9442	0.9389	0.9193	0.9345	0.9262	0.9077
KFCM_S	0.9594	0.9533	0.9369	0.9476	0.9437	0.9229	0.9358	0.9282	0.9119
EnFCM	0.9504	0.9459	0.9267	0.9393	0.9332	0.9134	0.9267	0.9207	0.9017
FGFCM	0.9232	0.9160	0.8952	0.9177	0.9113	0.8933	0.9073	0.9068	0.8879
NDFCM	0.9228	0.9158	0.8944	0.9165	0.9099	0.8887	0.9070	0.9053	0.8824
FLICM	0.9359	0.9284	0.9089	0.9387	0.9321	0.9036	0.9321	0.9197	0.8942
KWFLICM	0.9366	0.9289	0.9067	0.9283	0.9217	0.8979	0.9220	0.9123	0.8973
FCMSWI	0.9521	0.9507	0.9330	0.9281	0.9215	0.9057	0.8862	0.8880	0.8728
KGFCM	0.9559	0.9516	0.9306	0.9417	0.9355	0.9144	0.9302	0.9242	0.9041
FRFCM	0.9201	0.9112	0.8953	0.9134	0.9024	0.8841	0.9027	0.8960	0.8730
DSFCMN	0.9329	0.9272	0.9072	0.9318	0.9240	0.9079	0.9202	0.9148	0.8926
WRFCM	0.9387	0.9313	0.9127	0.9335	0.9264	0.9032	0.9232	0.9175	0.8959
IIFCM	0.9541	0.9513	0.9392	0.9397	0.9397	0.9243	0.9239	0.9241	0.9105
IFCMSNI	**0.9587**	**0.9553**	**0.9408**	**0.9484**	0.9388	**0.9341**	**0.9443**	**0.9401**	**0.9185**
IPFCM	0.9508	0.9481	0.9278	0.9395	0.9327	0.9127	0.9288	0.9226	0.9034
APFCMS	0.9301	0.9243	0.9065	0.9255	0.9198	0.9007	0.9181	0.9165	0.8961
AIPFCM	0.9321	0.9252	0.9053	0.9268	0.9196	0.8987	0.9192	0.9163	0.8927

Table 6.3 Dice score for WM BrainWeb dataset

Methods images	*Noise level 5*			*Noise level 7*			Noise level 9		
	INU 0	INU 20	INU 40	INU 0	INU 20	INU 40	INU 0	INU 20	INU 40
FCM_S	0.9636	0.9511	0.9251	0.9563	0.9512	0.9175	0.9511	0.9383	0.9123
FCM_SI	0.9651	0.9623	0.9436	0.9568	0.9517	0.9527	0.9464	0.9339	0.9267
FCM_S2	0.9709	0.9652	0.9480	0.9634	0.9570	**0.9602**	0.9503	0.9414	0.9332
KFCM_S	**0.9742**	0.9671	0.9558	0.9661	0.9618	0.9432	0.9584	0.9502	0.9350
EnFCM	0.9649	0.9607	0.9429	0.9573	0.9521	0.9338	0.9482	0.9427	0.9242
FGFCM	0.9528	0.9475	0.9291	0.9471	0.9418	0.9258	0.9398	0.9397	0.9215
NDFCM	0.9529	0.9476	0.9291	0.9475	0.9419	0.9234	0.9413	0.9395	0.9189
FLICM	0.9576	0.9509	0.9325	0.9568	0.9502	0.9199	0.9511	0.9395	0.9104
KWFLICM	0.9664	0.9591	0.9361	0.9595	0.9531	0.9288	0.9534	0.9474	0.9297
FCMSWI	0.9658	0.9636	0.9477	0.9486	0.9422	0.9274	0.9136	0.9142	0.9003
KGFCM	0.9693	0.9651	0.9463	0.9591	0.9546	0.9432	0.9525	0.9474	0.9269
FRFCM	0.9569	0.9489	0.9333	0.9518	0.9424	0.9242	0.9435	0.9366	0.9160
DSFCMN	0.9572	0.9532	0.9339	0.9557	0.9496	0.9318	0.9489	0.9463	0.9218
WRFCM	0.9613	0.9552	0.9395	0.9575	0.9522	0.9311	0.9511	0.9472	0.9273
IIFCM	0.9701	0.9674	**0.9569**	0.9603	0.9574	0.9434	0.9477	0.9464	0.9338
IFCMSNI	0.9729	**0.9686**	0.9562	**0.9661**	**0.9687**	0.9487	**0.9615**	**0.9548**	**0.9408**
IPFCM	0.9651	0.9621	0.9435	0.9574	0.9529	0.9339	0.9516	0.9465	0.9266
APFCMS	0.9552	0.9509	0.9361	0.9377	0.9328	0.9216	0.8996	0.9016	0.8919
AIPFCM	0.9573	0.9519	0.9344	0.9528	0.9477	0.9284	0.9476	0.9461	0.9244

Table 6.4 Dice score for GM BrainWeb dataset

Methods images	Noise level 5			Noise level 7			Noise level 9		
	INU 0	INU 20	INU 40	INU 0	INU 20	INU 40	INU 0	INU 20	INU 40
FCM_S	0.9039	0.8855	0.8902	0.8952	0.9011	0.8981	0.8903	0.8873	0.8858
FCM_S1	0.9322	0.9291	0.9033	0.9168	0.9043	**0.9102**	0.8960	0.8838	0.8718
FCM_S2	0.9387	0.9448	0.9351	0.9094	0.8929	0.8954	0.8858	0.8899	0.8778
KFCM_S	**0.9459**	0.9367	0.9150	**0.9303**	0.9247	0.8987	0.8843	**0.9050**	0.8843
EnFCM	0.9317	0.9262	0.9018	0.9076	0.9022	0.8927	0.8946	0.8916	0.8861
FGFCM	0.8537	0.8485	0.8389	0.8546	0.8506	0.8419	0.8426	0.8424	0.8393
NDFCM	0.8526	0.8473	0.8368	0.8502	0.8447	0.8304	0.8364	0.8362	0.8254
FLICM	0.8772	0.8742	0.8668	0.8917	0.8903	0.8856	0.8902	0.8817	0.8861
KWFLICM	0.8853	0.8832	0.8769	0.8791	0.8774	0.8715	0.8725	0.8645	0.8704
FCMSWI	0.9330	0.9316	0.9092	0.9019	0.8934	0.8741	0.8476	0.8514	0.8314
KGFCM	0.9382	0.9335	0.9069	0.9212	0.9134	0.8861	0.9067	0.8989	0.8731
FRFCM	0.8931	0.8826	0.8636	0.8857	0.8718	0.8496	0.8702	0.8643	0.8367
DSFCMN	0.9116	0.9052	0.8796	0.9128	0.8999	0.8795	0.8961	0.8908	0.8570
WRFCM	0.9191	0.9096	0.8872	0.9127	0.9043	0.8744	0.8989	0.8934	0.8650
IIFCM	0.9359	0.9331	0.9170	0.9168	0.9171	0.8982	0.8939	0.8955	0.8777
IFCMSNI	0.9378	**0.9529**	**0.9433**	0.9141	**0.9424**	0.9051	**0.9205**	0.9001	**0.8955**
IPFCM	0.9321	0.9291	0.9031	0.9091	0.8964	0.8915	0.8853	0.8815	0.8771
APFCMS	0.8704	0.8655	0.8551	0.8838	0.8765	0.8626	0.8183	0.8276	0.8125
AIPFCM	0.8697	0.8645	0.8549	0.8677	0.8596	0.8523	0.8588	0.8549	0.8452

Table 6.5 Dice score for CSF BrainWeb dataset

Methods images	Noise level 5			Noise level 7			Noise level 9		
	INU 0	INU 20	INU 40	INU 0	INU 20	INU 40	INU 0	INU 20	INU 40
FCM_S	0.9301	0.9108	0.8839	0.8952	0.9011	0.8981	0.8903	0.8873	0.8858
FCM_S1	0.9498	0.9515	0.9417	0.9107	0.8849	0.8976	0.8803	0.8898	0.8766
FCM_S2	0.9412	0.9341	0.9103	0.9266	0.9138	0.9209	0.9044	0.8959	0.8809
KFCM_S	0.9482	0.9516	0.9334	**0.9359**	0.9371	0.9248	0.9222	**0.9229**	0.9166
EnFCM	0.9424	0.9403	0.9312	0.9173	0.9102	0.8851	0.9007	0.8934	0.8694
FGFCM	0.8992	0.8903	0.8649	0.8901	0.8823	0.8597	0.8756	0.8766	0.8511
NDFCM	0.8991	0.8906	0.8646	0.8895	0.8817	0.8551	0.8776	0.8773	0.8478
FLICM	0.9152	0.9061	0.8822	0.9185	0.9105	0.8771	0.9096	0.8959	0.8654
KWFLICM	0.9277	0.9181	0.8912	0.9188	0.9103	0.8819	0.9114	0.9003	0.8797
FCMSWI	**0.9538**	**0.9558**	**0.9461**	0.9295	0.9283	0.9199	0.9027	0.9043	0.8972
KGFCM	0.9531	0.9534	0.9417	0.9264	0.9321	0.9253	0.8903	0.8861	0.8864
FRFCM	0.8373	0.8325	0.8286	0.8312	0.8254	0.8204	0.8267	0.8242	0.8110
DSFCMN	0.8773	0.8728	0.8676	0.8785	0.8726	0.8620	0.8648	0.8560	0.3712
WRFCM	0.8822	0.8782	0.8660	0.8795	0.8719	0.8609	0.8669	0.8612	0.8515
IIFCM	0.9443	0.9438	0.9368	0.9279	**0.9378**	**0.9288**	0.9179	0.9212	**0.9167**
IFCMSNI	0.9433	0.9380	0.9188	0.9311	0.9035	0.9116	**0.9252**	0.9208	0.8913
IPFCM	0.9488	0.9518	0.9413	0.9177	0.9102	0.8844	0.9041	0.8965	0.8719
APFCMS	0.9069	0.9004	0.8781	0.9186	0.9191	0.9098	0.8588	0.8874	0.8829
AIPFCM	0.9104	0.9025	0.8781	0.9032	0.8955	0.8684	0.8929	0.8915	0.8609

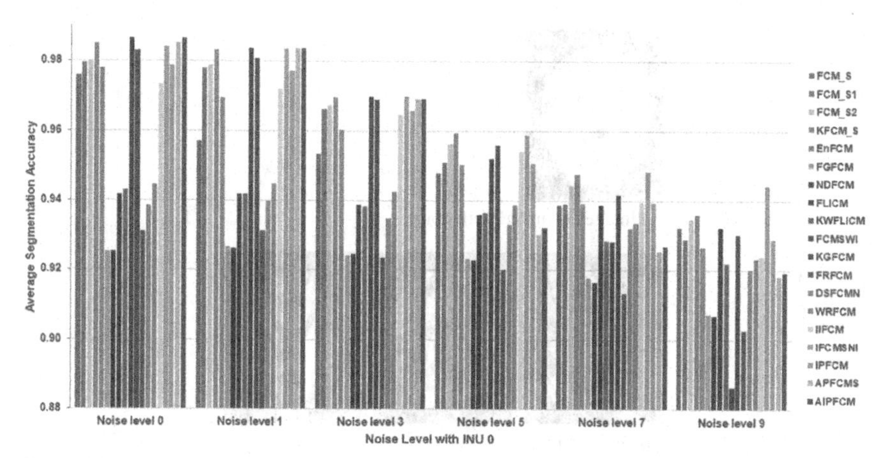

Figure 6.1 Variation in performance in terms of ASA on images with 0% INU.

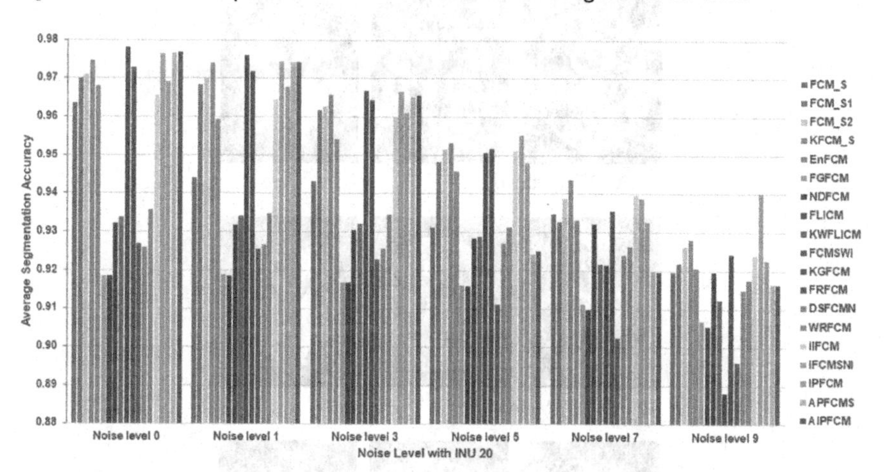

Figure 6.2 Variation in performance in terms of ASA on images with 20% INU.

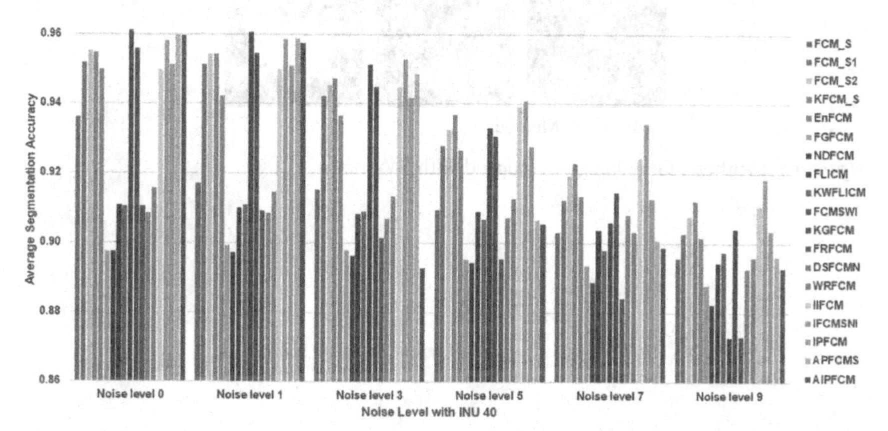

Figure 6.3 Variation in performance in terms of ASA on images with 40% INU.

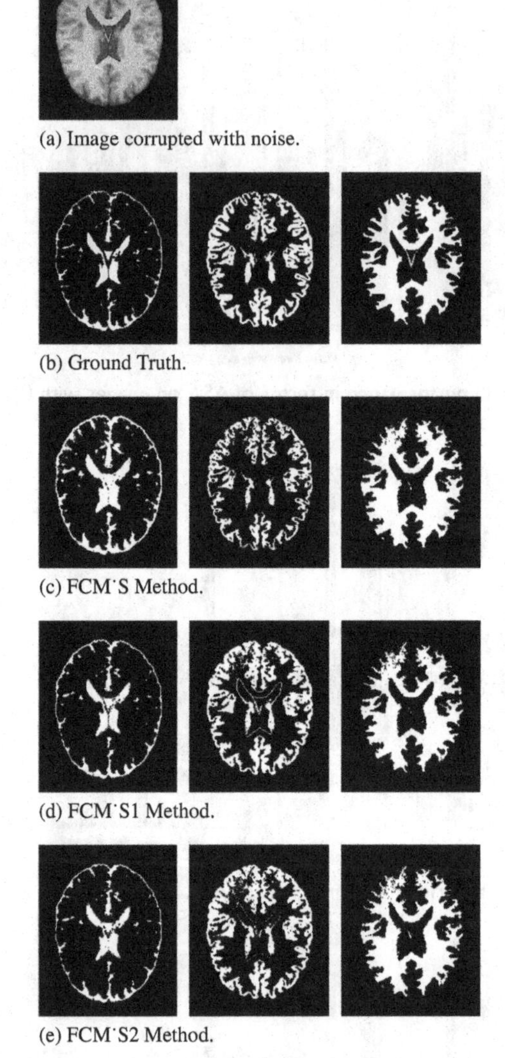

(a) Image corrupted with noise.

(b) Ground Truth.

(c) FCM'S Method.

(d) FCM'S1 Method.

(e) FCM'S2 Method.

Figure 6.4 Synthetic Gray image corrupted with BW noise.

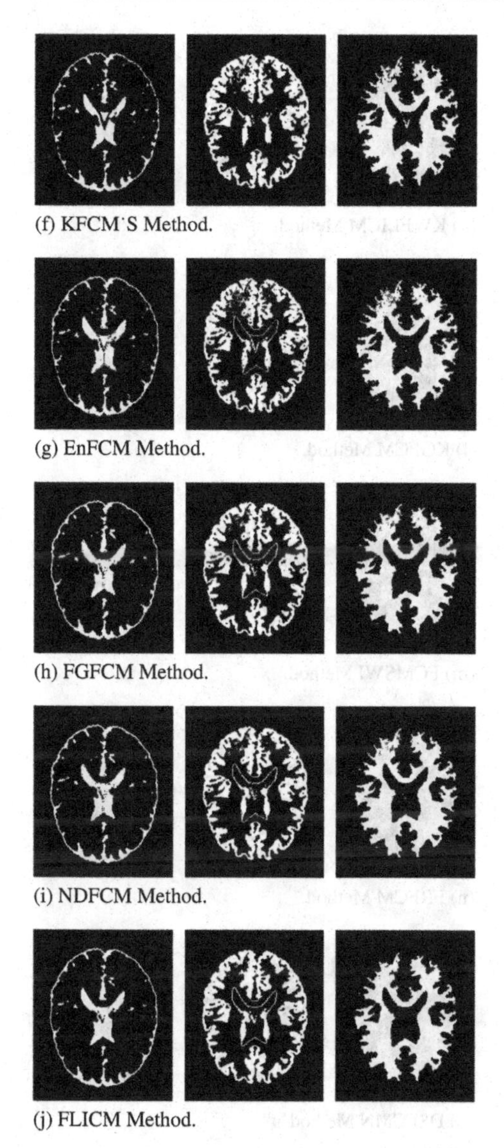

(f) KFCM'S Method.

(g) EnFCM Method.

(h) FGFCM Method.

(i) NDFCM Method.

(j) FLICM Method.

Figure 6.4 (Continued) Synthetic Gray image corrupted with BW noise.

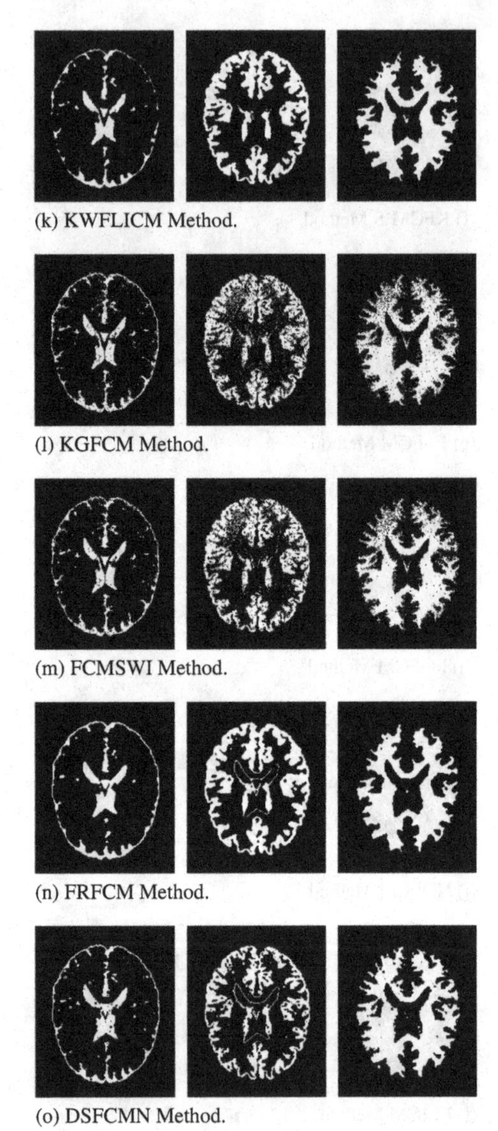

(k) KWFLICM Method.
(l) KGFCM Method.
(m) FCMSWI Method.
(n) FRFCM Method.
(o) DSFCMN Method.

Figure 6.4 (Continued) Synthetic Gray image corrupted with BW noise.

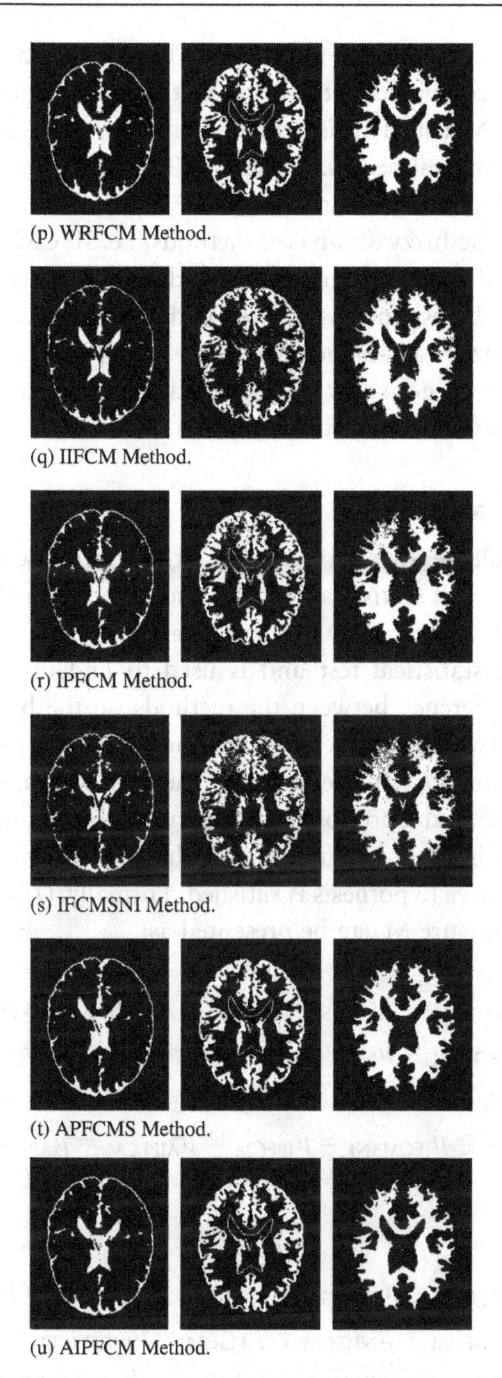

Figure 6.4 (Continued) Synthetic Gray image corrupted with BW noise.

2. The methods KFCM_S and KGFCM showed relatively good performance compared to the other methods indicating the efficiency of Kernel Metric. This is evident from their ASA and DS scores in the experimental results. Futher, KWFLICM kernel distance-based method did not show similar trend.
3. Intuitionistic fuzzy sets-based methods, i.e. IIFCM and IFCMSNI, were found to be best performing method indicating their capability to deal with hesitancy associated with noisy data.
4. Picture fuzzy sets-based methods, i.e. IPFCM, AIPFCM, and APFCMS, did not show the expected performance; they showed a similar performance to the fuzzy sets method.

6.4.3 Statistical test

To further evaluate the performance of the proposed KFCPFSKLD method, we conduct statistical tests for the different methods on Brainweb and IBSR dataset. We use Friedman test, which is a two-way parameter free statistical test and is used to find out if there is any considerable difference between the methods on the basis of observed results. It has two hypotheses, i.e. the null-hypothesis (H_0) and alternative hypothesis (H_1), respectively. If there is no major difference in the performance of the proposed method and other comparing methods then null-hypothesis is satisfied and if the performance gap is larger than the alternative hypothesis is satisfied. Formally, (H_0) and (H_1) for a performance measure M can be presented as:

$$\begin{aligned} H_0: \quad & \mu_{\mathrm{FCM\_S}} = \mu_{\mathrm{FCM\_S1}} = \mu_{\mathrm{FCM\_S2}} = \mu_{\mathrm{KFCM\_S}} = \mu_{\mathrm{EnFCM}} \\ & = \mu_{\mathrm{FGFCM}} = \mu_{\mathrm{NDFCM}} = \mu_{\mathrm{FLICM}} = \mu_{\mathrm{KWFLICM}} = \mu_{\mathrm{FCMSWI}} \\ & = \mu_{\mathrm{KGFCM}} = \mu_{\mathrm{FRFCM}} = \mu_{\mathrm{DSFCMN}} = \mu_{\mathrm{WRFCM}} = \mu_{\mathrm{IIFCM}} \\ & = \mu_{\mathrm{IFCMSNI}} = \mu_{\mathrm{IPFCM}} = \mu_{\mathrm{AIPFCM}} = \mu_{\mathrm{APFCMS}} \end{aligned} \tag{6.3}$$

$$\begin{aligned} H_1: \quad & \mu_{\mathrm{FCM\_S}} \neq \mu_{\mathrm{FCM\_S1}} \neq \mu_{\mathrm{FCM\_S2}} \neq \mu_{\mathrm{KFCM\_S}} \neq \mu_{\mathrm{EnFCM}} \\ & \neq \mu_{\mathrm{FGFCM}} \neq \mu_{\mathrm{NDFCM}} \neq \mu_{\mathrm{FLICM}} \neq \mu_{\mathrm{KWFLICM}} \neq \mu_{\mathrm{FCMSWI}} \\ & \neq \mu_{\mathrm{KGFCM}} \neq \mu_{\mathrm{FRFCM}} \neq \mu_{\mathrm{DSFCMN}} \neq \mu_{\mathrm{WRFCM}} \neq \mu_{\mathrm{IIFCM}} \\ & \neq \mu_{\mathrm{IFCMSNI}} \neq \mu_{\mathrm{IPFCM}} \neq \mu_{\mathrm{AIPFCM}} \neq \mu_{\mathrm{APFCMS}} \end{aligned} \tag{6.4}$$

We particularly use the average segmentation accuracy obtained from the different methods to rank them. In Friedman test, the average rank R_j of jth methods for a given N number of images is obtained with respect to a given performance measure as:

$$R_j = \frac{1}{N}\sum_{i=1}^{N} r_i^j \tag{6.5}$$

where $r_i^j \in \{1, 2, \ldots, k\}(1 \le i \le N, 1 \le j \le k)$ is rank value for i^{th} image and j^{th} method. Table 6.6 shows the average Friedman ranking of different segmentation methods corresponding to ASA for 9 BrainWeb brain images used for experiment [12, 15]. Lowest numerical value of rank for a segmentation method shows its better performance compared to other methods for a given performance measure. On the basis of Friedman ranking, the IFCMSNI method perform best in terms of ASA. The statistical hypothesis test proposed by Iman and Davenportis is used. The statistic F_{ID} is defined by Iman and Davenport[17] as:

$$F_{\text{ID}} = \frac{(N-1)\chi_F^2}{N(k-1) - \chi_F^2} \tag{6.6}$$

which is distributed according to F-distribution with $k-1$ and $(k-1)(N-1)$ degrees of freedom, where χ_F^2 is the Friedman's statistic defined as $\frac{12N}{k(k+1)}\left[\sum_j R_j^2 - \frac{k(k+1)^2}{4}\right]$. In our experiments $k = 19$ and $N = 9$. The p-values obtained by Iman and Davenport statistic are 2.12E-56. corresponding to the performance measures ASA, which advocate the

Table 6.6 Average Friedman ranking of algorithms.

Algorithms	*Ranking*	*Algorithms*	*Ranking*
IFCMSNI	1.44	WRFCM	10.89
KFCM_S	2.00	FCMSWI	12.33
FCM_S2	3.56	KWFLICM	12.89
IIFCM	4.33	DSFCMN	12.89
KGFCM	4.67	APFCMS	14.33
IPFCM	7.17	AIPFCM	14.78
FCM_S1	7.50	FGFCM	16.78
EnFCM	8.00	NDFCM	17.78
FCM_S	9.67	FRFCM	18.44
FLICM	10.56		

rejection of null hypothesis H_0 as there is significant difference among different segmentation methods at the significance level of 0.05.

However, these p-values so obtained are not suitable for comparison with the control method, i.e., the one that emerges with the lowest rank. So adjusted p-values [12] are computed which take into account the error accumulated and provide the correct correlation. This is done with respect to a control method which is the IFCMSNI (lowest rank for ASA). For this, a set of post-hoc procedures are defined and adjusted p-values are computed. The most widely used post-hoc method [12] to obtain adjusted p-values is Holm procedure. Table 6.7 shows the various value of adjusted p-values obtained. It could be inferred that higher the adjusted p-values for a method is more comparable it is to the contol methods. We could observe that KFCM_S has highest value in Table 6.7, hence it is the most effective algorithm after control method i.e. IFCMSNI. Similarly, other methods can also be ranked on the basis of adjusted p-value.

6.5 CONCLUSION

Medical image segmentation turns out to be a complex task because of the presence of several corruptions such as noises, intensity inhomogeneity, and partial volume effect. These corruptions tend to create ambiguities while segmentation which leads to inconsistency therefore in order to handle these ambiguities fuzzy set theory-based clustering is considered an effective method for medical image segmentation. In this chapter, we focused on the handling of noise corruption using spatial neighborhood information techniques. we analyzed 16 methods based on spatial information technique and used them for segmenting a publicly available dataset, i.e. Brain Web. The outcomes were further compared over performance metrics such as dice score and average image segmentation. The overview of observations can be that methods based on fuzzy set theory which used smoothing techniques to handle the problem of noise resulted in the loss of fine structures after segmentation, whereas IFS-based methods were able to preserve the boundary details. Also methods using Kernel distance showed a better performance in presence of noise compared to Euclidean distance-based method verifying the efficiency of Kernel metric to capture the nonlinearity in the data.

Table 6.7 Adjusted p-value (Friedman)

Algorithms	*Unadjusted p value*	p_Holm	*Algorithms*	*Unadjusted p value*	p_Holm
FRFCM	1.47E-10	2.65E-09	FLICM	5.93E-04	0.005
NDFCM	7.41E-10	1.26E-08	FCM_S	0.002	0.016
FGFCM	7.46E-09	1.19E-07	EnFCM	0.013	0.094
AIPFCM	5.00E-07	7.50E-06	FCM_S1	0.022	0.135
APFCMS	1.18E-06	1.65E-05	IPFCM	0.031	0.155
KWFLICM	1.60E-05	2.08E-04	KGFCM	0.224	0.898
DSFCMN	1.60E-05	2.08E-04	IIFCM	0.276	0.898
FCMSWI	4.05E-05	4.45E-04	FCM_S2	0.426	0.898
WRFCM	3.70E-04	0.003705	KFCM_S	0.834	0.898

REFERENCES

[1] Mohamed N Ahmed, Sameh M Yamany, Nevin Mohamed, Aly A Farag, and Thomas Moriarty. A modified fuzzy c-means algorithm for bias field estimation and segmentation of mri data. *IEEE Transactions on Medical Imaging*, 21(3):193–199, 2002.

[2] Alamgeer Ali and Kamal Kumar. Various noises in medical images and de-noising techniques. In *Proceedings of First International Conference on Computing, Communications, and Cyber-Security (IC4S 2019)*, pp. 303–315, 2020.

[3] Krassimir T Atanassov. Intuitionistic fuzzy sets. *Fuzzy Sets and Systems*, 20(1):87–96, 1986.

[4] Pavel Berkhin. A survey of clustering data mining techniques. In: Jacob Kogan and Charles Nicholas (Eds.), *Grouping Multidimensional Data*, pp. 25–71. Springer: Berlin, Germany, 2006.

[5] Weiling Cai, Songcan Chen, and Daoqiang Zhang. Fast and robust fuzzy c-means clustering algorithms incorporating local information for image segmentation. *Pattern Recognition*, 40(3):825–838, 2007.

[6] Mehmet Celenk. A color clustering technique for image segmentation. *Computer Vision, Graphics, and Image Processing*, 52(2):145–170, 1990.

[7] Songcan Chen and Daoqiang Zhang. Robust image segmentation using fcm with spatial constraints based on new kernel-induced distance measure. *IEEE Transactions on Systems, Man, and Cybernetics, Part B (Cybernetics)*, 34(4):1907–1916, 2004.

[8] P Chinmayi, Agilandeeswari Loganathan, and Manoharan Prabukumar. Survey of image processing techniques in medical image analysis: Challenges and methodologies. In: *Proceedings of the Eighth International Conference on Soft Computing and Pattern Recognition (SoCPaR 2016)*, pp. 460–471. Springer: Berlin, Germany, 2018.

[9] Keh-Shih Chuang, Hong-Long Tzeng, Sharon Chen, Jay Wu, and Tzong-Jer Chen. Fuzzy c-means clustering with spatial information for image segmentation. *Computerized Medical Imaging and Graphics*, 30(1):9–15, 2006.

[10] Chris A Cocosco, Vasken Kollokian, Remi K-S Kwan, G Bruce Pike, and Alan C Evans. Brainweb: Online interface to a 3d mri simulated brain database. In *NeuroImage*, Citeseer, 1997.

[11] Bui Cong Cuong and Vladik Kreinovich. Picture fuzzy sets-a new concept for computational intelligence problems. In *2013 Third World Congress on Information and Communication Technologies (WICT 2013)*, pp. 1–6. IEEE, 2013.

[12] Joaquín Derrac, Salvador García, Daniel Molina, and Francisco Herrera. A practical tutorial on the use of nonparametric statistical tests as a methodology for comparing evolutionary and swarm intelligence algorithms. *Swarm and Evolutionary Computation*, 1(1):3–18, 2011.

[13] Joseph C Dunn. A fuzzy relative of the isodata process and its use in detecting compact well-separated clusters. *Journal of Cybernetics*, 3:32–57, 1973

[14] Aarthipoornima Elangovan and T Jeyaseelan. Medical imaging modalities: A survey. In *2016 International Conference on Emerging Trends in Engineering, Technology and Science (ICETETS)*, pp. 1–4, 2016.

[15] Milton Friedman. The use of ranks to avoid the assumption of normality implicit in the analysis of variance. *Journal of the American Statistical Association*, 32(200):675–701, 1937.

[16] Maoguo Gong, Yan Liang, Jiao Shi, Wenping Ma, and Jingjing Ma. Fuzzy c-means clustering with local information and kernel metric for image segmentation. *IEEE Transactions on Image Processing*, 22(2):573–584, 2012.

[17] Ronald L Iman and James M Davenport. Approximations of the critical region of the fbietkan statistic. *Communications in Statistics-Theory and Methods*, 9(6):571–595, 1980.

[18] K Kameshwaran and K Malarvizhi. Survey on clustering techniques in data mining. *International Journal of Computer Science and Information Technologies*, 5(2):2272–2276, 2014.

[19] Myeongsu Kang and Jong-Myon Kim. Fuzzy c-means clustering with spatially weighted information for medical image segmentation. In *2014 IEEE Symposium on Computational Intelligence for Multimedia, Signal and Vision Processing (CIMSIVP)*, pp. 1–8, 2014.

[20] KVD Kiran and Katikireddy Srinivas. An efficient cluster system for bioinformatics data using amalgam of clustering methods. *European Journal of Molecular & Clinical Medicine*, 7(10):1958–1971, 2021.

[21] Vinay Kumar Kotte, Srinivasan Rajavelu, and Elijah Blessing Rajsingh. A similarity function for feature pattern clustering and high dimensional text document classification. *Foundations of Science*, 25(4):1077–1094, 2020.

[22] Stelios Krinidis and Vassilios Chatzis. A robust fuzzy local information c-means clustering algorithm. *IEEE Transactions on Image Processing*, 19(5):1328–1337, 2010.

[23] Dhirendra Kumar, Ramesh Kumar Agrawal, and Jyoti Singh Kirar. Intuitionistic fuzzy clustering method with spatial information for mri image segmentation. In *2019 IEEE International Conference on Fuzzy Systems (FUZZ-IEEE)*, pp. 1–7. IEEE, 2019.

[24] Lay Lee and Siau-Chuin Liew. A survey of medical image processing tools. In *2015 4th International Conference on Software Engineering and Computer Systems (ICSECS)*, 2015.

[25] Tao Lei, Xiaohong Jia, Yanning Zhang, Lifeng He, Hongying Meng, and Asoke K Nandi. Significantly fast and robust fuzzy c-means clustering algorithm based on morphological reconstruction and membership filtering. *IEEE Transactions on Fuzzy Systems*, 26(5):3027–3041, 2018.

[26] Geert Litjens, Thijs Kooi, Babak Ehteshami Bejnordi, Arnaud Arindra Adiyoso Setio, Francesco Ciompi, Mohsen Ghafoorian, Jeroen AWM van der Laak, Bram van Ginneken, and Clara I Sánchez. A survey on deep learning in medical image analysis. *Medical Image Analysis*, 42:60–88, 2017.

[27] SC Madeira and AL Oliveira. Biclustering algorithms for biological data analysis: a survey. *IEEE/ACM Transactions on Computational Biology and Bioinformatics*, 1(1):24–45, 2004.

[28] Alistair Moffat and Lang Stuiver. Exploiting clustering in inverted file compression. In *Proceedings of Data Compression Conference-DCC'96*, pp. 82–91. IEEE, 1996.

[29] H Oulhaj, Aouatif Amine, Mohammed Rziza, and Driss Aboutajdine. Noise reduction in medical images - comparison of noise removal algorithms. In *2012 International Conference on Multimedia Computing and Systems (ICMCS)*, pp. 344–349, 2012.

[30] Dzung Pham, Chenyang Xu, and Jerry Prince. A survey of current methods in medical image segmentation. *Annual Review of Biomedical Engineering*, 2:315–37, 02 2000.

[31] Cunyong Qiu, Jian Xiao, Long Yu, Lu Han, and Muhammad Naveed Iqbal. A modified interval type-2 fuzzy c-means algorithm with application in mr image segmentation. *Pattern Recognition Letters*, 34(12):1329–1338, 2013.

[32] Pradeep Rai and Singh Shubha. A survey of clustering techniques. *International Journal of Computer Applications*, 7(12):1–5, 2010.

[33] László Szilagyi, Zoltán Benyo, Sándor M Szilágyi, and HS Adam. Mr brain image segmentation using an enhanced fuzzy c-means algorithm. In *Proceedings of the 25th Annual International Conference of the IEEE Engineering in Medicine and Biology Society (IEEE Cat. No. 03CH37439)*, vo. 1, pp. 724–726. IEEE, 2003.

[34] Velmurugan Thambusamy. Applications of partition based clustering algorithms: A survey. In *IEEE Proceedings of International Conference on Computational Intelligence and Computing Research (ICCIC)*, pp. 703–707, 2013.

[35] Hanuman Verma, RK Agrawal, and Aditi Sharan. An improved intuitionistic fuzzy c-means clustering algorithm incorporating local information for brain image segmentation. *Applied Soft Computing*, 46:543–557, 2016.

[36] Uro Vovk, Franjo Pernus, and Botjan Likar. A review of methods for correction of intensity inhomogeneity in mri. *IEEE Transactions on Medical Imaging*, 26(3):405–421, 2007.

[37] Cong Wang, Witold Pedrycz, ZhiWu Li, and MengChu Zhou. Residual-driven fuzzy c-means clustering for image segmentation. *IEEE/CAA Journal of Automatica Sinica*, 8(4):876–889, 2020.

[38] Xiu-Xiu Wang and Fangfang Guo. Adaptive fuzzy c-means algorithm based on local noise detecting for image segmentation. *IET Image Processing*, 10:272–279 2016.

[39] Chengmao Wu and Yan Chen. Adaptive entropy weighted picture fuzzy clustering algorithm with spatial information for image segmentation. *Applied Soft Computing*, 86:105888, 2020.

[40] Chengmao Wu and Q Wu. A robust image segmentation algorithm based on modified picture fuzzy clustering method on picture fuzzy sets. *Journal of Xi'an University of Posts and Telecommunications*, 22(5):37–43, 2017.

[41] Lotfi A Zadeh. Fuzzy sets. *Information and Control*, 8(3):338–353, 1965.

[42] Yuxuan Zhang, Xiangzhi Bai, Ruirui Fan, and Zihan Wang. Deviation-sparse fuzzy c-means with neighbor information constraint. *IEEE Transactions on Fuzzy Systems*, 27(1):185–199, 2018.

[43] Feng Zhao, Licheng Jiao, and Hanqiang Liu. Kernel generalized fuzzy c-means clustering with spatial information for image segmentation. *Digital Signal Processing*, 23:184–199, 01 2013.

[44] Lin Zhu and Fu-Lai Chung. Generalized fuzzy c-means clustering algorithm with improved fuzzy partitions. *IEEE Transactions on Systems, Man, and Cybernetics, Part B: Cybernetics*, 39:578–591, 2009.

Chapter 7

Exploring the role of AI, IoT and BC during COVID-19

A bibliometric and network analysis

Parul Khurana
Lovely Professional University

Kiran Sharma
BML Munjal University

CONTENTS

7.1 INTRODUCTION

In 2019, the unprecedented outbreak of novel coronavirus (COVID-19) caused by an extremely contagious SARS-CoV-2 (severe acute respiratory syndrome coronavirus-2) has hounded the world [10]. With the proliferating spread of COVID-19 in quick succession and posing a severe infection, the world witnessed the adverse effects and found itself in an obnoxiously unexpected crisis. World Health Organization (WHO) at the start of 2020, declared this outbreak as a pandemic situation which raised a precarious situation and manifested tremendous pressure

DOI: 10.1201/9781003368342-7

globally [8, 46]. Most affected industries may include automotive, aviation, tourism, oil, construction, food, healthcare and telecommunications [12, 17]. This rapid outbreak adversely overburdened scientists, governments, medical personnel, health care institutions, researchers and laboratories to provide treatment strategies, develop vaccines and position a front line effort approach to confront and fight this pandemic globally [3, 33].

As a result, COVID-19 pandemic paradigm is expected to bring promising medical advancements, scientific discoveries and acceleration in knowledge acquisitions with the convergence of digital technologies [21]. Multitude of these digital approaches do play a vital role in order to unravel pandemic situations, address major diseases, generate new opportunities, project potential risks, collect real-time situation-centric data and produce cost-effective deliveries in a shared and distributed ledger-based networks [2, 39]. The WHO has also mitigated the confidence in the efficacy of digital technologies for tackling COVID-19 [20].

The decisive technological areas may include:

- *Artificial Intelligence (AI) (for screening during COVID-19):* AI is proved as an invigorating branch of rapidly emerging science used for simulations based on human intelligence [49]. Since its inception, this technology has been providing innumerable real-time solutions with the potential of screening, prediction and modeling [30]. The ideology of such developed platforms demonstrating natural intelligence gives AI an effective potential to combat the pandemic situation of COVID-19. Comprehensive analysis of data based on AI-based platforms is capable of forecasting disease outbreaks, infection risks and symptom susceptibility [19]. AI-based face cameras with multisensory technology can revolutionize the initial process of COVID-19 screening and quick examinations [36]. Data generated by such tools can be used for initial diagnostic testing to detect any unusual behaviors. AI-based medical imaging devices are developed to diagnose patient lungs for accelerating the examinations of patients [9, 48]. AI can also speed up the crucial process of drug discovery with the robust analysis and identification of existing research protocols, patient reports and potential treatment plans [4, 43]. With AI-based real-time analysis, clusters of patient health situations (with disease symptoms), virus progressions and detection of infectious patients, AI techniques can be concentrated as a first-aid calls in this pandemic outbreak [15]. AI-based patient flow platforms and robotic doctor–patient interactions are introduced to develop risk-free zones to minimize the spread of COVID-19 [22].

- *Internet of Things (IoT) (for surveillance during COVID-19):* IoT revolution is considered as an amalgamation of digital devices with mechanical devices over the internet offering features such as sensing, monitoring, communication, screening, tracing, alerting and controlling [23, 26]. In recent times, a surge in IoT-based everyday applications providing extensive support, services, ability to collect and transmit data efficiently is witnessed with transformative potential to reduce the burden of ongoing COVID-19 pandemic [5]. Transmitting IoT-based thermometer readings assimilated by medical authorities to identify fever hotspots in the region, IoT-based buttons to issue warnings, alerts, etc., to the management and personnel staff on duty, monitoring, evaluating and diagnosing patients remotely and avoiding physical interactions amid COVID-19 has reduced the risk of emanation to healthcare personnel [34, 45]. Without the involvement of humans, IoT is experimented widely in the form of CCTVs, powerful sensors, GPS-based wearable systems and smart phones uploading the recorded data for analysis and mass screening [7, 41]. IoT-based devices can be deployed easily at bus stations, airports, railway stations, borders, hospitals and at large crowded public areas for bulk screening and processing [35]. IoT is also used by medical experts and their teams for remote monitoring of temperatures, blood pressures, patient's physiology and symptom's progressions to collect vitals for COVID-19 treatments [16, 37]. Thus, IoT has a wide impact and can be seen as a prominent technology to battle against COVID-19 during screening, tracing, lockdown and quarantine [24, 29].
- *Blockchain (BC) (for data handling during COVID-19):* BC technology can be represented as an unique critical technology during COVID-19 outbreak to mitigate its impact and support health care systems for safer environments [27]. To combat COVID-19 challenges, BC serves as a facility for decision-making, providing efficient collaboration, shared repository, secured data acquisition and decentralized platform, to enable highly productive and sustainable environment [6]. The BC-based robust system exponen-

tially provides features such as immutability, easy accessibility and promising technology-driven frameworks with high level of secured trustworthy communications [42]. The combination of AI, IoT and BC can be seen as an envisioned softwarized solution in pandemic situation of COVID-19. AI and IoT-based applications can be combined with BC to battle against vivacious COVID-19 [1]. BC enables digital recording of medical data of patients with the concept of smart contracts and consensus algorithms, thus replicating such data between network users for secure exchange of information to fight current COVID-19 crisis globally [11, 40]. This also reduces the spread of false and fabricated data among individuals and organizations. All patient records on BC can be created with its secure distributed ledger convention system represented as an immutable records to overcome potential pandemics [13]. The ideology of BC is to convey data and act as an information highway to find the significant ways in pandemic situation to facilitate recording of patient details, to increase testing and reporting of patients and to enable secure environments for the payment of donations [25, 31].

The objectives of our study are outlined as:

- To perform bibliometric analysis of the publications to present a detailed overview of AI, IoT and BC literature amid COVID-19.
- To identify the relationship between all three themes (AI, IoT and BC).
- To investigate the pattern of open access publications.
- To investigate the team size, citation and funding pattern in AI, IoT and BC-based publications.
- To identify discipline-wise variations.
- To identify top countries based on their national and international collaborations theme-wise (AI, IoT and BC).
- To perform thematic analysis to demonstrate the usage of author keywords and research areas.
- To identify top journals and publishers based on all three themes (AI, IoT and BC).

Further, the study is organized as follows: Section 7.2 is on research methodology, divided into two subsections such as data description and its filtration. Section 7.3 presents the results divided into five broad perspectives. Initially the relationship between AI, IoT and BC is presented, followed by statistics relevant to number of authors, number of citations and number of funding organizations involved. Then discipline-wise patterns are presented for AI, IoT and BC. Top countries involved in national and international collaborations are also identified. Author keywords and research areas are presented with thematic analysis. At last, key journals and key publishers are presented. Finally, Section 7.4 concludes the study.

7.2 METHODOLOGY

Methodology covers two main stages such as (i) data description and (ii) data filtration to perform a conceptual review and present visual of study performed on the data collected amid COVID-19 wave in July 2021.

7.2.1 Data description

Data is collected from Clarivate (https://webofknowledge.com/). The choice is arbitrary and is based on the authenticity and genuineness of Clarivate as a data provider for analytics and trusted insights worldwide [28, 32]. The data extraction started with the query carrying three keywords such as *Artificial Intelligence*, *Internet of Things* and *Blockchain*. Artificial Intelligence-based query returned 1280 records, IoT-based query returned 251 records and Blockchain-based query returned 109 records, in total 1,640 records have been returned. The extracted data returned 66 fields carrying information of publication, author name, author affiliation, author orcid, author emails, document type, abstract content, author keywords, book details, conference details, funding information, citations, references, DOI numbers, research areas, journal details, publishers and unique WoS (Web of Science) IDs, etc. Table 7.1 presents the total number of publications (%) extracted year-month-wise for AI, IoT and BC.

7.2.2 Data filtration

In 1,640 records have been reviewed based on their title, duplicate WoS IDs and context of the subject. After initial review, 97 records are excluded resulting in a new total of 1,543 records such as AI (1,216), IoT

Table 7.1 A total number of publications year- and month-wise in (%) for AI, IoT and BC

Month	*No. of papers AI ([%)*		*No. of papers IoT (%)*		*No. of papers BC (%)*	
	2020	2021	2020	2021	2020	2021
Jan	2.9	15.5	6.5	15.9	0.0	13.0
Feb	0.0	16.9	0.0	16.7	0.0	14.5
Mar	1.5	19.0	1.1	15.9	0.0	21.7
Apr	2.0	14.0	1.1	16.7	3.0	23.2
May	5.5	18.8	4.3	10.1	6.1	10.1
Jun	8.6	11.8	7.5	20.3	6.1	10.1
Jul	9.3	4.1	9.7	4.3	3.0	7.2
Aug	11.5	-	6.5	-	15.2	-
Sep	13.4	-	14.0	-	9.1	-
Oct	15.2	-	10.8	-	15.2	-
Nov	12.8	-	17.2	-	21.2	-
Dec	17.4	-	21.5	-	21.2	-

(236) and BC (91). Document type of 1,543 records is article, correction, editorial material, letter, meeting abstract, news item and review. Based on document types, 163 studies are excluded, resulting in a final count of 1,380 (articles (1,189) and review (191)) records. In the last step of filtration, final categories such as AI, IoT, BC and Multiple (where subject context is of more than one type) have been created with counts such as AI (1,075), IoT(155), BC (66) and Multiple (84). Figure 7.1 describes the complete process of data filtration.

7.3 RESULTS

The results are presented in five phases. First phase is the temporal trend of publications which highlights the relationship between AI, IoT and BC with regard to publications and open access designations. This phase also highlights key aspects in terms of team sizes and citations received. Second phase presents discipline-wise analysis which highlights discipline-wise variations in the publications across AI, IoT and BC. Third phase highlights international and national collaboration among countries based on AI, IoT and BC. In the fourth phase, author keywords and research areas are analyzed and results are presented based on their keyword strengths. In the last phase, top journals along with publishers are summarized with their frequency of AI, IoT and BC-based publications.

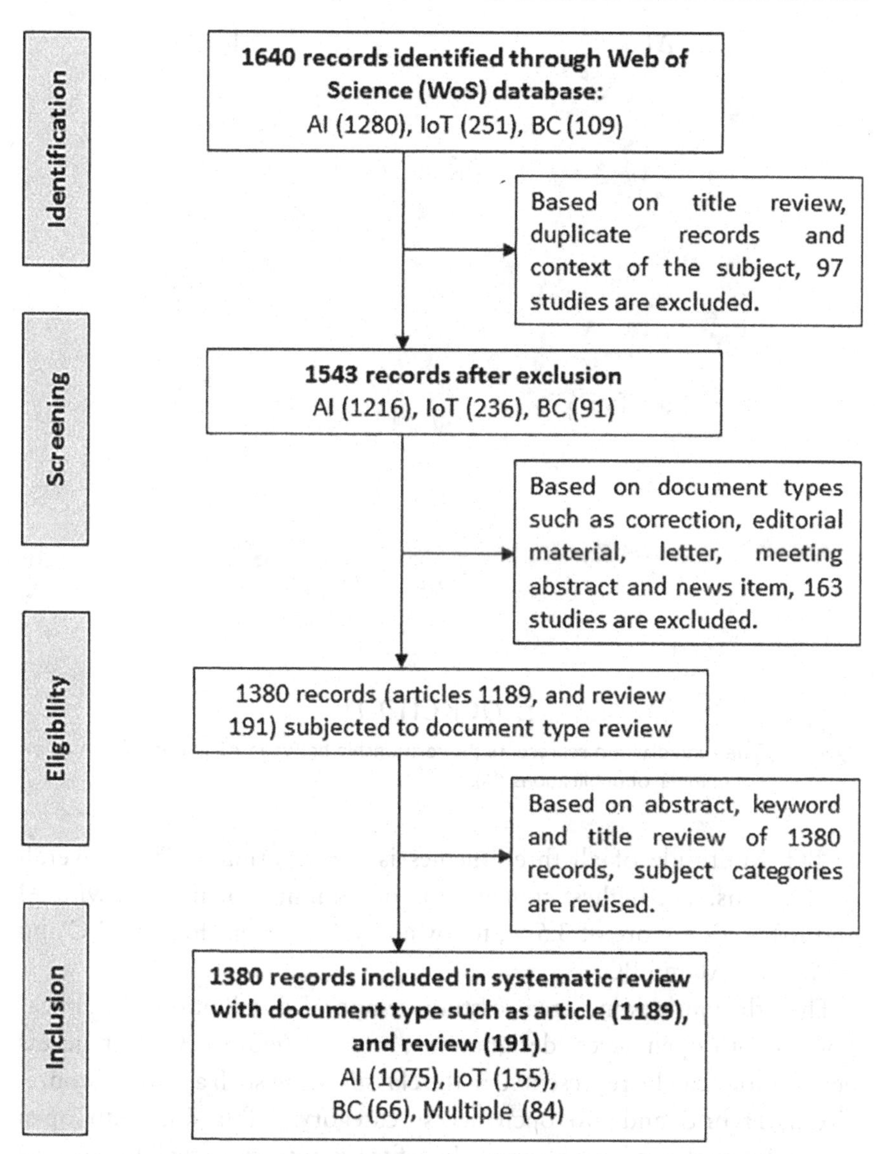

Figure 7.1 Flowchart describing the process of data extraction and filtration from WoS.

7.3.1 Temporal distribution of publications

Publications extracted with theme keywords (AI, IoT and BC) have a significant relationship among them. This temporal distribution presents such a relationship in the form of a venn diagram in Figure 7.2. In total, 1,380 publications are short listed for the study, among which 77.9%, a maximum one represents AI, followed by 11.2% as IoT and 4.8%

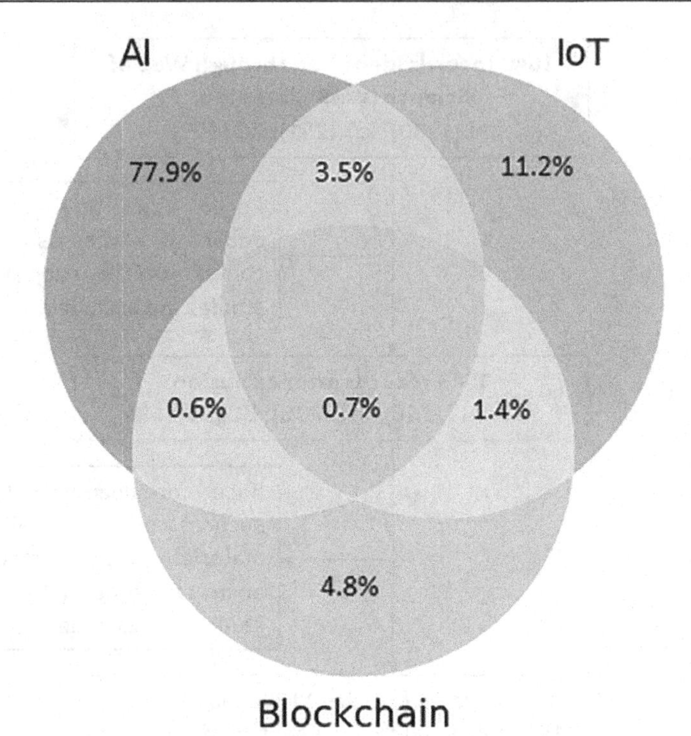

Figure 7.2 The venn diagram represents the relationship between AI, IoT and BC in terms of number of publications (%).

as BC. Multitude of all three themes is contributing <1% of overall publications. The highest contribution of combined themes lies with AI and IoT with a score of 3.5%, followed by 1.4% with IoT and BC and <1% with AI and BC.

The other interesting area to study temporal distribution of publications is with open access designations, refer to Figure 7.3. Open access designations can be represented in the classification such as Gold, Bronze, Green, Hybrid and No open access category. Publishing with open access designations has enormous benefits for authors as well for various stakeholders. Here, a major pie plot presents an overall distribution of AI, IoT and BC publications with various open access designations. Maximum publications are published in Hybrid mode 55%, followed by Gold 16%, NOA 12%, Bronze 11% and Green 6%. Hybrid here represents a mixture of various open access designations and NOA here represents- no open access categories specified or allocated by Clarivate.

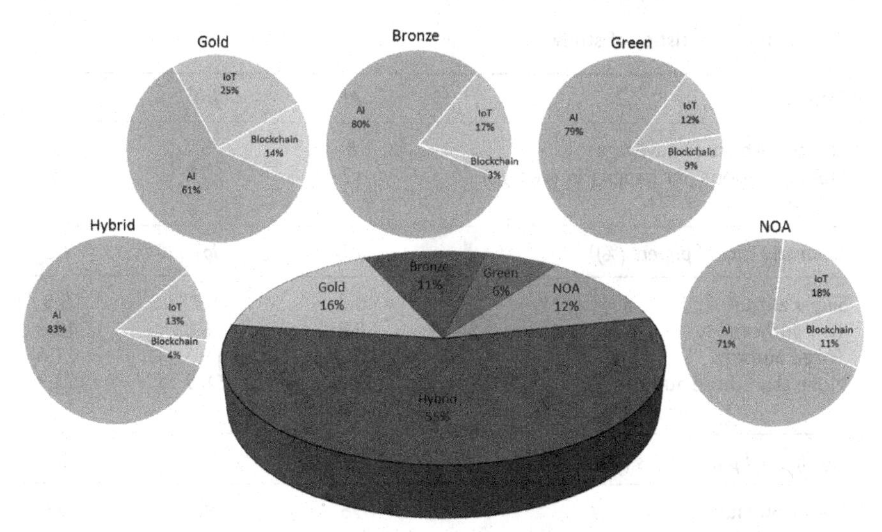

Figure 7.3 The major pie plot represents the distribution of open access publications for AI, IoT and BC broadly. Open access publications are categorized into Gold, Bronze, Green, Hybrid and NOA (No open access). Minor pie plots represent the distribution of AI, IoT and BC among various open access publications.

The contribution of AI, IoT and BC is also observed in comparison with various open access designations (in minor pie plots). Hybrid mode has received the highest contribution of theme AI with (83%), followed by Bronze (80%), Green (79%), NOA (71%) and Gold (61%). Gold mode has received the highest contribution of theme IoT (25%), followed by NOA (18%), Bronze (17%), Hybrid (13%) and Green (12%). BC has the highest contribution in Gold (14%), followed by NOA (11%), Green (9%), Hybrid (4%) and Bronze (3%).

Table 7.2 presents further statistics of initial study where highest average team size (8) and highest average citations (12) are received by AI theme. IoT has the same average number of authors (5) per paper in comparison with BC (5). Average number of citations per paper (7) for IoT are more than BC (6). All three themes (AI, IoT and BC) are compared on the basis of team size, where AI has 74.8% (highest among all themes) publications with more than three authors, followed by IoT (58.9%) and BC (53.9%). IoT has received the highest number of publications (8.7%) with a single author, followed by BC (5.9%) and AI (3.8%). BC has highest number of publications with two authors (18.6%) and three authors (21.6%), followed by IoT with (16.0%) with

Table 7.2 Initial statistics of study

Statistics	AI	IoT	BC
No. of authors (in average)	8	5	5
No. of citations per paper (in average)	12	7	6
Team size (no. of papers (%))	*AI*	*IoT*	*BC*
Single author	3.8	8.7	5.9
Two authors	8.8	16.0	18.6
Three authors	12.6	16.5	21.6
More than three authors	74.8	58.9	53.9
Highly cited publications (%)	*AI*	*IoT*	*BC*
Below 50 citations	96	97	97
Above 50 citations	4	3	3
Publications with funding (%)	58	52	53

two authors and (16.5%) with three authors, AI with (8.8%) with two authors and (12.6%) with three authors.

For both, IoT and BC, 97% of publications have received below 50 citations, whereas 4% of AI publications have received more than 50 citations. A total of 58% of AI publications (highest) have received funding, followed by BC (53%) and IoT (52%), which reflects that 50% publications of all themes have at least received funding for their work.

7.3.2 Discipline-wise analysis

Figure 7.4 presents discipline-wise analysis of all the publications of AI, IoT and BC. WoS category and Research Area information has been extracted for all 1380 publications. Based on the fields of science and technology classification available at (https://www.qnrf.org/en-us/FOS), all publications have been classified into four broad categories such as Engineering and Technology, Medical and Health Sciences, Natural Sciences and Social Sciences [18]. A measure of an interdisciplinary comparison has been done [38] and relationships among AI, IoT and BC across various disciplines have been identified and analyzed. Highest publications (%) of AI have been received in Medical and Health Sciences, followed by IoT in Engineering and Technology, BC in Social Sciences and Natural Sciences in Multiple (mixture of all themes) cate-

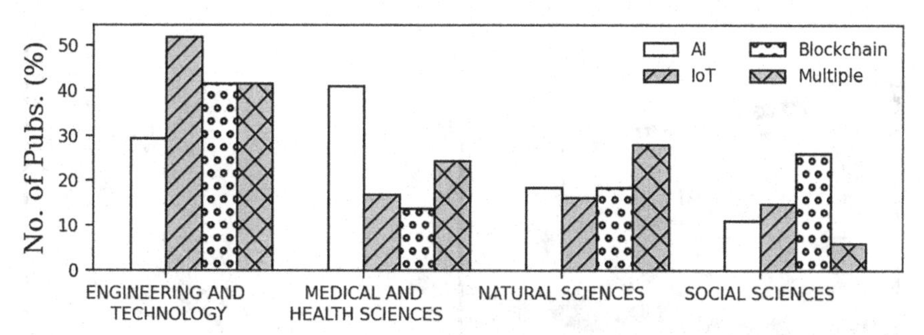

Figure 7.4 The bar plot represents the discipline-wise proportion of AI, IoT, BC and Multiple category publications (%).

gory. The lowest number of publications (%) have been received by AI in Engineering and Technology, followed by IoT in Natural Sciences, BC in Medical and Health Sciences and Multiple in Social Sciences. BC and Multiple have received an equal number of publications (%) Engineering and Technology.

7.3.3 Country-wise analysis

Figure 7.5 presents a trend of international collaboration based on AI, IoT, BC themes. During insight study of country-wise collaboration, 95 countries are identified, and a trend of their international collaboration is studied. It is analyzed that 169 unique county1-country2-theme (AI, IoT and BC) combinations exist with the highest number of unique combinations with AI (89), followed by IoT (54) and BC (26). Among all USA (sr. no. 15) has highest international collaborations followed by England (sr. no. 4), Peoples R China (sr. no. 11), India (sr. no. 7), Italy (sr. no. 8), Australia (sr. no. 1), Canada (sr. no. 2), Saudi Arabia (sr. no. 13), Egypt (sr. no. 3) and Pakistan (sr. no. 10).

Table 7.3 presents a list of countries with their serial numbers assigned in Figure 7.5.

Table 7.4 presents list of countries sorted on highest number of publications in national collaboration. Although Peoples R China has the highest number of publications in total but the USA has the highest publications in AI. Peoples R China has the highest number of publications in national collaboration in IoT and BC.

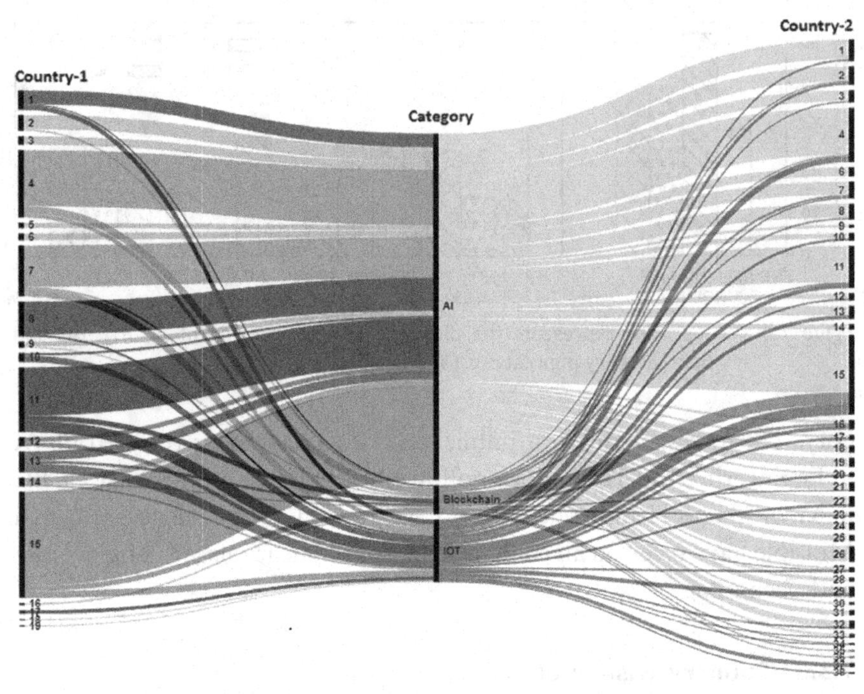

Figure 7.5 The alluvial diagram represents the ranking of top 19 countries based on their international collaboration for AI, IoT and BC.

Table 7.3 List of countries represented in Figure 7.5 (serial number wise)

Sr. No.	Country	Sr. No.	Country
1	Australia	20	Bangladesh
2	Canada	21	Taiwan
3	Egypt	22	Brazil
4	England	23	Norway
5	France	24	Scotland
6	Germany	25	Sweden
7	India	26	Switzerland
8	Italy	27	Qatar
9	Netherlands	28	Turkey
10	Pakistan	29	Vietnam
11	Peoples R China	30	Belgium
12	Portugal	31	Greece
13	Saudi Arabia	32	Japan
14	Spain	33	Ireland
15	USA	34	U Arab Emirates
16	Denmark	35	Wales
17	Iran	36	Finland
18	Singapore	37	Malaysia
19	South Korea	38	Tunisia

Table 7.4 List of countries with minimum ten papers in national collaboration

Country	*AI*	*IoT*	*BC*
Peoples R China	114	35	11
USA	119	16	4
India	51	10	7
Italy	42	5	5
South Korea	31	4	2
England	26	5	1
Spain	22	6	2
Saudi Arabia	14	6	2
Turkey	18	4	0
Canada	14	3	2
Brazil	13	2	0
Egypt	12	2	0
Australia	7	4	2
France	11	1	0
Taiwan	11	1	0
Singapore	9	2	0
Germany	10	0	0

7.3.4 Thematic analysis

Thematic analysis is one of the convenient ways to analyze the main features and flow of themes in publications [47]. To perform thematic analysis, author keywords are analyzed (theme-wise), and an overall view of authors in different publications has been retrieved. Author keywords also reflect the idea of subject understanding by the author in terms of visibility of publication at various platforms, areas supported by the study of the author, important trends followed during the study and distribution of an idea in a wide range of solutions. Figure 7.6 presents a thematic analysis of AI theme where 3,071 unique author keywords are identified with a total frequency of 6,361 in AI-based publications. The top identified keyword is COVID-19 with a repetition range of 663, which is almost 10.4% of total author keyword strength in AI-based publications, followed by artificial intelligence (5.0%), deep learning (2.3%), machine learning (2.2%) and sars-cov-2 (2.1%). Figure 7.7 presents thematic analysis of the theme IoT. A total of 926 unique authors' keywords have been extracted from the publications relevant to the theme IoT. The most used author keyword is COVID-19 with strength of 121 which is almost 8% of available keywords in total, followed by IoT 3%, pandemic 1.3% and coronavirus 1.3% as well. There are 772 keywords which have been used exactly once by the authors. Figure 7.8

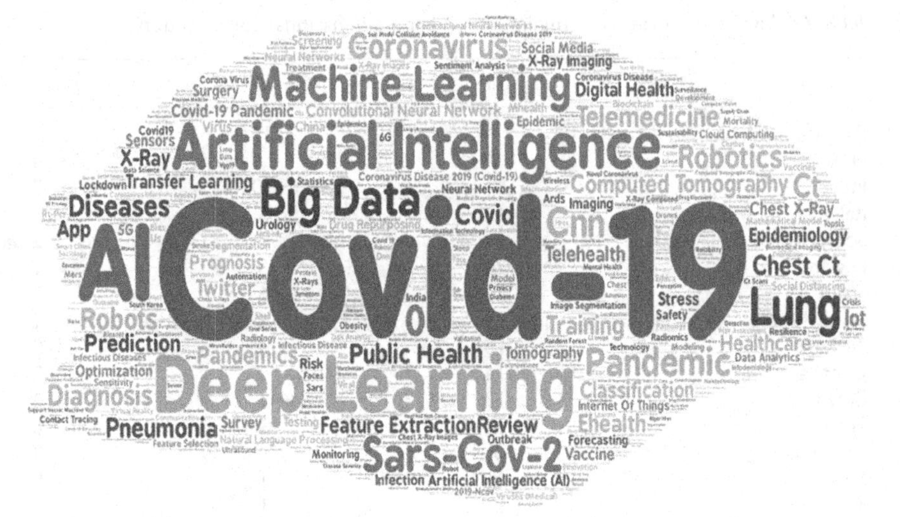

Figure 7.6 Word cloud of author's keywords for AI-based publications. The size of the keyword is proportional to the frequent use of the keyword.

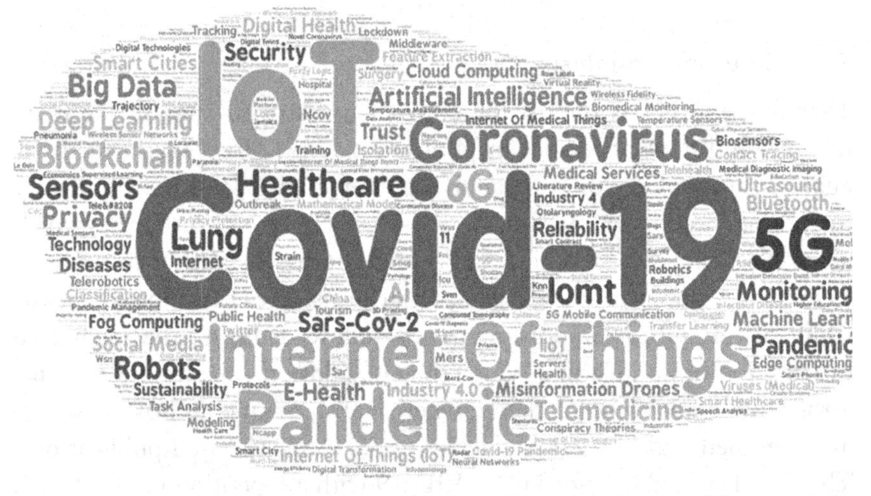

Figure 7.7 Word cloud of author's keywords for IoT-based publications. The size of the keyword is proportional to the frequent use of the keyword.

is presenting thematic analysis of BC-based publications. It carries 461 unique keywords with blockchain as a keyword on the top with strength of 9.0%, followed by COVID-19 (7.4%), privacy (1.4%), coronavirus (1.2%) and smart contracts (1.1%). The total keyword strength is 725 words. There are 71 keywords which are used at least two times by the authors, followed by 390 keywords which have been used only once by

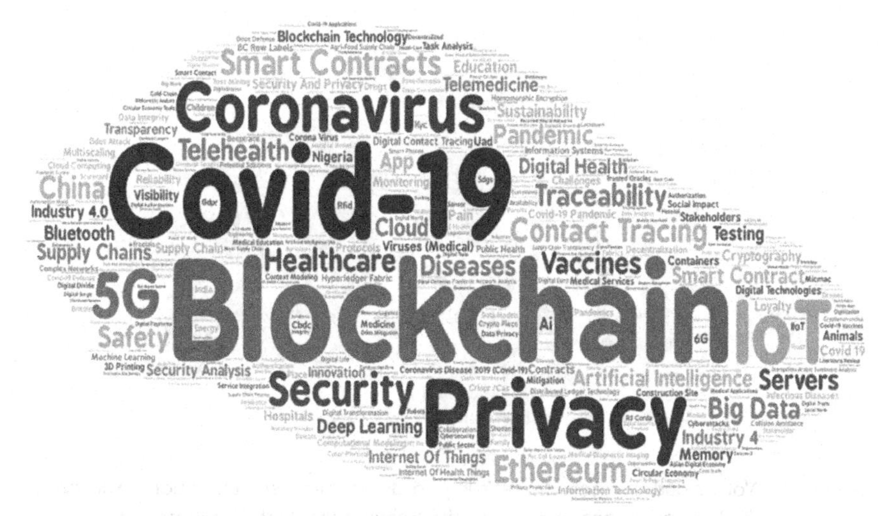

Figure 7.8 Word cloud of author's keywords for BC-based publications. The size of the keyword is proportional to the frequent use of the keyword.

the authors. Top ten author keywords in combined pattern i.e. AI, IoT and BC are COVID-19, artificial intelligence, deep learning, machine learning, sars-cov-2, coronavirus, blockchain, pandemic, IoT and big data. Figure 7.9 presents the thematic pattern of AI-based publications in relevance to the research areas associated with publications. Research areas are generally assigned by Clarivate for the key categorization of the publications. This thematic analysis has presented AI, IoT and BC separately. For AI-based publications, 232 unique research area-based keywords exist with computer science with highest frequency of 7.9%, followed by health care sciences & services; medical informatics (5.9%), general & internal medicine (4.8%), science & technology - other topics (4.7%), radiology, nuclear medicine & medical imaging (4.0%). There have been at least 26 keywords which are used ten or more than ten times by the authors based on AI publications and there are 112 keywords which are used only once by the authors.

Figure 7.10 presents a thematic pattern based on IoT publications. A total of 74 unique keywords have been used by the authors with computer science; engineering; telecommunications at the top with the highest frequency of 17.3%, followed by computer science (9.5%), chemistry; engineering; instruments & instrumentation (4.8%), computer science; telecommunications (3.9%), health care sciences & services; medical informatics (3.9%), science & technology - other topics; environmental

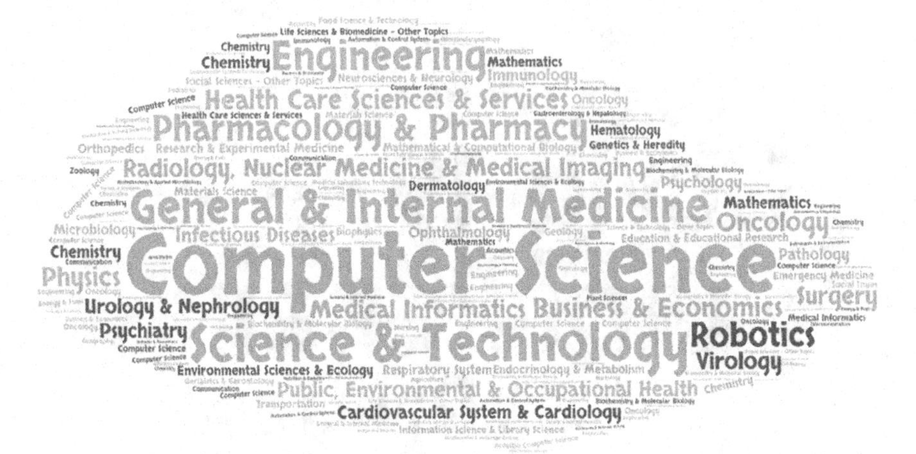

Figure 7.9 Word cloud of research area's keywords for AI-based publications. The size of the keyword is proportional to the frequent use of the keyword.

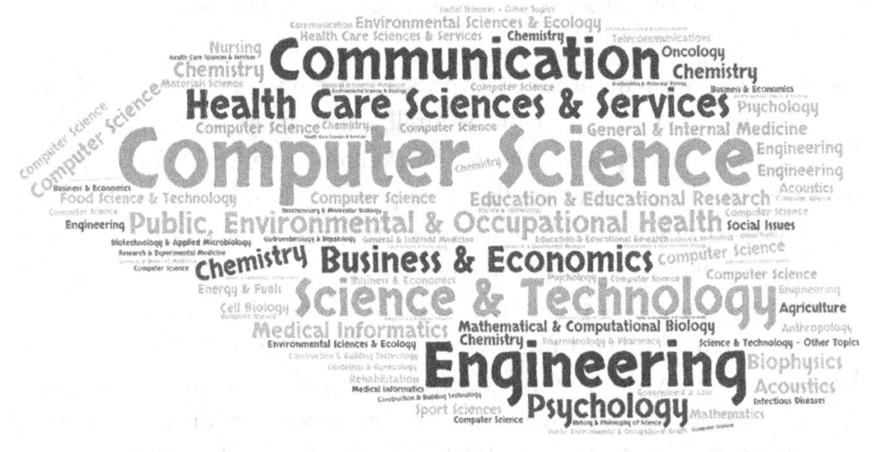

Figure 7.10 Word cloud of research area's keywords for IoT-based publications. The size of the keyword is proportional to the frequent use of the keyword.

sciences & ecology (3.9%). A total of 42 keywords have been used only once by the authors in IoT-based publications.

Figure 7.11 presents thematic analysis of BC-based publications where 38 unique keywords are used. Computer Science; Engineering; Telecommunications is at the top with 23.5% frequency strength of overall keywords used in BC-based publications, followed by science & technology - other topics; environmental sciences & ecology (6.9%), computer science (5.9%), information science & library science (5.9%), science & technology - other topics (4.9%), environmental sciences & ecology; public,

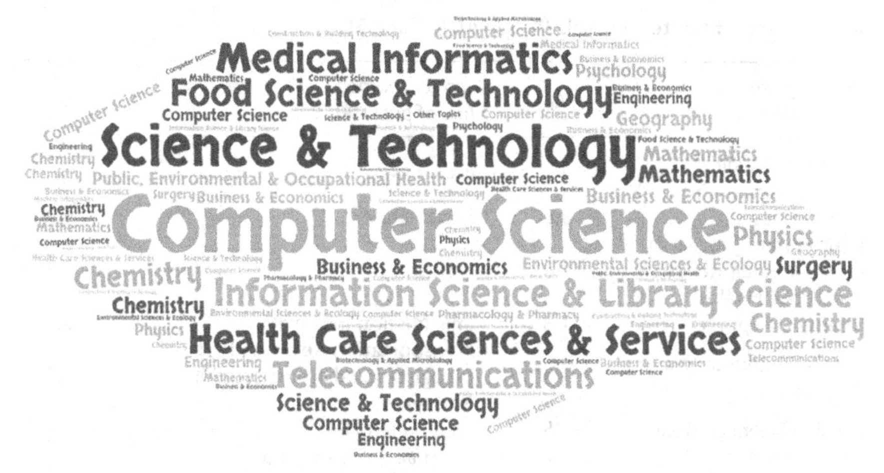

Figure 7.11 Word cloud of research area's keywords for BC-based publications. The size of the keyword is proportional to the frequent use of the keyword.

environmental & occupational health (2.9%), health care sciences & services (2.9%), food science & technology (2.9%), medical informatics (2.9%),chemistry; engineering; instruments & instrumentation (2.9%), business & economics; engineering; operations research & management science; transportation (2.9%), public, environmental & occupational health (2.9%). Nineteen keywords are used only once by the authors with publications based on BC. Top ten research area keywords combined with AI, IoT and BC are computer science, health care sciences & services; medical informatics, general & internal medicine, science & technology - other topics, radiology, nuclear medicine & medical imaging, computer science; engineering; telecommunications, computer science; engineering; telecommunications, environmental sciences & ecology; public, environmental & occupational health, pharmacology & pharmacy, computer science; engineering; telecommunications.

7.3.5 Publication analysis

Table 7.5 presents the journal-wise analysis based on AI, IoT and BC-based publications. In total 599 journals have published the papers for all themes together with IEEE Access with highest publications (together for all themes), followed by journal of medical internet research, international journal of environmental research and public health, sustainability, cmc-computers materials & continua, sensors, scientific reports, applied sciences-basel, plos one and diagnostics. Theme-wise top ten

Table 7.5 List of top ten journals (%) for AI, IoT and BC

Top ten journals (no. of pubs. %)	*AI*	*Top ten journals (no. of pubs. %)*	*BC*
Journal of Medical Internet Research	4.2	IEEE Access	18.6
IEEE Access	3.8	Sustainability	6.9
International Journal of Environmental Research and Public Health	2.4	Sensors	2.9
Scientific Reports	1.8	Jmir Medical Informatics	2.9
CMC-Computers Materials & Continua	1.8	Transportation Research Part E-Logistics and Transportation Review	2.9
Applied Sciences-Basel	1.5	IEEE Network	2.9
Sustainability	1.3	International Journal of Environmental Research and Public Health	2.9
Diagnostics	1.1	International Journal of Information Management	2.9
Sensors	1.1	Technological Forecasting and Social Change	2.0
PLoS One	1.1	Journal of Cleaner Production	2.0
		Information Technology & People	2.0
Top ten journals (no. of pubs. in %)	IoT	Electronics	2.0
IEEE Access	9.5	Journal of Network and Computer Applications	2.0
Sensors	4.8	Applied Sciences-Basel	2.0
Sustainability	3.5	Information Processing & Management	2.0
Journal of Medical Internet Research	3.0	Computer Standards & Interfaces	2.0
Electronics	2.6		
CMC-Computers Materials & Continua	2.2		
IEEE Internet of Things Journal	2.2		
Omics-A Journal of Integrative Biology	1.7		
Journal of Intelligent & Fuzzy Systems	1.7		
IEEE Network	1.7		

journals have been presented in Table 7.5. Table 7.6 presents the list of top ten publishers theme-wise. A total of 143 publishers have published the papers, including prominent publishers such as MDPI, Elsevier, IEEE, Springer, Wiley, Jmir, Nature research and Frontiers media. Table 7.6 presents theme-wise top ten publishers with their number of publications (%).

Table 7.6 List of top ten publishers (%) for AI, IoT and BC

Top ten publishers (No. of pubs. %)	AI	Top ten publishers (No. of pubs. %)	BC
Elsevier	17.7	Elsevier	25.5
Springer	12.5	IEEE	23.5
MDPI	11.0	MDPI	21.6
IEEE	7.5	Springer	5.9
Wiley	6.8	Wiley	3.9
Jmir Publications, Inc	5.5	Emerald Group Publishing Ltd	3.9
Taylor & Francis Ltd	3.6	Jmir Publications, Inc	3.9
Nature Research	3.4	Nature Research	2.0
Frontiers Media Sa	3.0	Mary Ann Liebert, Inc	2.0
Tech Science Press	2.0	Frontiers Media Sa	2.0
Top ten publishers (no. of pubs. %)	IoT		
IEEE	17.7		
Elsevier	16.5		
MDPI	16.5		
Springer	12.1		
Wiley	9.1		
Jmir Publications, Inc	4.3		
Tech Science Press	2.6		
Mary Ann Liebert, Inc	2.6		
Sage Publications Ltd	2.2		
Ios Press	1.7		

7.4 DISCUSSION AND CONCLUSION

COVID-19 pandemic has created a grappling impact on medical, financial and social situations of the countries all over the world [14]. To curb the impact of this pandemic, various technologies such as AI, IoT and BC are endeavoring to act as a core technologies for prediction, surveillance and sharing of data [44]. This study starts with the introduction of AI, IoT and BC in which their features, applications and various capabilities are focused. Following this, we discussed the course of data extraction and its filtration. In the thorough discussion, post introduction and methodology, we dissect the comprehensive review into five segments, we explored the relationship between AI, IoT and BC-based publications, we also listed the impact of various open access designations such as Gold, Green, Bronze, Hybrid and NOA following all three themes (AI, IoT and BC). We also listed the key statistics related to authors team size, their publications, citations, funding, etc. In the next segment, we primarily focused on the impact of AI, IoT and BC in various disciplines such as engineering and technology, medical and health sciences, natural sciences and social sciences. To calibrate the encounter of COVID-19 across different countries, we performed network analysis in which the interventions are presented in which countries are working together in collaboration based on AI, IoT and BC to provide technological interventions. National-level collaboration is also studied to provide the foundation for AI, IoT and BC at individual country level. Following this, we presented the thematic trend of author keywords and research areas with the selection of AI, IoT and BC. This comprehensive overview provides the extreme insight of all three themes (AI, IoT and BC) that how these have empowered the thoughts of authors and how noticeably they have performed the continuous monitoring to interact with COVID-19 literature. Finally, in the last segment, we focused on the key players in terms of journals and publishers who have the vision to develop a successful literature of COVID-19 in order to productively analyze and inhibit the spread further.

7.4.1 Limitations and future work

The limitations and further possibilities of the above study can be discussed as:

- The data is extracted from Clarivate but as the number of publications varies from database to database, this study can be extended further with the use of other databases such as Scopus, Google Scholar, etc.
- Just like AI, IoT and BC, this study can be extended with various other technologies in trend such as Big data, robotics, machine learning, deep learning, drones, 5G, etc.
- The characteristics and implementations of AI, IoT and BC-based applications can be added to extend the context of technical discoveries in the existing study for actual development of healthcare procedures.

7.5 DISCLOSURE STATEMENT

The author declares that they have no conflict of interest.

7.6 NOTES ON CONTRIBUTOR(S)

Both the authors conceived and designed the analysis, collected the data, performed the analysis and wrote the draft.

REFERENCES

[1] Alaa A Abd-Alrazaq, Mohannad Alajlani, Dari Alhuwail, Aiman Erbad, Anna Giannicchi, Zubair Shah, Mounir Hamdi, and Mowafa Househ. Blockchain technologies to mitigate Covid-19 challenges: A scoping review. *Computer Methods and Programs in Biomedicine Update*, 1:100001, 2021.

[2] Mohamed Abdel-Basset, Victor Chang, and Nada A Nabeeh. An intelligent framework using disruptive technologies for Covid-19 analysis. *Technological Forecasting and Social Change*, 163:120431, 2021.

[3] Shiva Ahir, Dipali Telavane, and Riya Thomas. The impact of artificial intelligence, blockchain, big data and evolving technologies in coronavirus disease-2019 (Covid-19) curtailment. In *2020 International Conference on Smart Electronics and Communication (ICOSEC)*, pp. 113–120. IEEE, 2020.

[4] Mukhtar AL-Hashimi and Allam Hamdan. The applications of artificial intelligence to control Covid-19. In *Advances in Data Science and Intelligent Data Communication Technologies for COVID-19*, pp. 55–75. Springer, 2022.

[5] Abdulqader M Almars, Ibrahim Gad, and El-Sayed Atlam. Applications of ai and IoT in Covid-19 vaccine and its impact on social life. In *Medical Informatics and Bioimaging Using Artificial Intelligence*, pp. 115–127. Springer, 2022.

[6] Saeed Hamood Alsamhi, Brian Lee, Mohsen Guizani, Neeraj Kumar, Yuansong Qiao, and Xuan Liu. Blockchain for decentralized multi-drone to combat Covid-19 and future pandemics: Framework and proposed solutions. *Transactions on Emerging Telecommunications Technologies*, 32(9):e4255, 2021.

[7] Joseph Bamidele Awotunde, Rasheed Gbenga Jimoh, Muyideen AbdulRaheem, Idowu Dauda Oladipo, Sakinat Oluwabukonla Folorunso, and Gbemisola Janet Ajamu. IoT-based wearable body sensor network for Covid-19 pandemic. In: Aboul-Ella Hassanien, Sally M. Elghamrawy, and Ivan Zelinka (Eds.), *Advances in Data Science and Intelligent Data Communication Technologies for COVID-19*, pp. 253–275. Springer: Cham, 2022.

[8] Mahmood A Bazel, Fathey Mohammed, Mogeeb Alsabaiy, and Hussein Mohammed Abualrejal. The role of internet of things, blockchain, artificial intelligence, and big data technologies in healthcare to prevent the spread of the Covid-19. In *2021 International Conference on Innovation and Intelligence for Informatics, Computing, and Technologies (3ICT)*, pp. 455–462. IEEE, 2021.

[9] Sanjay Chakraborty and Lopamudra Dey. The implementation of ai and ai-empowered imaging system to fight against Covid-19: a review. *Smart Healthcare System Design: Security and Privacy Aspects*, pp. 301–311, 2022.

[10] Vinay Chamola, Vikas Hassija, Vatsal Gupta, and Mohsen Guizani. A comprehensive review of the Covid-19 pandemic and the role of IoT, drones, ai, blockchain, and 5g in managing its impact. *IEEE Access*, 8:90225–90265, 2020.

[11] Min Cheol Chang and Donghwi Park. How can blockchain help people in the event of pandemics such as the Covid-19? *Journal of Medical Systems*, 44(5):1–2, 2020.

[12] Sarat Chettri, Dipankar Debnath, and Pooja Devi. Leveraging digital tools and technologies to alleviate Covid-19 pandemic. *SSRN Electronic Journal*, 1–10, 2020.

[13] Hong-Ning Dai, Muhammad Imran, and Noman Haider. Blockchain-enabled internet of medical things to combat Covid-19. *IEEE Internet of Things Magazine*, 3(3):52–57, 2020.

[14] Ashok Kumar Das, Basudeb Bera, and Debasis Giri. Ai and blockchain-based cloud-assisted secure vaccine distribution and tracking in iomt-enabled Covid-19 environment. *IEEE Internet of Things Magazine*, 4(2):26–32, 2021.

[15] Gauri Deshpande, Anton Batliner, and Björn W Schuller. Ai-based human audio processing for Covid-19: A comprehensive overview. *Pattern Recognition*, 122:108289, 2022.

[16] Yudi Dong and Yu-Dong Yao. IoT platform for Covid-19 prevention and control: A survey. *IEEE Access*, 9:49929–49941, 2021.

[17] Farshad Firouzi, Bahar Farahani, Mahmoud Daneshmand, Kathy Grise, Jae Seung Song, Roberto Saracco, Lucy Lu Wang, Kyle Lo, Plamen Angelov, Eduardo Soares, et al. Harnessing the power of smart and connected health to tackle Covid-19: IoT, ai, robotics, and blockchain for a better world. *IEEE Internet of Things Journal*, 8(16):12826–12846, 2021.

[18] Qatar Foundation. The fields of science and technology classification, 2021.

[19] Awishkar Ghimire, Surendrabikram Thapa, Avinash Kumar Jha, Amit Kumar, Arunish Kumar, and Surabhi Adhikari. Ai and IoT solutions for tackling Covid-19 pandemic. In *2020 4th International Conference on Electronics, Communication and Aerospace Technology (ICECA)*, pp. 1083–1092. IEEE, 2020.

[20] Deepti Gupta, Smriti Bhatt, Maanak Gupta, and Ali Saman Tosun. Future smart connected communities to fight Covid-19 outbreak. *Internet of Things*, 13:100342, 2021.

[21] Wu He, Zuopeng Justin Zhang, and Wenzhuo Li. Information technology solutions, challenges, and suggestions for tackling the Covid-19 pandemic. *International Journal of Information Management*, 57:102287, 2021.

[22] Mohamed Yaseen Jabarulla and Heung-No Lee. A blockchain and artificial intelligence-based, patient-centric healthcare system for combating the Covid-19 pandemic: Opportunities and applications. *Healthcare (Basel)*, 9:1019, 2021.

[23] Garima Jain, Garima Shukla, Priyanka Saini, Anubha Gaur, Divya Mishra, and Shyam Akashe. Secure Covid-19 treatment with blockchain and IoT-based framework. In Jennifer S. Raj, Yong Shi, Danilo Pelusi, and Valentina Emilia Balas (Eds.), *Intelligent Sustainable Systems*, pp. 785–800. Springer: Berlin/Heidelberg, Germany, 2022.

[24] Mohd Javaid and Ibrahim Haleem Khan. Internet of things (IoT) enabled healthcare helps to take the challenges of Covid-19 pandemic. *Journal of Oral Biology and Craniofacial Research*, 11(2):209–214, 2021.

[25] Anshuman Kalla, Tharaka Hewa, Raaj Anand Mishra, Mika Ylianttila, and Madhusanka Liyanage. The role of blockchain to fight against Covid-19. *IEEE Engineering Management Review*, 48(3):85–96, 2020.

[26] Mohsin Kamal, Abdulah Aljohani, and Eisa Alanazi. IoT meets Covid-19: Status, challenges, and opportunities. arXiv preprint arXiv:2007.12268, 2020.
[27] Mousa Mohammed Khubrani and Shadab Alam. A detailed review of blockchain-based applications for protection against pandemic like Covid-19. *Telkomnika*, 19(4):1185–1196, 2021.
[28] Abhaya V Kulkarni, Brittany Aziz, Iffat Shams, and Jason W Busse. Comparisons of citations in web of science, scopus, and google scholar for articles published in general medical journals. *JAMA*, 302(10):1092–1096, 2009.
[29] Krishna Kumar, Narendra Kumar, and Rachna Shah. Role of IoT to avoid spreading of Covid-19. *International Journal of Intelligent Networks*, 1:32–35, 2020.
[30] Shashank Kumar, Rakesh D Raut, and Balkrishna E Narkhede. A proposed collaborative framework by using artificial intelligence-internet of things (AI-IoT) in Covid-19 pandemic situation for healthcare workers. *International Journal of Healthcare Management*, 13(4):337–345, 2020.
[31] Dounia Marbouh, Tayaba Abbasi, Fatema Maasmi, Ilhaam A Omar, Mazin S Debe, Khaled Salah, Raja Jayaraman, and Samer Ellahham. Blockchain for Covid-19: Review, opportunities, and a trusted tracking system. *Arabian Journal for Science and Engineering*, 45(12):9895–9911, 2020.
[32] Alberto Martín-Martín, Enrique Orduna-Malea, Mike Thelwall, and Emilio Delgado López-Cózar. Google scholar, web of science, and scopus: A systematic comparison of citations in 252 subject categories. *Journal of Informetrics*, 12(4):1160–1177, 2018.
[33] Zahra Mastaneh and Ali Mouseli. Technology and its solutions in the era of Covid-19 crisis: A review of literature. *Evidence Based Health Policy, Management and Economics*, 4(2):138–149, 2020.
[34] Mohammed N. Abdulrazaq, Halim Syamsudin, Salah Salman Al-Zubaidi, Sairah Abdul Karim, Rusyaizila Ramli, and Eddy Yusuf. Novel Covid-19 detection and diagnosis system using IoT based smart helmet. *International Journal of Psychosocial Rehabilitation*, 24(7):2296–2303, 2020.
[35] Musa Ndiaye, Stephen S Oyewobi, Adnan M Abu-Mahfouz, Gerhard P Hancke, Anish M Kurien, and Karim Djouani. IoT in the wake of Covid-19: A survey on contributions, challenges and evolution. *IEEE Access*, 8:186821–186839, 2020.
[36] Dinh C Nguyen, Ming Ding, Pubudu N Pathirana, and Aruna Seneviratne. Blockchain and ai-based solutions to combat coronavirus (Covid-19)-like epidemics: A survey. *IEEE Access*, 9:95730–95753, 2021.
[37] Mwaffaq Otoom, Nesreen Otoum, Mohammad A Alzubaidi, Yousef Etoom, and Rudaina Banihani. An IoT-based framework for early identification and monitoring of Covid-19 cases. *Biomedical Signal Processing and Control*, 62:102149, 2020.
[38] Alan Porter, Alex Cohen, J David Roessner, and Marty Perreault. Measuring researcher interdisciplinarity. *Scientometrics*, 72(1):117–147, 2007.
[39] Ignacio Rodríguez-Rodríguez, José-Víctor Rodríguez, Niloofar Shirvanizadeh, Andrés Ortiz, and Domingo-Javier Pardo-Quiles. Applications of artificial intelligence, machine learning, big data and the internet of things to the Covid-19 pandemic: A scientometric review using text mining. *International Journal of Environmental Research and Public Health*, 18(16):8578, 2021.

[40] Abhishek Sharma, Shashi Bahl, Ashok Kumar Bagha, Mohd Javaid, Dinesh Kumar Shukla, and Abid Haleem. Blockchain technology and its applications to combat Covid-19 pandemic. *Research on Biomedical Engineering*, 38(1):173, 2022.

[41] Arjun Sharma, B Nagajayanthi, A Chaitanya Kumar, and Shirish Dinakaran. IoT-based Covid-19 patient monitor with alert system. In: A Sivasubramanian, Prasad N Shastry, and Pua Chang Hong (Eds.), *Futuristic Communication and Network Technologies*, pp. 1019–1027. Springer Nature: Berlin, Germany, 2022.

[42] Kiran Sharma and Parul Khurana. Emerging trends and collaboration patterns unveil the scientific production in blockchain technology: A bibliometric and network analysis from 2014-2020. arXiv preprint arXiv:2110.01871, 2021.

[43] Yu-Ting Shen, Liang Chen, Wen-Wen Yue, and Hui-Xiong Xu. Digital technology-based telemedicine for the Covid-19 pandemic. *Frontiers in Medicine*, 8:933, 2021.

[44] Pranav Kumar Singh, Sukumar Nandi, Kayhan Zrar Ghafoor, Uttam Ghosh, and Danda B Rawat. Preventing Covid-19 spread using information and communication technology. *IEEE Consumer Electronics Magazine*, 10(4):18–27, 2020.

[45] Ravi Pratap Singh, Mohd Javaid, Abid Haleem, and Rajiv Suman. Internet of things (IoT) applications to fight against Covid-19 pandemic. *Diabetes & Metabolic Syndrome: Clinical Research & Reviews*, 14(4):521–524, 2020.

[46] Daniel Shu Wei Ting, Lawrence Carin, Victor Dzau, and Tien Y Wong. Digital technology and Covid-19. *Nature Medicine*, 26(4):459–461, 2020.

[47] A Velez-Estevez, Pablo García-Sánchez, José Antonio Moral-Muñoz, and Manuel J Cobo. Thematical and impact differences between national and international collaboration on artificial intelligence research. In *2020 IEEE Conference on Evolving and Adaptive Intelligent Systems (EAIS)*, pp. 1–8. IEEE, 2020.

[48] Robin Wang, Zhicheng Jiao, Li Yang, Ji Whae Choi, Zeng Xiong, Kasey Halsey, Thi My Linh Tran, Ian Pan, Scott A Collins, Xue Feng, et al. Artificial intelligence for prediction of Covid-19 progression using ct imaging and clinical data. *European Radiology*, 32(1):205–212, 2022.

[49] Qingpeng Zhang, Jianxi Gao, Joseph T Wu, Zhidong Cao, and Daniel Dajun Zeng. Data science approaches to confronting the Covid-19 pandemic: a narrative review. *Philosophical Transactions of the Royal Society A*, 380(2214):20210127, 2022.

Chapter 8

Biomedical named entity recognition using natural language processing

Shaina Raza
University of Toronto

Syed Raza Bashir
Ryerson University

Vidhi Thakkar
University of Victoria

Usman Naseem
The University of Sydney

CONTENTS

8.1 INTRODUCTION

In the last few years, there has been a dramatic increase in biomedical articles and resources. There are many scientific articles related

DOI: 10.1201/9781003368342-8

to biomedical research published daily in various journals (Tsatsaronis et al. 2012). For example, MEDLINE, a large-scale resource for medical articles, contains around 28 million articles (MEDLINE 2021). This expansion of biomedical information necessitates large-scale management to provide biomedical knowledge to the research community on time. Recently, due to the surge of COVID-19, there are thousands of articles get published in just 2 years, which are also accessible through CORD-19 (Lu Wang et al. 2020), LitCOVID (Chen et al. 2021a), and other initiatives (Wang and Lo 2021; Chen et al. 2021b; Raza et al. 2022). Researchers find it hard to manage such a gigantic amount of unstructured text data that is exponentially increasing and to transform it into refined knowledge (Campos et al. 2012). As a result, efficient and accurate natural language processing (NLP) techniques are becoming increasingly important for use in computational data analysis, and advanced text mining techniques are required to analyse biomedical literature and extract useful information from the texts automatically.

In addition to an increase in scholarly literature, there has been an increase in electronic health record (EHR) data in recent years (Meystre et al. 2010). An unusually high hospitalization rate during COVID-19 has also increased the EHR data (Estiri et al. 2021). An EHR is an electronic version of a patient's medical history, which may include patient conditions, medications, demographics, past medical history, and laboratory radiology reports (Schulte 2009). These EHRs also contain detailed information about the patients, such as personal information, medical history, and social status. To protect patients' privacy, the patients' records should be de-identified (Kushida et al. 2012).

In the biomedical domain, a fundamental task of named entity recognition (NER) is the recognition of named entities, such as genes, diseases, species, chemicals, drug names, and related entity types (Cho and Lee 2019). Biomedical NER (BioNER) can play a critical role in a variety of downstream NLP tasks, including information extraction, question answering, drug-drug interaction analysis, and gene identification among others (Rebholz-Schuhmann et al. 2010; Efroni et al. 2020). The state-of-the-art work (Lee et al. 2020; Efroni et al. 2020) in BioNER mostly focus on limited named entities. Different from previous works, we intend to use advanced computational methods to automatically identify numerous types of clinical entities from texts. We also aim to de-identify the patients' records in such a way that re-establishing a link between the individual and his or her data becomes difficult.

This study aims to propose an end-to-end solution for identifying clinically named entities from the biomedical text. We propose a trainable BioNER pipeline that leverages many components, such as a preprocessor and tokenizer to prepare the data into a readable format; an embedding lookup component that can load any pre-trained embedding models; a state-of-the-art model based on Bidirectional Long Short-Term Memory (Bi-LSTM) with Convolution Neural Network (CNN) and Conditional Random Field (CRF) for the task of NER; and a de-identifier to de-identify patients' personal information; all these components are stacked together to train the pipeline to support new entity types with no code change. Our goal is to help provide better patient care by identifying clinical entities associated with patients' data and to help improve overall population health by assisting researchers, clinicians, and biomedical experts in analysing biomedical data on time without going into the extensive details of sifting through the text data. The specific contributions of this work are as:

1. We propose and develop an accessible BioNER pipeline that is focused on identifying clinically named entities from biomedical text-based data. We aim to consolidate and explain essential Machine Learning (ML) best practices as well as to provide a complete pipeline with numerous convenient features that can be used as it is or as a starting point for further customization and improvement.
2. We organize this pipeline for the following basic stages including data pre-processing, tokenization, and feature transformation; embedding lookup to load any pre-trained embedding models; NER modelling and de-identification of the patients' personal information.
3. We demonstrate the efficacy and utility of this pipeline by comparing it with the state-of-the-art methods on public benchmark datasets. We also describe how to apply this pipeline to documents from the CORD-19 dataset.

The rest of the chapter is organized as: Section 8.2 is the related work; Section 8.3 is the methodology; Section 8.4 is the experimental setup; Section 8.5 is the results and analysis, and Section 8.6 is the conclusion.

8.2 RELATED WORK

The related work section is discussed here.

Named entity recognition (NER): NER is the task of identifying a named entity (a real-world object or concept) in unstructured text and then classifying the entity into a standard category (Nadeau and Sekine 2007). Traditional NER methods only consider names, places, and organizations. However, there can be more entities, depending on the domain being used. In the last few years, there has been a dramatic increase in biomedical data. There are many new articles related to biomedical research published daily in various journals (Tsatsaronis et al. 2012). This expansion of biomedical information necessitates large-scale management to provide knowledge in a timely manner. Recently, as a result of COVID-19, there has been a massive increase in biomedical data that is difficult to read, even more so when the urgency of time and the surge of patients are increasing exponentially. Due to the critical nature of comprehending and fully utilizing this biomedical data, several NLP tasks are initiated. These tasks include Biomedical Question Answering (Tsatsaronis et al. 2012), CORD-19 challenge (Allen Institute 2020; Ngai et al. 2021), and TREC-COVID challenge (Voorhees et al. 2020). To perform these tasks, it is, therefore, necessary to accommodate a prior process of BioNER. BioNER is the task of identifying named entities in the biomedical domain, such as diseases, proteins, viruses, disorders, drugs, or so. The existing BioNER methods (Nadeau and Sekine 2007; Goyal et al. 2018; Efroni et al. 2020) mainly focus on general approaches to named entities that are not specific to the biomedical field. On the other hand, there are some works (Leser and Hakenberg 2005; Eltyeb and Salim 2014; Lee et al. 2020; Saad et al. 2020) that focus solely on clinical NER, which is also a motivation for this research.

De-identification of patients' records: According to a 2016 survey, nearly 95% of eligible hospitals in the United States use an EHR (Toscano et al. 2018); with that figure expected to rise by 2022. The standard EHRs contain 18 categories of critical private information about patients (e.g., name, age, and address), which must be removed before they are made public, as required by the Health Insurance Portability and Accountability Act (HIPPA) (Fernández-Calienes 2013). De-identification is the process of removing sensitive information from EHRs (Meystre et al. 2010). For the de-identification purpose, researchers used a variety of methods, including rule-based methods, machine learning-based methods, and hybrid methods that combine both approaches. Researchers used rule-based methods to match common patterns in patients' records by manually curating rules and using medical vocabularies (Meystre et al. 2010). The rules were usually implemented using regular expressions.

Research in BioNER and de-identification: The majority of studies employ de-identification as a task of the BioNER task (Fabregat et al. 2019) in which first the patient-related entities are identified and are then de-identified. The CRF models (Lafferty et al. 2001), and Structured Support Vector (SVM) (Tsochantaridis et al. 2005) are some of the commonly used models for NER tasks and for the de-identification of patients' records. In recent years, deep learning models have been applied to BioNER and patient de-identification tasks, which achieve better performance in the clinical domain (Yang et al. 2019). Deep learning models based on recurrent neural networks (RNN) and CNN models (Raza and Ding 2021) are also used for biomedical named entities and de-identification of clinical notes (Yang et al. 2019). In this work, we also use deep learning-based methods to build a pipeline for the BioNER task, which additionally includes a component for the de-identification of patients' records.

8.3 METHODOLOGY

In this study, we propose and develop a BioNER pipeline that takes raw data as input, pre-processes it, and applies ML techniques to recognize and classify clinical entities into predefined classes (such as disease disorder, diagnosis, medication dosage, symptoms, etc.). We build this pipeline[1] following the Spark ML pipeline format, which provides a default solution to scalable solutions without requiring much computation power (Kocaman and Talby 2021). Our goal is to automate

[1] https://spark.apache.org/docs/latest/ml-pipeline.html.

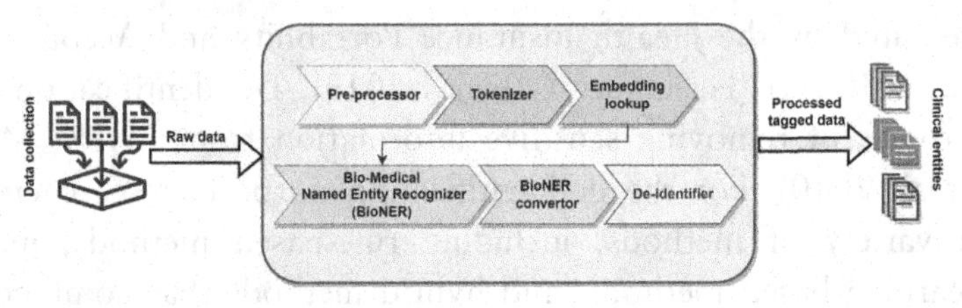

Figure 8.1 BioNer pipeline.

the ML workflow by allowing data to be transformed into a model (or a set of multiple models) that can be analysed to achieve outputs. The workflow of this pipeline is shown in Figure 8.1.

Next, we explain each phase of this pipeline:

> *Data collection:* The input to the model is the data that can be collected from different sources. In this work, we input some benchmark biomedical datasets and a portion of the latest publications data from the CORD-19 (Allen Institute 2020) source. We discuss datasets in Section 8.4.

8.3.1 BioNER pipeline

We develop a pipeline that consists of various components, each of which represents a stage in the pipeline. Each component inputs the text data performs some processing (either training or data transformation) and then produces an output. These components are discussed next:

> *Pre-processor:* The pre-processor takes an input of the raw data obtained through the data collection phase, pre-processes it, detects the sentence boundaries in each record (document) and then transforms the data into the format that is readable by the next stage (i.e., tokenizer) in the pipeline. Transforming the data means adding a new column containing the result of the current stage without modifying or replacing the current information. The output from the pre-processor is the set of records that are pre-processed.
>
> *Tokenizer:* The pre-processed data from the pre-processor goes into the tokenizer. Tokenization is the process of breaking the input text into smaller chunks (words, or sentences) called tokens (Webster and Kit 1992). These tokens aid in comprehending the context and in developing the NLP model. The output from the tokenizer

is transformed data, containing the tokens (words in this work) corresponding to each document.

Embedding lookup component: The tokenized data from the tokenizer goes into the embedding lookup component, which maps tokens to vectors. We have used the word embeddings from the BlueBERT model (https://github.com/ncbi-nlp/bluebert) that is trained on PubMed abstracts and MIMIC-III. This component can download any pre-trained model (such as Glove, BERT, BioBERT) for embeddings, which can be used in the next phase (BioNER) in the pipeline.

Bio-Medical Named Entity *Recognizer (BioNER)*: BioNER is a component that identifies clinical entities in the text. We introduce our BioNER model in Figure 8.2 and explain its work below.

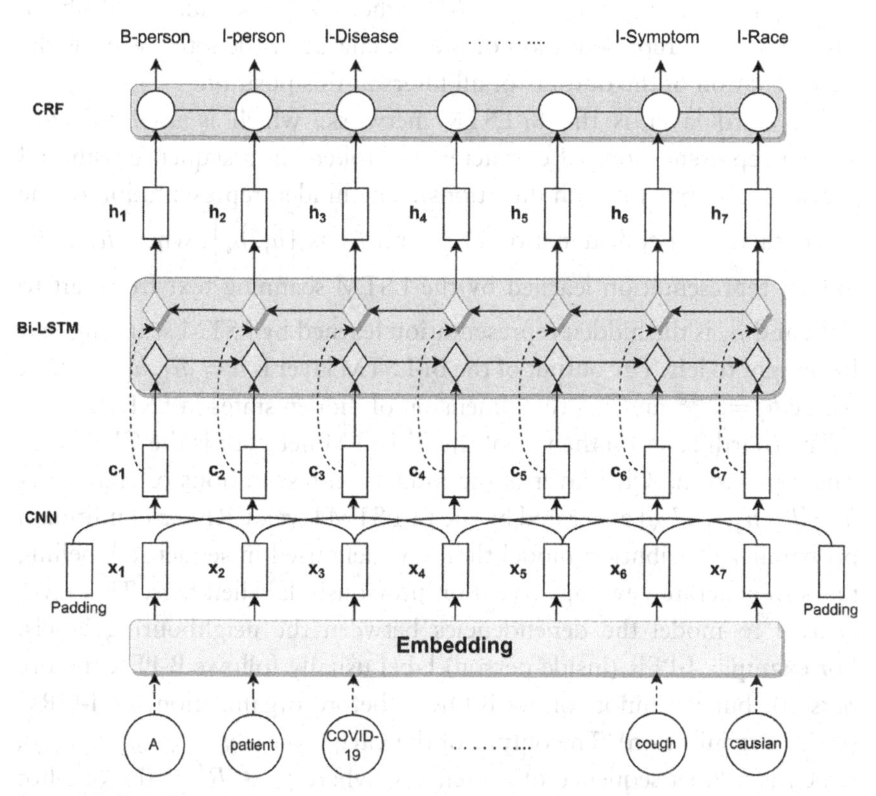

Figure 8.2 BioNER model.

As shown in Figure 8.2, the BioNER takes as input the sequence of words as $s = [w_1, w_2, \dots, w_N]$, where N is the sentence length and $w_i \in R^V$ is the one-hot representation of the ith character in the sequence. This input goes to the character embedding layer.

The embedding layer is the first layer in the model that converts a sentence from a sequence of characters into a sequence of dense vectors. In this work, we use the pre-trained embeddings that are loaded and provided by the embedding lookup component in the pipeline. The output of this layer is a sequence of vectors $x = [x_1, x_2, \dots, x_N]$, where $x_i = Ew_i \in R^D$, E is for embedding and x_i is the into a dense vector representation of w_i.

The second layer in this model is a CNN network that is used to capture local information within the given words in biomedical contexts. Each position in the sequence has sliding windows, and CNN performs a transformation for each sliding window. The output of the CNN layer is $c = [c_1, c_2, \dots, c_N]$, where $c_i \in R^M$, where M is the number of filters. The contextual representation of the ith, character (denoted as c_i) is the concatenation of the outputs of all filters at this position.

The third layer is the Bi-LSTM network, which is used to learn hidden representations of characters for tokens in a sequence using all previous contexts (in both directions). The hidden representation of the ith character is a concatenation of $\vec{h}_i$ and $\overleftarrow{h}_i$ as $\left[\vec{h}_i, \overleftarrow{h}_i\right]$, where $\vec{h}_i$ is the hidden representation learned by the LSTM scanning text from left to right and $\overleftarrow{h}_i$ is the hidden representation learned by LSTM scanning text from right to left. The output of the Bi-LSTM layer is $h = [h_1, h_2, \dots, h_N]$, where $h_i = R^{2S}$ and S is the dimension of hidden states in LSTM.

The fourth layer on the top of the Bi-LSTM network is the CRF layer. The input to the CRF layer is the hidden representations of characters $h = [h_1, h_2, \dots, h_N]$ generated by the Bi-LSTM layer. CRF is a conditional probability distribution model that is widely used in sequence labelling tasks to generate new tags based on previously labelled tags. This layer is used to model the dependencies between the neighbouring labels. For example, I-PER (inside person) label usually follows B-PER (before person), but it cannot follow B-ORG (before organization) or I-ORG (inside organization). The output of the CRF layer is $y = [y_1, y_2, \dots, y_N]$, which is a label sequence of sentence s, where $y_i \in R^L$ is the one-hot representation of the ith character's label and L is the number of labels. In this work, the clinical entities are the labels.

In the training procedure, we use the negative loglikelihood function over all training samples to calculate the loss function $\mathcal{L}$, which can be formulated as:

$$\mathcal{L}_{\text{BioNER}} = -\sum_{s \in S} \log \left(p \left(y_s | h_s; \, \theta \right) \right)$$

where p is the probability, θ is the parameter set, S is the set of sentences in training data, y_s and h_s are the hidden representations and label sequence of sentence *s* respectively.

BioNER converter: This annotator converts an inside-outside-beginning (IOB) format representation of named entities to a user-friendly representation, by associating the tokens of recognized entities and their label. IOB (Hacioglu et al. 2004) is a common method for formatting tags in chunking tasks such as named entity recognition. The output from this annotator is the 'chunk'. A chunk is a tagged portion of the sentence into named entities.

De-identifier: In this component, we employ the data obfuscation technique, which is a process that obscures the meaning of data (Bakken et al. 2004). For example, to replace identified names with different fake names or to mask some data value. This component provides the HIPPA (Nosowsky and Giordano 2006) compliance when dealing with text documents that may contain protected health information. We use the pre-trained de-identification model inside the pipeline to de-identify the personal records of the patients.

8.3.2 Clinical entities

The output of the pipeline is the clinical entities. In this work, we incorporate the following clinical entities that we collected after analysing the pertinent literature (Caufield et al. 2019; Johnson et al. 2016):

Admission (patient admission status), oncology (tumour/cancer), blood pressure, respiration (e.g., shortness of breath), dosage (amount of medicine/drug taken), diet (food type, nutrients, minerals), alcohol, smoking, vital signs, symptom, kidney disease, temperature (body), diabetes, vaccine, time (days, weeks or so), obesity (status), pregnancy, BMI, height (of the patient), heart disease, pulse, hypertension, drug name, hyperlipidaemia, date, cerebrovascular disease, disease, syndrome

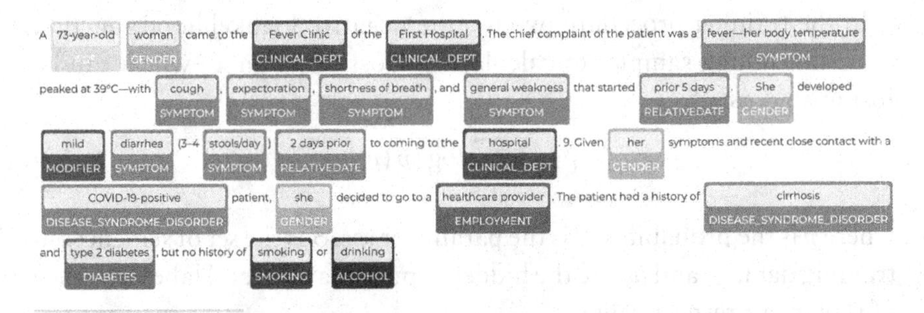

Figure 8.3 The clinical entities recognized by BioNER pipeline.

index	sentence	deidentified
0	A 73-year-old woman came to the Fever Clinic of the First Hospital.	A 73-year-old woman came to the Fever Clinic of the GENESYS REGIONAL MEDICAL CENTER - HEALTH PARK.
1	The name of patient is Oliveira who lives in Cocke County Baptist Hospital .	The name of patient is Rayna Buttery who lives in CHRISTUS MOTHER FRANCES HOSPITAL - SULPHUR SPRINGS .
2	0295 Keats Street.	P.O. Box 101.
3	Phone 111-347-837.	Phone 06435 14 64 15.

Figure 8.4 De-identification of patient record.

disorder, symptom, treatment, clinical department, name (patient), age (of the patient), relative date, weight (of the patient), admission or discharge (from the hospital), gender, modifier (modifies the current state).

Sample Prediction: A sample prediction from one COVID-19 document taken from our dataset is shown in Figure 8.3.

As shown in Figure 8.3, we identify many clinical entities from the given text. We also show the de-identification of personal information in Figure 8.4).

8.4 EXPERIMENTS

8.4.1 Datasets

In this study, we train our BioNER pipeline on the following datasets as shown in Table 8.1.

Except for the CORD-19 dataset, which we manually prepared for the NER task, all other datasets are publicly available benchmark datasets. These datasets JNLPBA are NCBI Disease, which can be obtained from

Table 8.1 Datasets used in this work

Dataset	*Entity type*	*Sentences*	*Annotations*	*Data size*
JNLPBA (Collier and Kim 2004)	Gene/proteins	22,562	35,336	2,404 abstracts
NCBI disease (Dogan et al. 2014)	Disease	7,639	6,881	793 abstracts
CORD-19 (Lu Wang et al. 2020)	Manually annotated	~20,000	~2,500	10k collected publications, 500 annotated

here. These datasets are already in the IOB scheme for encoding entity annotations as token tags. However, we further process these datasets to prepare in CONLL-2003 format.[2] We also prepare our CORD-19 dataset in CONLL format for the training purpose.

CORD-19 dataset preparation: COVID-19 Open Research Dataset (CORD-19) (Lu Wang et al. 2020) is an open-access repository of tens of thousands of research publications on COVID-19, SARS-CoV-2, and related coronaviruses for use by the global academic community. The dataset was first released on March 16, 2020, and is updated on daily basis. In this work, we collect a sample of 10,000 publications on COVID-19 chronologically arranged by date. We obtain these files in Portable Document Format (PDF) and parse and convert the text from each document to generate a textual representation for each document. We annotate around 500 parsed documents from CORD-19 using the clinical entities (mentioned in Section 8.3.2) using the JohnSnowLabs annotation tool[3] and prepare it in the CONLL (Tjong Kim Sang and de Meulder 2003) format.

We have divided all datasets into training, validation, and test sets, with a 75:15:15 ratio for all experiments. We used the Stratified 5-Folds cross-validation (CV) strategy for train/test split if original datasets do not have an official train/test split.

[2] https://docs.allennlp.org/main/api/data/dataset_readers/conll2003/.
[3] https://www.johnsnowlabs.com/annotation-lab/.

Table 8.2 Baseline methods used in this work

Method	*Description*
SciSpacy	A python library that offers biomedical natural language, processing models. We use the full spaCy pipeline[4] for biomedical data with ~785k vocabulary and allenai/scibert-base as the transformer model
BioBert	A pre-trained biomedical language model for biomedical text mining. We use the BioBert-based-cased v1.0[1] that is pre-trained on 200k PubMed articles
Stanza	Stanza offers NER functionality with native python support. We use the biomedical pipeline of[5] Stanza that are already trained on all the benchmark datasets (mentioned above) and can detect diseases, chemical, genes, etc.

[1] https://github.com/dmis-lab/biobert.

8.4.2 Evaluation metrics

Following the standard practice (Chen et al. 2015; Tsai et al. 2006) to evaluate NER tasks, we use the following metrics:

- *Micro-average F1-score measures the F1-score of aggregated contributions of all classes.*
- *Macro-average F1-score adds all the measures (Precision, Recall, or F-Measure) and divides with the number of labels, which is more like an average.*

8.4.3 Baseline methods for comparison

We compare our BioNER pipeline approach against the following state-of-the-art baseline methods shown in Table 8.2.

All of the baselines are trained on the aforementioned datasets. The experimental results are based on the optimal hyperparameter setting and the best results for each baseline.

8.4.4 Experimental setup and hyperparameters

We use PyTorch for the model implementation. We also use the Spark NLP pipeline to build our biomedical pipeline. We run our experiments on Google Colab Pro[6] (NVIDIA P100 or T4, 24 GB RAM, 2 x vCPU)

4 https://s3-us-west-2.amazonaws.com/ai2-s2-scispacy/releases/v0.5.0/en_core_sci_scibert-0.5.0.tar.gz.
5 https://stanfordnlp.github.io/stanza/available_biomed_models.html.
6 https://colab.research.google.com/.

Table 8.3 Hyperparameters used

Hyperparameter	*Optimal value (values used)*
Learning rate	1.E-03 (1.E-02, 1.E-03, 1.E-05, 2.E-05, 5.E-05, 3.E-04)
Batch size	64 (8, 16, 32, 64, 128)
Epochs	30 ({2, 3, ..., 30})
LSTM state size	200 (200, 250)
Dropout rate	0.5 ({0.3, 0.35, ..., 0.7})
Optimizer	Adam
Embedding dimension	768
CNN filters	2 (2,3,4,5)

and used Apache Spark NLP in local mode (no cluster) to integrate the components of the ML pipeline.

In this work, we try different pre-trained embedding methods in the embedding lookup component, such as glove_100d,[7] word2vec[8] embeddings and BERT-based embeddings and find better performance with BlueBERT embeddings (Peng et al. 2019), so we use this pre-trained model in our pipeline.

We specify the following set of hyperparameters in Table 8.3, with optimal hyperparameter value and values within the parenthesis represent the parameter ranges tested. We use Grid search to get the optimal values for the hyperparameters. We also use early stopping to overcome possible overfitting.

8.5 RESULTS AND ANALYSIS

The results and analysis are given below.

8.5.1 Comparison with baseline methods

We report the Marco-average F1 (macro) and Micro-average F1 (micro) scores on each dataset in Table 8.4. The best scores are in bold.

Overall, these results show that our BioNER approach achieves state-of-the-art performance on public biomedical benchmarks (NCBI Disease, JNLPDP) as well as on a new dataset designed specifically for biomedical named entities. This demonstrates the generalizability of our

7 https://nlp.stanford.edu/projects/glove/.
8 https://fasttext.cc/docs/en/english-vectors.html.

Table 8.4 Test results on all datasets using different methods

Methods	*Metric*	*Datasets*		
		NCBI (disease)	JNLPDP (gene/proteins)	Our dataset (36 entities)
SciSpacy	Micro	81.15	77.13	76.23
	Macro	82.13	80.65	78.29
Stanza	Micro	83.32	79.23	81.23
	Macro	84.12	83.56	78.10
BioBERT	Micro	88.52	79.39	86.27
	Macro	85.89	87.18	87.78
BioNER (ours)	Micro	91.12	87.13	91.34
	Macro	92.14	88.01	92.78

pipeline across different domains. The superiority of this approach is attributed to its pipeline design, which consists of various components and phases, such as different data pre-processing, tokenization, and embedding lookup prior to the BioNER stage.

Our approach achieves the best micro F1 score of 91.34 on our dataset (36 entities), 91.12 on NCBI Disease (disease entity), and 87.13 on JNLPDP (gene/proteins) dataset. We see similar patterns of highest performance by our pipeline for macro F1 scores.

The BioBERT model also shows a competitive performance (after our model) in these results. Overall, we observe that BioBERT achieves better micro F1 and macro F1 scores on disease entities (NCBI), followed gene/proteins entities (JNLPDP). The better performance of BioBERT attributes to its training method, which is trained on PubMed abstracts. In this work, we use the BlueBERT embedding pre-trained on PubMed abstracts and clinical notes (MIMIC-III), which shows at least 1%–2% better results than BioBERT pre-trained on PubMed abstracts.

The default biomedical pipeline of Stanza (as mentioned in the original paper (Zhang et al. 2021)) is trained on many datasets listed here.[9] We also observe that Stanza performs better in identifying many diseases and gene/protein entities. In our experiments, Stanza performs better than SciSpacy. SciSpacy is pre-trained on SciBERT (Beltagy et al. 2020), that's why its performance is somehow compromised on the biomedical entities, however, it still achieves a performance above 75% in these experiments. Our BioNER approach performs better than Stanza, but Stanza performs better than SciSpacy. SciSpacy's relatively lower

9 https://stanfordnlp.github.io/stanza/available_biomed_models.html.

performance here could be attributed to the fact that it does not cover as much training and inference on biomedical entities as Stanza. However, because our pipeline is quite generic, it is quite possible to train it on any named entity type. As a result, it performs better with almost every dataset that is used to train the BioNER model. In comparison to previous research, our method is capable of recognising a wide variety of clinical entity types.

8.5.2 Human evaluation

We conduct a human baseline to determine the efficacy of our pipeline on the datasets. We randomly selected 20 documents from each dataset. Two medical doctors were asked to manually annotate the named entities on the documents independently. Since accuracy and F1 score do not take into account the expected chance agreement, so we choose Cohen's kappa coefficient (Scarpellini 2020) which measures the agreement between two annotators who classify N items into mutually exclusive categories.

Cohen's kappa coefficient from our annotation, based on 20 shared documents between the annotators was 0.898, which according to Cohen is a very strong level of agreement. From these human evaluation scores, we infer that our approach can provide clinically informative and human-like response.

8.5.3 Effectiveness of the BioNER on CORD-19 data

We show the most frequent five clinical entity types predicted through parsing 100 CORD-19 documents using our approach and show results in Table 8.5.

As can be seen in Table 8.5, we can get some valuable information regarding the most frequent clinical entities, such as diseases, symptoms, and drugs, as mentioned in COVID-19-related publications. According

Table 8.5 Most used clinical entities from random 100 case reports

Admission	*Drug*	*Heart disease*	*Disease*	*Symptom*
Admission	Antibiotics	Acute	Coronavirus	Cough
Admitted	Dobutamine	Bi-ventricular	Cardiogenic	Cold
Hospitalized	Oseltamivir	Cardiogenic	COVID-19	Flu
Pre-admission	Fluids	ESC	Gastroenteritis	Abdominal
Discharged	Saline	ECG	Hepatitis	Critically ill

to this table, the most common symptom is cough and cold while the most common diseases mentioned is a coronavirus and cardiogenic.

8.5.4 Application of proposed research to the health care professionals and policymakers

The implications of these findings to the field of health sciences are multi-factorial. For example, these types of clinical evaluation scores and human evaluation scores can help doctors, nurses, and other healthcare professionals align symptoms to diagnosis, treatment, and follow-up. Human and computer interactions have been studied by many health services researchers and data scientists to characterize the true value of medical records for clinical implications (Bologva et al. 2017). As the field of NLP advances, there are also opportunities for policymakers to understand the value that is within electronic medical records and clinical records to understand the cost-effectiveness and cost-saving implications of health systems planning. For example, having an idea of the number of clinically informative, human diagnoses within a population can help health systems design in planning a healthy human workforce. If it is known that there is a city or area with an increased area of cardiopathies, then policymakers can ensure that hospitals have a stable budget to hire interventional cardiologists.

Tracking health disparities can also lead to the reduction of inequities through NLP. For example, multiple research studies have shown that the application of NLP in the health sciences has led to a reduction of bias and enabled better science (Farley et al. 2020; Brakefield et al. 2021). While this originates from the field of Computer Science more broadly, NLP and the development of pipelines to predict clinical entities is a valuable next step in advancing the frontier in innovative data sciences research. The field of data science has advanced significantly in a learning health system, where data practices translate into knowledge, evidence, and clinical impact. Further research is required to better understand and evaluate the dataset.

8.6 CONCLUSION

In conclusion, this chapter presents BioNER pipeline, an approach to train models for the clinically named entity using the Bi-LSTM-CNN-CRF model plus BERT-based embeddings. This chapter shows that using contextualized word embedding pre-trained on biomedical corpora significantly improves the results of BioNER tasks. We evaluated the performance of BioNER on five datasets (two benchmark datasets and one of our own) and our approach achieves the state-of-the-art results compared to the baselines. Further through human evaluation, we conclude that the predicted entities are accurate, informative, and clinical. For future study, we plan to train our pipeline with a big annotated biomedical corpus. For this, we plan to annotate our dataset in large numbers to train the model.

REFERENCES

Allen Institute. 2020. "COVID-19 Open Research Dataset Challenge (CORD-19)." *Semantic Scholar*. https://www.kaggle.com/datasets/allen-institute-for-ai/CORD-19-research-challenge.

Bakken, David E., R. Rarameswaran, Douglas M. Blough, Andy A. Franz, and Ty J. Palmer. 2004. "Data Obfuscation: Anonymity and Desensitization of Usable Data Sets." *IEEE Security & Privacy* 2(6), 34–41.

Beltagy, Iz, Kyle Lo, and Arman Cohan. 2020. "SCIBERT: A Pretrained Language Model for Scientific Text." In *EMNLP-IJCNLP 2019-2019 Conference on Empirical Methods in Natural Language Processing and 9th International Joint Conference on Natural Language Processing, Proceedings of the Conference*, pp. 3615–3620. doi:10.18653/v1/d19-1371.

Bologva, Ekaterina V, Diana I Prokusheva, Alexey V Krikunov, Nadezhda E Zvartau, and Sergey V Kovalchuk. 2017. "Human-Computer Interaction in Electronic Medical Records: From the Perspectives of Physicians and Data Scientists." *Procedia Computer Science* 121, 469–474.

Boudjellal, Nada, Huaping Zhang, Asif Khan, Arshad Ahmad, Rashid Naseem, Jianyun Shang, and Lin Dai. 2021. "ABioNER: A BERT-Based Model for Arabic Biomedical Named-Entity Recognition." *Complexity* 2021. doi:10.1155/2021/6633213.

Brakefield, Whitney S, Nariman Ammar, Olufunto A Olusanya, and Arash Shaban-Nejad. 2021. "An Urban Population Health Observatory System to Support COVID-19 Pandemic Preparedness, Response, and Management: Design and Development Study." *JMIR Public Health and Surveillance* 7(6). doi:10.2196/28269.

Campos, David, Sérgio Matos, and José Luis Oliveira. 2012. "Biomedical Named Entity Recognition: A Survey of Machine-Learning Tools." In: Shigeaki Sakurai (Ed.), *Theory and Applications for Advanced Text Mining*. InTech: Rijeka, Croatia, pp. 175–195.

Caufield, J Harry, Yichao Zhou, Yunsheng Bai, David A Liem, Anders O Garlid, Kai-Wei Chang, Yizhou Sun, Peipei Ping, and Wei Wang. 2019. "A Comprehensive Typing System for Information Extraction from Clinical Narratives." MedRxiv, 19009118. https://www.medrxiv.org/content/10.1101/19009118v1%0Ahttp://files/803/.

Chen, Qingyu, Alexis Allot, and Zhiyong Lu. 2021a. "LitCovid: An Open Database of COVID-19 Literature." *Nucleic Acids Research* 49(D1), D1534–D1540. doi:10.1093/nar/gkaa952.

Chen, Qingyu, Robert Leaman, Alexis Allot, Ling Luo, Chih-Hsuan Wei, Shankai Yan, and Zhiyong Lu. 2021b. "Artificial Intelligence in Action: Addressing the COVID-19 Pandemic with Natural Language Processing." *Annual Review of Biomedical Data Science* 4(1), 313–339. doi:10.1146/annurev-biodatasci-021821-061045.

Chen, Yukun, Thomas A Lasko, Qiaozhu Mei, Joshua C Denny, and Hua Xu. 2015. "A Study of Active Learning Methods for Named Entity Recognition in Clinical Text." *Journal of Biomedical Informatics* 58, 11–18. doi:10.1016/j.jbi.2015.09.010.

Cho, Hyejin, and Hyunju Lee. 2019. "Biomedical Named Entity Recognition Using Deep Neural Networks with Contextual Information." *BMC Bioinformatics* 20(1), 1–11. doi: 10.1186/s12859-019-3321-4.

Collier, Nigel and Jin-Dong Kim. 2004. "Introduction to the Bio-Entity Recognition Task at JNLPBA." In *Proceedings of the International Joint Workshop on Natural Language Processing in Biomedicine and Its Applications (NLP-BA/BioNLP)*, Geneva, Switzerland, pp. 73–78.

Doğan, Rezarta Islamaj, Robert Leaman, and Zhiyong Lu. 2014. "NCBI Disease Corpus: A Resource for Disease Name Recognition and Concept Normalization." *Journal of Biomedical Informatics* 47, 1–10. doi: 10.1016/j.jbi.2013.12.006.

Efroni, Sol, Min Song, Vincent Labatut, Frank Emmert-Streib, Nadeesha Perera, and Matthias Dehmer. 2020. "Named Entity Recognition and Relation Detection for Biomedical Information Extraction." *Frontiers in Cell and Developmental Biology* 1, 673. doi: 10.3389/fcell.2020.00673.

Eltyeb, Safaa, and Naomie Salim. 2014. "Chemical Named Entities Recognition: A Review on Approaches and Applications." *Journal of Cheminformatics* 6(1), 1–12.

Estiri, Hossein, Zachary H Strasser, Jeffy G Klann, Pourandokht Naseri, Kavishwar B Wagholikar, and Shawn N Murphy. 2021. "Predicting COVID-19 Mortality with Electronic Medical Records." *NPJ Digital Medicine* 4(1). doi: 10.1038/s41746-021-00383-x.

Fabregat, Hermenegildo, Andres Duque, Juan Martinez-Romo, and Lourdes Araujo. 2019. "De-Identification through Named Entity Recognition for Medical Document Anonymization." In *CEUR Workshop Proceedings*, vol. 2421, pp. 663–670.

Farley, John H, Jeffrey Hines, Nita K Lee, Sandra E Brooks, Navya Nair, Carol L Brown, Kemi M Doll, Ellen J Sullivan, and Eloise Chapman-Davis. 2020. "Clinical Practice Statement Promoting Health Equity in the Era of COVID-19." *Gynecologic Oncology* 158, 25–31. doi: 10.1016/j.ygyno.2020.05.023.

Fernández-Calienes, Raúl. 2013. "Health Insurance Portability and Accountability Act of 1996." *Encyclopedia of the Fourth Amendment*. doi: 10.4135/9781452234243.n359.

Goyal, Archana, Vishal Gupta, and Manish Kumar. 2018. "Recent Named Entity Recognition and Classification Techniques: A Systematic Review." *Computer Science Review* 29, 21–43.

Hacioglu, Kadri, Sameer Pradhan, Wayne Ward, James H Martin, and Dan Jurafsky. 2004. "Semantic Role Labeling by Tagging Syntactic Chunks." In *Proceedings of the Eighth Conference on Computational Natural Language Learning (CoNLL-2004)* at HLT-NAACL 2004, pp. 110–113.

Johnson, Alistair E W, Tom J Pollard, Lu Shen, Li Wei H Lehman, Mengling Feng, Mohammad Ghassemi, Benjamin Moody, Peter Szolovits, Leo Anthony Celi, and Roger G Mark. 2016. "MIMIC-III, a Freely Accessible Critical Care Database." *Scientific Data* 3. doi: 10.1038/sdata.2016.35.

Kocaman, Veysel, and David Talby. 2021. "Spark NLP: Natural Language Understanding at Scale." *Software Impacts* 8, 100058.

Kushida, Clete A, Deborah A Nichols, Rik Jadrnicek, Ric Miller, James K Walsh, and Kara Griffin. 2012. "Strategies for De-Identification and Anonymization of Electronic Health Record Data for Use in Multicenter Research Studies." *Medical Care* 50, S82.

Lafferty, John, Andrew Mccallum, and Fernando Pereira. 2001. "Conditional Random Fields : Probabilistic Models for Segmenting and Labeling Sequence Data Abstract." In *Proceedings of the Eighteenth International Conference on Machine Learning*, San Francisco, CA, pp. 282–289.

Lee, Jinhyuk, Wonjin Yoon, Sungdong Kim, Donghyeon Kim, Sunkyu Kim, Chan Ho So, and Jaewoo Kang. 2020. "BioBERT: A Pre-Trained Biomedical Language Representation Model for Biomedical Text Mining." *Bioinformatics* 36(4), 1234–1240. doi: 10.1093/bioinformatics/btz682.

Leser, Ulf, and Jörg Hakenberg. 2005. "What Makes a Gene Name? Named Entity Recognition in the Biomedical Literature." *Briefings in Bioinformatics* 6(4), 357–369.

Lu Wang, Lucy, Kyle Lo, Yoganand Chandrasekhar, Russell Reas, Jiangjiang Yang, Darrin Eide, Kathryn Funk, et al. 2020. CORD-19: The *Covid-19 Open Research Dataset. ArXiv.* http://www.ncbi.nlm.nih.gov/pubmed/32510522/; http://www.pubmedcentral.nih.gov/articlerender.fcgi?artid=PMC7251955/.

Ma, Xuezhe, and Eduard Hovy. 2016. "End-to-End Sequence Labeling via Bi-Directional Lstm-Cnns-Crf." ArXiv Preprint ArXiv:1603.01354.

MEDLINE. 2021. "MEDLINE Overview." *U.S. National Library of Medicine.* https://www.nlm.nih.gov/medline/medline_overview.html; https://www.nlm.nih. gov/.

Meystre, Stephane M, F Jeffrey Friedlin, Brett R South, Shuying Shen, and Matthew H Samore. 2010. "Automatic De-Identification of Textual Documents in the Electronic Health Record: A Review of Recent Research." *BMC Medical Research Methodology* 10(1), 1–16.

Nadeau, David, and Satoshi Sekine. 2007. "A Survey of Named Entity Recognition and Classification." *Lingvisticae Investigationes* 30(1), 3–26.

Naseem, Usman, Imran Razzak, Matloob Khushi, Peter W Eklund, and Jinman Kim. 2021a. "Covidsenti: A Large-Scale Benchmark Twitter Data Set for COVID-19 Sentiment Analysis." *IEEE Transactions on Computational Social Systems* 99, 1–13.

Naseem, Usman, Matloob Khushi, Vinay Reddy, Sakthivel Rajendran, Imran Razzak, and Jinman Kim. 2021b. "Bioalbert: A Simple and Effective Pre-Trained Language Model for Biomedical Named Entity Recognition." In *2021 International Joint Conference on Neural Networks (IJCNN)*, pp. 1–7.

Ngai, Hillary, Yoona Park, John Chen, and Mahboobeh Parsapoor. 2021. "Transformer-Based Models for Question Answering on COVID19," 1–7. http://arxiv.org/abs/2101.11432.

Nosowsky, Rachel, and Thomas J Giordano. 2006. "The Health Insurance Portability and Accountability Act of 1996 (HIPAA) Privacy Rule: Implications for Clinical Research." *Annual Reviews*, 57, 575–590.

Peng, Yifan, Shankai Yan, and Zhiyong Lu. 2019. "Transfer Learning in Biomedical Natural Language Processing: An Evaluation of BERT and ELMo on Ten Benchmarking Datasets." ArXiv Preprint ArXiv:1906.05474.

Raza, Shaina, and Chen Ding. 2021. "News Recommender System: A Review of Recent Progress, Challenges, and Opportunities." *Artificial Intelligence Review* 55, 749–800. doi: 10.1007/s10462-021-10043-x.

Raza, S., Schwartz, B. & Rosella, L.C. "CoQUAD: a COVID-19 question answering dataset system, facilitating research, benchmarking, and practice." *BMC Bioinformatics* 23, 210 (2022). https://doi.org/10.1186/s12859-022-04751-6.

Rebholz-Schuhmann, Dietrich, Antonio José Jimeno Yepes, Erik M. Van Mulligen, Ning Kang, Jan Kors, David Milward, Peter Corbett, et al. 2010. "The CALBC Silver Standard Corpus for Biomedical Named Entities: A Study in Harmonizing the Contributions from Four Independent Named Entity Taggers." *Proceedings of the 7th International Conference on Language Resources and Evaluation, LREC 2010*, pp. 568–573.

Saad, Farag, Hidir Aras, and René Hackl-Sommer. 2020. "Improving Named Entity Recognition for Biomedical and Patent Data Using Bi-LSTM Deep Neural Network Models." In *International Conference on Applications of Natural Language to Information Systems*, 25–36.

Scarpellini, G. 2020. "Cohen's Kappa Free Calculator - IDoStatistics." https://idostatistics. com/cohen-kappa-free-calculator/.

Schulte, Margaret F. 2009. "Electronic Health Records." *Frontiers of Health Services Management*. doi:10.1097/01974520-200907000-00001.

Tjong Kim Sang, Erik F, and Fien de Meulder. 2003. "Introduction to the CoNLL-2003 Shared Task: Language-Independent Named Entity Recognition." *Proceedings of the 7th Conference on Natural Language Learning, CoNLL 2003* at HLT-NAACL 2003, 142–147.

Toscano, F, E O'Donnell, M A Unruh, D Golinelli, G Carullo, G Messina, and L P Casalino. 2018. "Electronic Health Records Implementation: Can the European Union Learn from the United States?" *European Journal of Public Health* 28, 213–401.

Tsai, Richard Tzong-Han, Shih-Hung Wu, Wen-Chi Chou, Yu-Chun Lin, Ding He, Jieh Hsiang, Ting-Yi Sung, and Wen-Lian Hsu. 2006. "Various Criteria in the Evaluation of Biomedical Named Entity Recognition." *BMC Bioinformatics* 7(1), 1–8.

Tsatsaronis, George, Michael Schroeder, Georgios Paliouras, Yannis Almirantis, Ion Androutsopoulos, Eric Gaussier, Patrick Gallinari, et al. 2012. "BioASQ: A Challenge on Large-Scale Biomedical Semantic Indexing and Question Answering." In *AAAI Fall Symposium: Information Retrieval and Knowledge Discovery in Biomedical Text*.

Tsochantaridis, Ioannis, Thorsten Joachims, Thomas Hofmann, Yasemin Altun, and Yoram Singer. 2005. "Large Margin Methods for Structured and Interdependent Output Variables." *Journal of Machine Learning Research* 6(9), 1453–1484.

Voorhees, Ellen, Tasmeer Alam, Steven Bedrick, Dina Demner-Fushman, William R Hersh, Kyle Lo, Kirk Roberts, Ian Soboroff, and Lucy Lu Wang. 2020. "TREC-COVID: Constructing a Pandemic Information Retrieval Test Collection," 1–10. http://arxiv.org/abs/2005.04474.

Wang, Lucy Lu, and Kyle Lo. 2021. "Text Mining Approaches for Dealing with the Rapidly Expanding Literature on COVID-19." *Briefings in Bioinformatics* 22(2), 781–799. doi: 10.1093/bib/bbaa296.

Webster, Jonathan J, and Chunyu Kit. 1992. "Tokenization as the Initial Phase in NLP." In *COLING 1992 Volume 4: The 14th International Conference on Computational Linguistics*.

Yang, Xi, Tianchen Lyu, Qian Li, Chih Yin Lee, Jiang Bian, William R Hogan, and Yonghui Wu. 2019. "A Study of Deep Learning Methods for De-Identification of Clinical Notes in Cross-Institute Settings." *BMC Medical Informatics and Decision Making* 19(Suppl 5), 1–9. doi: 10.1186/s12911-019-0935-4.

Zhang, Yuhao, Yuhui Zhang, Peng Qi, Christopher D Manning, and Curtis P Langlotz. 2021. "Biomedical and Clinical English Model Packages for the Stanza Python NLP Library." *Journal of the American Medical Informatics Association* 28(9), 1892–1899. doi: 10.1093/jamia/ocab090.

[illegible] Learning, [illegible] Machine Learning Research [illegible]
148.

[illegible] Wang, [illegible]
[illegible]

[illegible] 2021 [illegible] Application [illegible]
[illegible]

[illegible]

[illegible]

[illegible]

[illegible]

Chapter 9

Image segmentation of skin disease using deep learning approach

Manbir Singh and Maninder Singh
Punjabi University Patiala

CONTENTS

9.1 INTRODUCTION

Skin diseases affect people of all ages, including children and pose a psychological and financial burden on patients. Clinicians can diagnose some skin disorders by visual inspection of lesions and evaluation of features, which includes size, shape, color, location and patterns. Correct diagnosis also depends upon the experience and expertise of the clinicians. Further, the correct identification of a skin disease requires specific clinical tests, depending on the type of skin disorder. For example, autoimmune blistering skin diseases (AIBD) are rare skin disorders in which the immune system attacks proteins that bind multiple layers of

DOI: 10.1201/9781003368342-9

skin together and cause blistering lesions. There are several types of AIBD, which can be accurately diagnosed based on various clinical tests among which direct immunofluorescence is a gold standard test for the confirmation. Tests that confirm the skin diseases are costly and are available in multi-specialty hospitals and hence, cause delay in diagnosis. Working in this direction, research is being done for the diagnosis of skin diseases using artificial intelligence-based computerized systems. It is a very challenging task to classify skin diseases from clinical/non-dermoscopic images of skin diseases as these images have very less information as compared to dermoscopic images because usually the setting in which clinical images are captured is non-uniform and has background artifacts. In literature, various architecture of convolution neural network (CNN) were used for the classification of non-dermoscopic images which provides end-to-end solutions, requires very minimal pre-processing and automatically extracts most appropriate features by themselves. During classification, it is observed that CNN classified images based on coarse similarity rather than looking into detailed features of lesions. Therefore, to improve the accuracy, segmentation of skin lesions prior to classification is required, which can provide the ability to deep learning algorithms to extract only relevant features from the input image.

Manual segmentation of medical images is very time-consuming, tiresome, possibility of human error and irreproducible. Therefore, end-to-end trainable segmentation methods are required. Traditional machine learning-based approaches for segmentation, such as region-based segmentation and thresholding are not reliable and require pre-processing, image processing, extraction of hand-driven features and domain experts for appropriate feature extraction depending upon the types of diseases. Nowadays deep learning-based algorithms are being used in the field of image classification, object detection and segmentation, but approaches based on deep learning require large labeled dataset size. Some popular datasets related to skin diseases are shown in Table 9.1.

9.2 RELATED WORK

Ali et al. (2021) proposed U-Net based architecture for the segregation of cardiac boundary from cardiac echocardiographic images. ResNet, which is a residual network, was modified for the encoder part. ResNet

Table 9.1 Skin diseases dataset

Dataset	Number of images	Number of classes	Type of images
XiangyaDerm (Dong et al., 2017)	107,565	541	Clinical
Dermofit Image Library	1,300	10	
ISIC dataset comes from the International Skin Imaging Collaboration (ISIC) (Cassidy et al., 2022)	44,108 (year 2020)		Dermoscopic (year 2020)
(Dermnet - skin disease atlas)	23,000	23	Clinical and dermoscopic
Dermnet NZ	25,000	-	Dermoscopic, histological clinical images
DermIS (Dermatology Information System)	7,172	735	Clinical
MED-NODE (Giotis et al., 2016)	170	2	Dermoscopic
HAM10000 (Human Against Machine with 10,000 training images) (Tschandl et al., 2018)	10,015	7	Dermoscopic
PH2 (Mendonça et al., 2013)	200	3	Dermoscopic
Derm7pt (Kawahara et al., 2018)	1,011	2	Dermoscopic and clinical
SD-198 (Sun et al., 2016)	6,584	198	Dermoscopic and clinical

consists of multiple layers, each layer has multiple blocks and each block of the network receives two inputs which are the output from the previous layer and the output from the second to the previous layer. In the proposed model, the input of the first block of each layer is propagated to every block, which helps in dealing with the noise. The model was trained on the publicly available CAMUS (Cardiac Acquisitions for Multi-Structure Ultrasound Segmentation) dataset. Experimental results show the Dice score of 0.97%.

Saood and Hatem (2021) evaluated two deep neural networks, SegNet and U-Net for segmentation from CT lung image for the identification of COVID-19 severity. SegNet is primarily used for scene segmentation and U-Net for the segmentation of medical images. The results of this chapter showed that in binary segmentation, SegNet outperformed U-Net, whereas in multi-class segmentation the performance of U-Net was better.

Wang et al. (2021) proposed a model based on a fully convolutional network that used prediction-aware one-to-one label assignment and a 3D Max Filtering for end-to-end object detection.

Kalane et al. (2021) presented the end-to-end deep learning model based on U-Net architecture for the detection of COVID-19 from clinical images. Model was trained on 1,000 images, which include CT images, some of which are single-slice CT images and Chest X-rays. The U-Net architecture is altered, each block of contraction path comprising two 3×3 convolutional layers with the same padding, and each layer is followed by ReLU and after activation function 2×2 max pooling layer with stride 2 is used. The expansive part comprised up-sampling layers followed by a convolutional operation of 2×2. Resulting feature maps after convolutions are combined using concatenation with corresponding feature maps from the contraction path. After merging the feature, two 3×3 convolution operations, each one of it followed by ReLU, are applied. Finally, in the end, 1×1 convolution was used which reduced the channels of the feature map according to desired segmentation map. The proposed architecture has achieved a sensitivity of 94.86% and specificity of 93.47% and overall accuracy of 94.10%.

Yuan (2017) proposed FCN-based architecture for skin lesion segmentation from dermoscopic images. Dataset comprised 2,000 images and corresponding masks. The network architecture consists of four groups of two convolutional layers followed by a pooling layer after that one convolution layer in the encoder path. Decoder part consists of a deconvolution layer and upsampling layer followed by three groups of two deconvolution layers and upsampling layer and in the end, one deconvolution layer is used. In the decoder path, both up-sampling and deconvolutional layers are used to recover the information which was lost in the encoder path. The model achieved an average Jaccard index of 0.784.

Dong et al. (2017) proposed the U-Net-based architecture for automatic brain tumor detection and segmentation from MRI images. During contraction, the size of feature maps decreased from 240 × 240 (input image) to 15 × 15 (feature maps size) and the up-sampling path recovered the feature maps back to 240 × 240 (segmentation map). Finally, a 1 × 1 convolutional layer is used to reduce the number of channels of feature maps to two, which represent the foreground and background segmentation map, respectively. The model was evaluated on the BRATS 2015 datasets.

Díaz-Pernas et al. (2021) proposed a deep learning-based approach for brain tumor segmentation and classification from MRI images. The proposed network has three parallel paths, each path having three scales, and each path comprises a group of two convolution layers and max pooling layer, followed by another convolution layer, which concatenates all features of three paths and at last fully connected layer for classification. Segmentation of tumor is based on the region that contains all pixels identified as a given tumor type. In this approach, each pixel is classified according to a predefined input window of size 65 × 65 pixels. This approach achieved a dice index of 0.828, pttas value of 0.967 and sensitivity of 0.940.

In another study, the U-Net-based architecture was used for lung segmentation from CT images. The label data, masks and corresponding images, for training, are prepared by manual process. Some modification was done to the existing U-Net architecture. Pre-trained CNN, ResNet-34, was used as a base network (encoder part) and to fuse the features of the encoder layer with the corresponding decoder layer bidirectional convolutional long short-term memory is used. The proposed model achieved a dice coefficient index of 97.31%, accuracy of 97.83%, precision of 99.93%, recall of 97.45%, and F1-score of 98.67% (Jalali et al., 2021).

Existing architecture of U-Net was modified for the segmentation of skin lesions from dermoscopic images. Group Normalization (GN) between layers of encoder and decoder, Attention Gates (AG) and Tversky Loss (TL) as loss function was used to enhance the performance. AG provides the ability to focus on certain regions while providing less attention to insignificant regions. The model tested on ISIC 2018 dataset and achieved the accuracy of 0.95 (Arora et al., 2021).

Quantitative results of deep learning-based object detection and segmentation techniques are summarized in Table 9.2.

9.3 CONVOLUTION NEURAL NETWORK

CNN has been used in several fields including the medical domain and achieved human-level accuracy to identify diseases from clinical images. A typical architecture of CNN consists of convolution layers, to perform convolution operation on the input image with a number of filters/kernels, pooling layer, activation layer, fully connected layer and softmax layer for final prediction as shown in Figure 9.1. Several CNN networks are being designed to obtain excellent results for the classification of skin diseases from clinical images. There exist countless ways by which a CNN can be designed depending on the number and position of the layers. Usually, these types of networks use fully connected (FC) layers at the end, which increase the number of parameters and force users to use fixed size images for classification. We may also use as many layers in a network to make the network deeper. The vanishing gradient problem may occur in deeper networks, which decreases the network accuracy. However, several approaches and different CNN architectures such as ResNet (He et al., 2016) and GoogleNet (Szegedy et al., 2015) have been developed to solve this problem. CNN is mainly used for classification tasks in which output is probabilities value of classes and the value with a high score is chosen as the predicted label of the input image. The classification analyzes the entries image, but it does not localize the objects present in the image, object detection algorithms give the location of objects along with associate class label and probability. The location of an object in the object detection algorithm is in the form of a rectangular bounded box, but the exact shape/outline and area of the objects present in the image cannot be determined. In some applications of the medical domains, precise shape of an object is very important for further analysis i.e. for the classification of benign and melanoma from the skin images

Table 9.2 Results of deep learning architecture for object detection and segmentation

Sr. No	Author	Architecture	Problem	Accuracy
1	Ali et al. (2021)	U-Net	Segmentation	0.97% (dice score)
2	Saood and Hatem (2021)	SegNet and U-Net	Segmentation	-
3	Wang et al. (2021)	Fully convolutional network	Object detection	-
4	Kalane et al. (2021)	U-Net	Segmentation	94.10%
5	Yuan (2017)	Fully convolutional network	Segmentation	0.784 (Jaccard index)
6	Dong et al. (2017)	U-Net	Segmentation	-
7	Díaz-Pernas Convolutional Neural Networks et al. (2021)	Convolutional Neural Networks	Segmentation and classification	0.828 (dice index) and 0.973 (classification accuracy)
8	Jalali et al. (2021)	U-Net	Segmentation	97.83%
9	Arora et al. (2021)	U-Net	Segmentation	0.95%

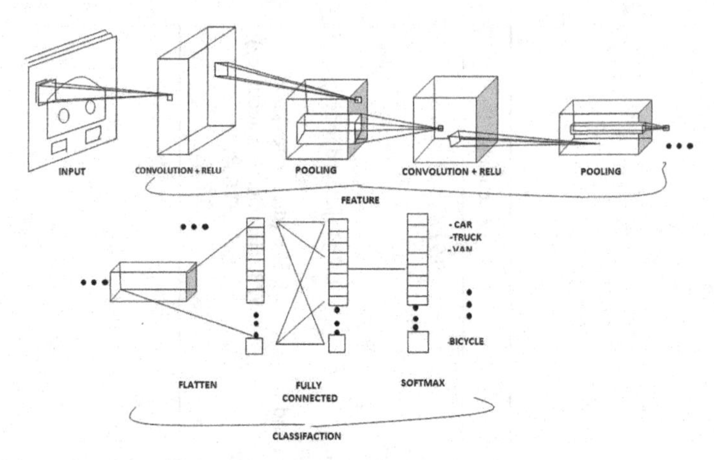

Figure 9.1 A typical convolution neural network architecture.

shape of lesions is considered to be very important. Image segmentation is one step ahead of object detection, which determines the exact shape of objects present in the image. Segmentation algorithms can estimate the area and perimeter of an object present in the input image. Deep learning-based segmentation approaches use both image classification and object detection techniques in their algorithm.

It is also noticed that without segmenting the image CNN only picks the images with a coarse similarity and doesn't look into the details (Liao et al., 2016). When we use segmentation before classification, then CNN extracts those features, which provide better representation. During classification using CNN, an input image's size decreases as it goes through the convolution layers, and in the end, the softmax layer is used for the prediction of label for the input image. In CNN, features at each successive convolutional layer increase while spatial and boundary information is lost which is essential for the segmentation. To preserve this information, we need an upsampling of feature maps produced by convolutional layers. Therefore, deep neural network-based segmentation has up-sampling layers, which increase the spatial resolution to make the size of the output the same as the size of the input image.

9.4 OBJECT DETECTION

Object detection algorithms detect the instances of all objects and their associated class from the input image. Over time, various methods for object detection have been developed.

9.4.1 Sliding window

In this approach, a rectangular window, which slides all over the image from left to right and top to bottom, extracts the region from the input image. To locate objects of different sizes, image pyramids are used; image pyramids represent an image at different scales. In this approach, a window slides over every layer of the image pyramid to identify the objects. We can convert any CNN into an object detection algorithm by using an image pyramid and sliding window. During sliding over the input image, regions are extracted from the image, which is then passed to a classifier, which can be a classical or deep learning classifier, for the prediction of object. In this way, objects from the image can be located by exploring every region of the input image. This approach is computationally expensive because each area of the input image needs to be processed as the object can be at any location. We need to choose the size of the sliding window while considering the aspect ratio of different objects. This is not an end-to-end trainable solution.

To solve the problem of sliding windows, in place of sliding windows, selective search algorithms have been developed that generate regions from the input image that are likely to contain objects. Selective Search (Uijlings et al., 2013) is computationally more efficient than image pyramids and sliding windows. This approach merges superpixels and over-segmented the image based on the similarity of texture, size, color and shape and identifies locations in an image that may contain objects. Selective search generates candidate regions without any knowledge about the object itself in that region. The regions then pass to the classifier for final output. The output may be numerous bounding boxes that represent an object and may overlap, which can be converted into a single bounded box for each object using non-maxima suppression (NMS).

9.4.2 Region-based Convolutional Neural Networks

Region-based Convolutional Neural Networks (R-CNNs) are a family of machine learning models for object detection. To locate the objects from the input image, In R-CNN selective search is used for regions proposal, CNN for features extraction from each region, support vector machine process the features extracted by the CNN and outputs a confidence score of the presence of an object in that region and bounding-box regressor is used to accurately locate the bounding box (Girshick et al., 2014).

Training of R-CNN required training data, which comprised a set of images and bounded box coordinates of objects presented in the images. For feature extraction, we can use any pre-trained networks or fine-tune the networks using the transfer learning approach. R-CNN uses selective search to generate candidate regions without any learning. To implement this algorithm, we need to train CNN, SVM and bounding box regressor individually which is very time-consuming. The shortcoming of R-CNN is solved in another R-CNN that is Fast R-CNN. The architecture of this is similar to R-CNN except instead of input every region generated by region proposal to CNN, the entire image is input into CNN to generate the feature map and generated feature maps are then used to identify the region proposals. After the region proposal, the region of interest (RoI) pooling layer is used to reshape the feature map to a fixed size as required by fully connected layers which are passed to fully connected layers. In the end, a softmax layer is used which gives the prediction of the region's class and offset values for the bounding box (Girshick, 2015). RoI pooling layer accepts two inputs which are feature maps extracted using CNN and candidate region. Both R-CNN and Fast R-CNN used a selective search algorithm, which is very time-consuming. Faster R-CNN, which is another R-CNN, fixes this problem by using convolutional neural network instead of using a selective search for candidate regions (Ren et al., 2015). CNN specifically used to generate candidate regions in Faster R-CNN is called Region Proposal Network (RPN). RPN in Faster R-CNN is used to generate candidate regions where there is possibility of objects. In RPN, input image is passed through CNN, which gives the feature maps. After the extraction of feature maps, a sliding window at every step is used to generate anchors having three different aspect ratios and three different scales. This process generated the nine anchors for every position in feature maps corresponding to the sliding window. All anchors generated by RPN may not have an object in them; therefore, we need to train RPN to automate the process of identifying foreground versus background anchors and offsets for the foreground boxes. This is achieved by two using convolution layers that are bounding box regressor and bounding box classifier used to generate the offset and classify the anchor having object or not respectively using learning from ground truth training data. The RPN is a trainable and end-to-end solution to generate the region proposal. We can also minimize the region proposals based on a cutoff of IoU values.

9.5 IMAGE SEGMENTATION

Image segmentation is one step ahead of object detection, which finds out the exact shape of objects from the image. There are many image segmentation approaches based on deep learning that are reviewed in this paper.

Segmentation labels every pixel of an image based on some attributes and the whole image is divided into various regions based on the grouping of pixels. Segmented images are easy to analyze and can be used in many applications including medical domain.

9.5.1 Type of segmentation

Segmentation divides the image into different segments based on certain characteristics for further processing of the image. The division is broadly divided into two subtypes:

a. *Semantic segmentation*: Semantic segmentation assigned a label to every pixel of the image in such a way that all pixels belong to a similar object assigned a single label. All instances belong to an object considered as a single entity and a single label is assigned to them.
b. *Instance segmentation*: It is one step ahead of semantic segmentation and it treats multiple instances of an object as a separate entity and assigns different labels to each instance.
c. *Panoptic segmentation*: It combines the concept of semantic segmentation and Instance segmentation (Kirillov et al., 2019). In this type, every pixel of the image is assigned two labels i.e. semantic label and instance id. A semantic label is assigned to every individual object present in the image while a unique instance id is assigned to every instance belonging to an object. All pixels belong to uncountable regions such as background and pavement not assigned any instance id. A valid instance id is assigned only to countable regions.

9.6 DEEP LEARNING METHODS FOR SEGMENTATION

Image segmentation based on deep learning is an end-to-end trainable solution. Deep learning-based segmentation makes use of classification and object detection algorithms as during segmentation classification and object detection is performed and after the prediction of a bounded box precise shape of object is computed. Various approaches to segmentation have been developed. The basic methods on the basis of which other advanced methods are being developed are listed below.

9.6.1 Sliding window approach

Deep learning-based segmentation can be achieved by using CNN. One approach, which is based on a sliding window, divides the input image into various patches and CNN classifies each pixel of image based on the classification of the central pixel of each patch. This approach is very computationally expensive and time-consuming because we need to label every pixel of the input image, which requires patches for every central pixel of the image. Furthermore, the overlapping patches in this approach do not share the features that make this approach highly inefficient.

9.6.2 Fully convolutional network

The shortcomings of the sliding window approach are overcome by modifying the existing CNN architecture in which only convolutional layers are retained and fully connected layers are removed from the network. It makes convolutional layers to make prediction for the entire input image rather than making predictions for every individual pixel of the image. This type of architecture is called fully convolutional network (FCN) (Chen et al., 2017; Long et al., 2015; Wang et al., 2021). The CNN can be converted into FCN by replacing fully connected layers by 1×1 convolutional layer, which enables the network to make predictions on inputs of arbitrary size. Any pre-trained classification network can be converted into FCN for segmentation. In FCN, dimension of input image is preserved throughout the network by using convolution layers having the same padding. The output of the network is a segmentation mask in which every pixel is classified (Figure 9.2).

The use of convolution layers with the same padding, to keep the output the same size as the input, makes the network computationally expensive and to resolve this issue FCN uses down-sampling and up-sampling layers in the architecture. During down-sampling, the first part of FCN has architecture similar to CNN without fully connected layers that convert input images into feature maps. In the second part of the

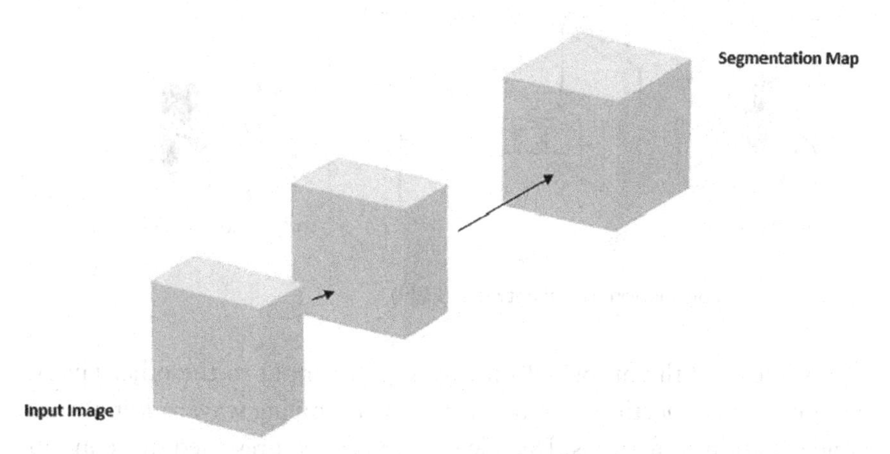

Figure 9.2 Fully connected Network used the convolution layers with the same padding to preserve the output and model learns from input images and corresponding masks.

network that consists of up-sampling layers, feature maps are up-sample in which the spatial resolution of the feature maps is increased to make the output image to be the same size as the input image. The feature maps after downsampling have smaller size but larger number of channels. In this form of FCN, rather than using all convolution layers of the same padding which preserved the dimension of output, in downsampling part there is a choice of using convolution layers with the same padding or without the same padding and max pooling layers to down-sampled the feature maps which are then up-sampled by up-sampling layers in the second part of the network as shown in Figure 9.3. The down-sampling part of the network extracts contextual information which focuses on what is present in the input image (what), while the focus of the up-sampling layers is on the precise location (where) of objects. After up-sampling, the feature maps are the same size as the input and the number of channels is based on the objects that need to be segmented from the input image.

Spatial information is lost by down-sampling layers and to recover that up-sampling layers are used. Initially as shown in Figure 9.3, only one layer is used in the up-sample part of the network to recover the size of feature maps. The major limitation of this network is that during up-sampling it becomes very difficult to recover the spatial information. To recover this information skip connections are used. A skip connection is an alternate path in the network through which we can bypass some

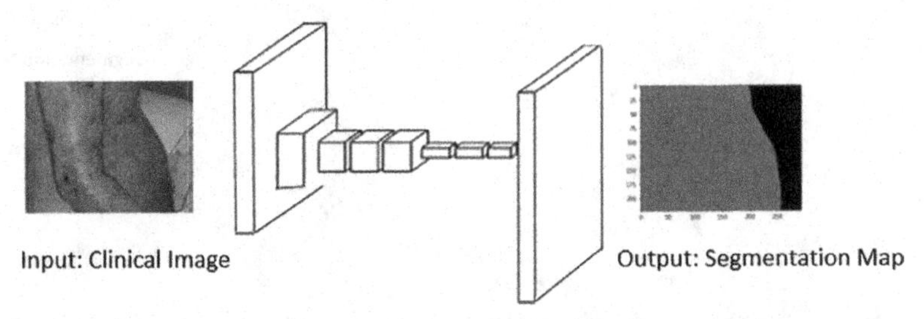

Figure 9.3 Fully convolution neural network (FCN).

layers and feed the output of one layer as the input to the other layers. Mainly skip connections can be used in the following ways: addition and concatenation of features. Deep learning architectures used this concept to solve various problems. For example, the skip connections are used to solve the vanishing gradient problem in the residual network. In FCN, skip connections are used to combine the feature maps from the contracting path with feature maps from the expansive path to recover the original image resolution by merging the context information from the contracting path with the spatial information from the expansive path.

There variants of FCN, based on the position of the skip connection, are i.e. FCN 32, FCN 16 and FCN 8 based on the position of skip connection. In another form of FCN, multiple down-sampling and up-sampling layers are used. This makes the network very deep and computationally efficient as in the network several layers work at lower resolution. In addition to multiple layers, we can also use skip connections, which combine the feature maps of down-sampling layers with feature maps of up-sampling layers. The fusion of feature maps enhances the performance of FCN. Based on the FCN architecture, various network models have been proposed by the researcher like U-Net and SEGnet. In addition to that, experimental modifications are being done on these models for further improvement. In addition to that, experimental modifications are being done on these models for further improvement. Since dense layers (fully connected layers) are not used in FCN, this reduces the number of parameters and computation time and enables FCN to operate on images of arbitrary size. U-Net, which is a convolutional network for image segmentation is symmetrical and features of down-sampling layers are merged with corresponding up-sampling layers using concatenation while in FCN features are merged using summation. Due to symmetrical architecture, in the U-Net number of layer layers in the up-sampling path are equal to the number of layers in down-sampling path.

9.6.3 U-Net architecture

U-Net, based on deep neural networks, is primarily designed for medical image segmentation (Ronneberger et al., 2015). The network mainly contained two sections: contraction and expansion. The architecture of U-Net as specified by Ronneberger et al., comprised contraction (down-sampling) at the left side, bottleneck at middle and expansive part (up-sampling) at the right side. The U-Net has a u-shape structure as shown in Figure 9.4. Contracting/down-sampling path, which is similar to a convolutional network that consist of four blocks and each block has two 3 × 3 convolutional layers with the same padding, followed by ReLU (nonlinear activation function) and 2 × 2 Max Pooling with stride 2. After every block in the contracting path, feature information increases while the semantic information reduces. The feature map doubles after every block while the resolution of the feature map decreases.

Expanding/up-sampling path is also consisting of four blocks, and each block consists of 2 × 2 up-convolution layer, which up-sample the resolution and reduces the channels of feature maps by halves and two 3 × 3 convolution layers followed by ReLU (non-linear activation function). In addition to these two paths, skip connections are also used to concatenate the features of the contracting path with the features of expanding path. The skip connections in the network combine the information related to the location of objects with the contextual information

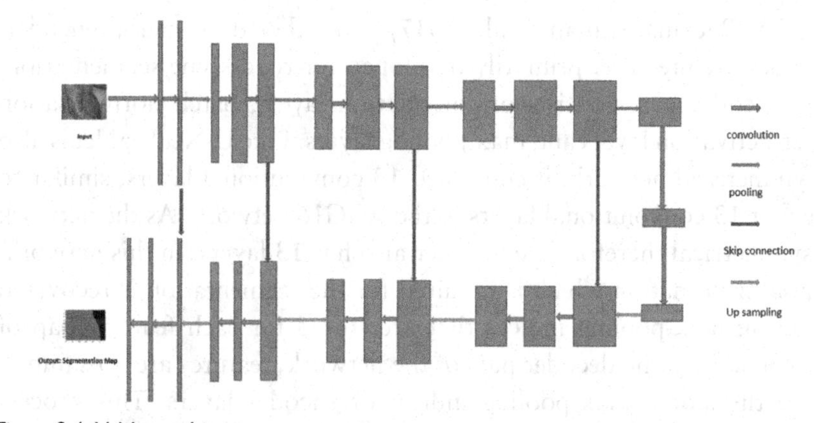

Figure 9.4 U-Net architecture.

coming from the contracting path and generate a segmentation map. The concatenation/combination of the features from the contracting path and expanding path helps to retain the spatial information, which is important for segmentation. In contraction, the image progressively goes down with respect to size and goes up with respect to the number of features, whereas in expansion, the number of the features decreases while the size of images progressively increases.

This architecture can be trained and gives good results on a dataset having very few images. As shown in Figure 9.4, contraction is implemented by many successive up-sampling layers, which progressively increase the resolution of the feature maps. The network recovers the spatial information, which is lost in the contracting path, by combining the features from layers of encoder with the corresponding decoder's layers by using skip connections.

Similar to FCN, this network also does not have any fully connected layers, but one major modification made in the architecture is that the up-sampling part comprises many up-sampling layers, which makes the expansive path symmetrical to the contracting path.

The architecture produces segmentation map using end-to-end learning. This is not a universal architecture; we can modify the network as per the requirement based on the problem. There exist many ways by which we can improve or modify the network, which include the number of layers, type of layers, sequence of layers, etc. we can also use the existing pre-trained CNN architecture for the contraction part.

9.6.4 SegNet architecture

SegNet (Badrinarayanan et al., 2017) is another deep neural encoder-decoder architecture, primarily developed for road scene segmentation. The encoder part consists of convolution layers, batch normalization layer, activation layers and max pooling layers. Like U-Net SegNet is also a symmetrical network. It contained 13 convolutional layers, similar to the first 13 convolutional layers in the VGG16 network. As the network is symmetrical therefore the decoder also has 13 layers. In this network, spatial information which is required for the segmentation is recovered by using max-pooling indices that are stored for each feature map of the encoder. In the decoder part of the network, features are up-samples using the stored max-pooling indices of encoder layers. This process creates sparse feature maps, which are then converted into dense feature maps by convolutional layers, but in the U-Net entire feature maps from the encoder path are concatenated with up-sampled feature maps.

The final layer of decoder in this network generates feature maps having multiple channels fed to the softmax classifier, which gives class probability for each pixel of image.

9.7 UP-SAMPLING

In a convolutional neural network, the size of the input image progressively decreases while the number of feature maps increases causing the spatial information in the input images to disappear which is necessary for segmentation. To recover this information up-sampling is required.

The up-sampling layers are used to increase the resolution of feature maps received from the contraction path. There exist many techniques of up-sampling, but transposed convolution and unpooling are widely used in designing a deep neural architecture for segmentation.

Unpooling, which is an up-sampling technique, is based on polling. In pooling (max pooling) maximum value from each window is selected for down-sampling the feature maps. Unpooling operation converts the feature map back to its original size. Unpooling can be performed in various ways: Nearest-Neighbor, Bed of Nails and Max unpooling. Nearest-Neighbor unpooling copies the pixel value from the input feature map to all positions in the corresponding sub window. Bed of Nails unpooling shifts the pixel value of input feature map to top-left position and all other positions in the corresponding sub-window are filled with zero. The max unpooling operation which is another unpooling technique is similar to Bed of Nails but in this operation, position of pixel value is memorized and recalled during the operation. In all unpooling operations no learning/training is performed.

Transpose convolution or de-convolution is a type of up-sampling layer in which learning/training is performed during the network development and it up-samples the feature map to a desired size based on some trainable parameter. In transpose convolution, every pixel value starting from the upper left element is multiplied by the kernel value to produce the up-sampled feature map. During this process some values may overlap which can be solved by adding all overlap values.

9.8 PERFORMANCE MATRIX FOR EVALUATING THE SEGMENTATION

There are several matrices used to evaluate the performance. Most commonly used matrices are recall, precession, Intersection over Union (IoU) or Jaccard Index, average precision, mean average precision (mAP), Dice similarity coefficient (DSC) or F1 score (Setiawan, 2020). Recall measures the ability of a network to correct the identification of true positive samples. Precision measures the percentage of predictions that are correct. In the case of segmentation, we calculate the recall and precision based on the threshold IoU value. The IoU or Jaccard Index is calculated as the intersection or overlapping area of the ground truth bounded box and predicated bounded box divided by the union of their area. The Average precession which is the mean of all precision areas computed by measuring the area under the precision-recall curve and the mean average precision (mAP) is calculated by taking the average AP over all classes. The ground-truth bounding boxes are manually labeled bonded boxes. The predicted bounded boxes are predicted by the model. Along with the bonded boxes, label classes to which they belong are also required to calculate the matrixes. Dice similarity coefficient (DSC), is a statistic used to measure the performance of segmentation (Zou et al., 2004). DSC is calculated by multiplying 2 with the number of similar pixels in ground truth mask and predicted segmentation map and dividing it by the total number of pixels in both images. These matrices are mathematically expressed as follows:

$$\text{Precision} = \frac{\text{True positive}}{\text{True positive} + \text{false poitive}} \tag{9.1}$$

$$\text{Recall} = \frac{\text{True positive}}{\text{True positive} + \text{false negtive}} \tag{9.2}$$

$$\text{Intersection over union} = \frac{\text{Overlapping area}}{\text{Total area}} \tag{9.3}$$

$$\text{Dice similarity coefficient} = 2 \times \frac{|A \cap B|}{A \cup B} \tag{9.4}$$

where A is ground truth and B is predicted segmentation map.

9.9 CONCLUSION

Deep learning networks are an end-to-end solution that requires very minimal pre-processing and automatically extracts most appropriate features by themselves. CNN, a deep neural network, achieved an excellent result in skin disease classification. The performance of such networks can be higher than the experts in their field. To further improve the classification performance of deep learning models, sometimes we need to perform segmentation prior to the classification. Clinical images that are usually captured using different gadgets, i.e. mobile phones and cameras, have noise and background objects. In some cases, it is observed that CNN has classified images based on overall resemblance rather than looking into fine details. Therefore, we have to force the CNN to extract relevant features only from certain regions of the input images and discard features from irrelevant regions such as background and other artifacts presented in the input image. Deep learning-based segmentation can be trained to extract regions of interest from the input clinical skin images. After that, the segmented regions can be input into CNN for classification and in this way we can restrict our algorithm to classify skin images based on the features that are necessary, which will reduce the features to participating in the decision process. Implementation of segmentation along with classification in deep learning models makes the model computationally efficient, reduced training time, overfitting and increases classification accuracy. Therefore, to improve the accuracy, segmentation of skin lesions before classification is can be very useful. Various deep learning-based segmentation networks are available and can be used by some modification in their architecture for skin disease segmentation and classification from clinical images.

AUTHORS CONTRIBUTION

Manbir Singh: Writing – original draft, Visualization. Maninder Singh: Writing – review & editing, Supervision.

REFERENCES

Ali Y, Janabi-Sharifi F, Beheshti S. 2021. Echocardiographic image segmentation using deep Res-U network. *Biomedical Signal Processing and Control* 64:102248.

Arora R, Raman B, Nayyar K, Awasthi R. 2021. Automated skin lesion segmentation using attention-based deep convolutional neural network. *Biomedical Signal Processing and Control* 65:102358.

Badrinarayanan V, Kendall A, Cipolla R. 2017. Segnet: A deep convolutional encoder-decoder architecture for image segmentation. *IEEE Transactions on Pattern Analysis and Machine Intelligence* 39:2481–2495.

Cassidy B, Kendrick C, Brodzicki A, Jaworek-Korjakowska J, Yap MH, 2022. Analysis of the ISIC image datasets: Usage, benchmarks and recommendations. *Medical Image Analysis* 75:102305.

Chen Q, Xu J, Koltun V. 2017. Fast image processing with fully-convolutional networks. In *Proceedings of the IEEE International Conference on Computer Vision*, pp. 2497–2506.

DermIS (Dermatology Information System), http://www.dermis.net.

Dermnet - skin disease atlas, http://www.dermnet.com.

Dermnet NZ, https://www.dermnetnz.org.

Dermofit Image Library, https://licensing.edinburgh-innovations.ed.ac.uk/product/dermofit-image-library

Díaz-Pernas FJ, Martínez-Zarzuela M, Antón-Rodríguez M, González-Ortega D. 2021. A deep learning approach for brain tumor classification and segmentation using a multiscale convolutional neural network. *Healthcare*, 9(2):153.

Dong H, Yang G, Liu F, Mo Y, Guo Y. 2017. Automatic brain tumor detection and segmentation using U-Net based fully convolutional networks. In *Annual Conference on Medical Image Understanding and Analysis*. Springer, pp. 506–517.

Giotis NM, Land S, Biehl M, Jonkman MF, Petkov N, 2016. MED-NODE: A computer-assisted melanoma diagnosis system using non-dermoscopic images. *Expert Systems with Applications*, 42:6578–6585.

Girshick R. 2015. Fast r-cnn. In *Proceedings of the IEEE International Conference on Computer Vision*, pp. 1440–1448.

Girshick R, Donahue J, Darrell T, Malik J. 2014. Rich feature hierarchies for accurate object detection and semantic segmentation. In *Proceedings of the IEEE Conference on Computer Vision and Pattern Recognition*, pp. 580–587.

He K, Zhang X, Ren S, Sun J. 2016. Deep residual learning for image recognition. In *Proceedings of the IEEE Conference on Computer Vision and Pattern Recognition*, pp. 770–778.

Jalali Y, Fateh M, Rezvani M, Abolghasemi V, Anisi MH. 2021. ResBCDU-Net: A deep learning framework for lung CT image segmentation. *Sensors* 21:268.

Kalane P, Patil S, Patil B, Sharma DP. 2021. Automatic detection of COVID-19 disease using U-Net architecture based fully convolutional network. *Biomedical Signal Processing and Control* 67:102518.

Kawahara J, Daneshvar S, Argenziano G, Hamarneh G. 2018. Seven-point checklist and skin lesion classification using multitask multimodal neural nets. *IEEE Journal of Biomedical and Health Informatics* 23(2):538–546.

Kirillov A, He K, Girshick R, Rother C, Dollár P. 2019. Panoptic segmentation. In *Proceedings of the IEEE/CVF Conference on Computer Vision and Pattern Recognition*, pp. 9404–9413.

Liao H, Li Y, Luo J. 2016. Skin disease classification versus skin lesion characterization: Achieving robust diagnosis using multi-label deep neural networks. *2016 23rd International Conference on Pattern Recognition (ICPR)*. IEEE, pp. 355–360.

Long J, Shelhamer E, Darrell T. 2015. Fully convolutional networks for semantic segmentation. In *Proceedings of the IEEE Conference on Computer Vision and Pattern Recognition*, pp. 3431–3440.

Mendonça T, Ferreira PM, Marques JS, Marcal AR, Rozeira J. 2013. PH 2-A dermoscopic image database for research and benchmarking. In *2013 35th Annual International Conference of the IEEE Engineering in Medicine and Biology Society (EMBC)*, pp. 5437–5440.

Ren S, He K, Girshick R, Sun J. 2015. Faster r-cnn: Towards real-time object detection with region proposal networks. *Advances in Neural Information Processing Systems* 28:91–99.

Ronneberger O, Fischer P, Brox T. 2015. U-net: Convolutional networks for biomedical image segmentation. In *International Conference on Medical Image Computing and Computer-Assisted Intervention*. Springer, pp. 234–241.

Saood A, Hatem I. 2021. COVID-19 lung CT image segmentation using deep learning methods: U-Net versus SegNet. *BMC Medical Imaging* 21:1–10.

Setiawan AW. 2020. Image segmentation metrics in skin lesion: Accuracy, sensitivity, specificity, dice coefficient, Jaccard index, and Matthews correlation coefficient. In *2020 International Conference on Computer Engineering, Network, and Intelligent Multimedia (CENIM)*. IEEE, pp. 97–102.

Sun X, Yang J, Sun M, Wang K. 2016. A benchmark for automatic visual classification of clinical skin disease images. In *European Conference on Computer Vision*. Springer, Cham, pp. 206–222.

Szegedy C, Liu W, Jia Y, Sermanet P, Reed S, Anguelov D, Erhan D, Vanhoucke V, Rabinovich A. 2015. Going deeper with convolutions. In *Proceedings of the IEEE Conference on Computer Vision and Pattern Recognition*, pp. 1–9.

Tschandl P, Rosendahl C, Kittler H. 2018. The HAM10000 dataset, a large collection of multi-source dermatoscopic images of common pigmented skin lesions. *Scientific Data* 5(1):1–9.

Uijlings JR, Van De Sande KE, Gevers T, Smeulders AW. 2013. Selective search for object recognition. *International Journal of Computer Vision* 104:154–171.

Wang J, Song L, Li Z, Sun H, Sun J, Zheng N. 2021. End-to-end object detection with fully convolutional network. In *Proceedings of the IEEE/CVF Conference on Computer Vision and Pattern Recognition*, pp. 15849–15858.

Yuan Y. 2017. Automatic skin lesion segmentation with fully convolutional-deconvolutional networks. arXiv preprint arXiv:1703.05165.

Zou KH, Warfield SK, Bharatha A, Tempany CM, Kaus MR, Haker SJ, Wells III WM, Jolesz FA, Kikinis R. 2004. Statistical validation of image segmentation quality based on a spatial overlap index1: Scientific reports. *Academic Radiology* 11:178–189.

Chapter 10

Multimodality dementia detection system using machine and deep learning

Shruti Srivatsan and Sumneet Kaur Bamrah
Sri Venkateswara College of Engineering, Sriperumbudur

K. S. Gayathri
Sri Sivasubramaniya Nadar College of Engineering

CONTENTS

10.1 INTRODUCTION

Every individual values health. Healthcare includes issues related to the brain as well. Older people are subject to risks of memory loss and succumb to dementia. Several organizations take initiatives to promote healthcare and well-being. There are global and national institutions at the forefront that address the concerns of dementia prevention and its detection. Various officials and experts have described and defined the syndrome [1, 3, 4, 8, 14, 19, 21, 34]. According to the WHO, the rise in individuals succumbing to the condition is projected to be 78 million by 2030 and 139 million by 2050 [35]. The National Health Portal (NHP) in India indicates that 2.7% of the 65 million citizens senior citizens are subject to the risk of dementia. 20% of the individuals above the age of 80 are in need of immediate geriatric care for the same. Identifying the onset is critical since relevant information is shared among researchers,

DOI: 10.1201/9781003368342-10

experts, clinicians, and caretakers to devise novel and patient-friendly techniques of detection.

Dementia is caused by a multitude of factors and varies accordingly [10, 15]. Behavior and cognition are correlated. Since dementia is related to cognition, the brain cells are prone to function irregularly or get damaged [20]. When the brain's cells are not able to communicate effectively behavioral and thinking patterns are influenced. The brain has different sections responsible for distinct activities [33]. Various types of dementia can be identified based on understanding how particular brain cells have been damaged in a specific region.

Dementia is exhibited in several different forms showcased by varied symptoms as follows:

- *Creutzfeldt-Jakob disease*: Symptoms include slowness in thinking, planning, and judgment capabilities with the weakening of the memory.
- *Lewy body dementia*: Standard symptoms of memory loss are displayed. The additional distinctive symptoms are related to body balance and movement, stiffness, and trembling.
- *Down Syndrome and Alzheimer's disease*: Noticeable switch in personality is visible because of irregular behavior. Later stages are identified by memory loss issues.
- *Fronto-temporal dementia*: Varied parts of the brain are affected leading to behavioral and personality redevelopment.
- *Mixed dementia*: Multiple forms of dementia are detected at the same time. Patients above the age of 80 are more susceptible to it.
- *Vascular dementia*: Caused by issues in blood flow to the brain.

Speech and language impairment, gait, posture, sleep patterns, abnormalities in daily routine activities, and memory impairment are identified with newer and sophisticated sensors in a smart environment.

The use of a variety of modalities provides detailed information about the patient's overall health using sensors, video feeds, text, and audio samples. Researchers are able to extract relevant information for diagnosis and detection of early stages of dementia or Mild Cognitive Impairment (MCI). Medical experts further use brain scans extensively to identify and detect the progression of the disease.

Machine and deep learning are applied vastly for various healthcare tasks [27]. Detection of dementia is complex and intricate as it tends to the elderly population. Being able to identify unique symptoms not coinciding with normal-aging factors is a challenge faced by the experts. With the use of a different set of modalities as seen in Figure 10.1, there is a wider scope of understanding unique aspects of the individual showcasing symptoms of dementia. Capturing a wide variety of pattern variations assists in deploying suitable and effective mechanisms in inpatient and assistive care.

The chapter is divided into broad sections. Section 10.2 highlights and expands in-depth about the different forms of information processed for the detection of dementia. A variety of machine and deep learning techniques are used in the detection process with individual modalities in Section 10.3. In addition, the use of natural language processing (NLP) and transfer learning (TL) are included. Multiple modalities can

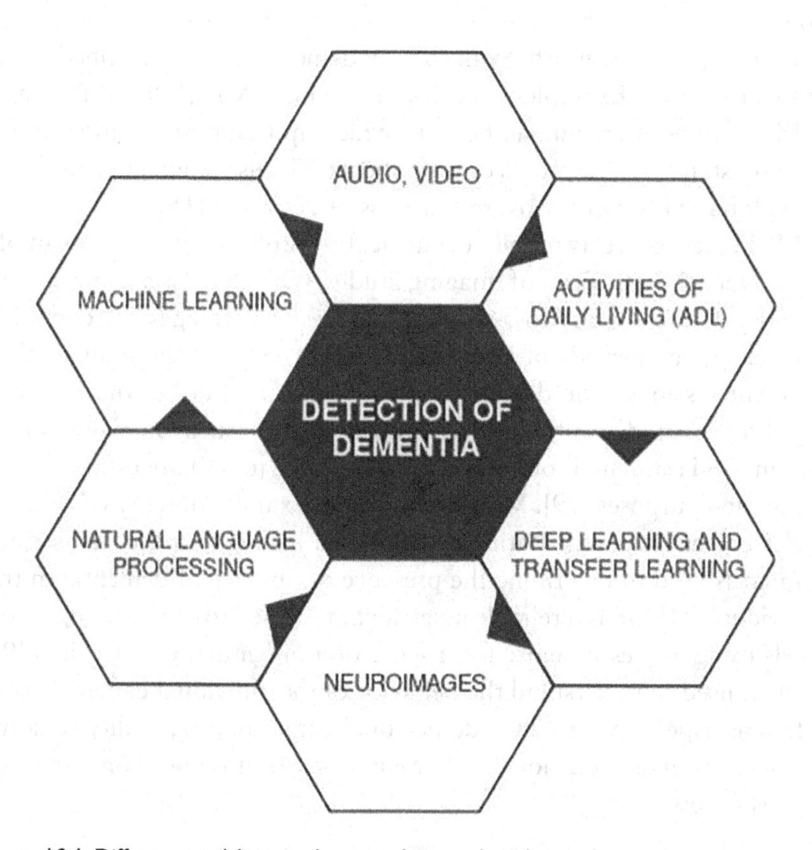

Figure 10.1 Different modalities and approaches used to detect dementia.

be integrated to improve the overall dementia detection process, which is showcased as well.

10.2 MODALITIES USED TO DETECT DEMENTIA

There are several forms of data used to identify symptoms of dementia. Different forms of data include neuroimages, daily routine information, videos, audio samples, and speech data.

Detection of dementia and MRIs go hand in hand when discussed in the field of healthcare research. Clinicians use sophisticated and detailed imaging techniques for medical diagnosis of the condition. Brain scans are widely used in the process. CT scans use X-rays to detect the structure of the brain. MRI scans use magnetic fields to detect the hydrogen atoms in the tissues of the body. In addition, functional brain imaging displays how the brain functions. It is not used as a diagnostic tool exclusively but is used largely for research. Symptoms of dementia can be identified much more in advance. Examples of such scans include fMRI, SPECT, PET, and MEG. Tissues of the human body provide important information useful to understand the symptoms of the patients. The use of imaging modality is explored widely in the overall process of detection [15].

MRI datasets are available for medical researchers, one such example is the Open Access Series of Imaging Studies (OASIS). It is a combination of MRI datasets with cross-sectional images. The images are compiled over elongated periods of time with frequent visits of the individual in different sessions. The data is used to classify and detect the presence or absence of dementia in individuals. Values such as whole-brain volume and estimated total intracranial volume (eTIV) are estimated for evaluation purposes [29]. Mini-Mental State Examination (MMSE) score and Clinical Dementia Rating (CDR) scale included in the dataset are standards used to determine the presence or absence of dementia in the individual. MMSE is a reliable assessment test used to evaluate cognition levels using a questionnaire for a score of a maximum of 30 points [9]. CDR is used to understand the behavior of the individual encompassing different aspects, which include personal care, hobbies, ability to solve problems or judge, memory, and orientation [5]. It is based on a scale of 0–3 as follows:

0 - state of no dementia
0.5 - state of questionable dementia

1 - state of Mild cognitive impairment (MCI)
2 - state of moderate cognitive impairment
3 - state of severe cognitive impairment

The project is further extended to include longitudinal images in Ref. [2]. CDR is used as a baseline to characterize the subjects in the study. A voxel is a unit measurement used in 3D imaging. Normalized whole-brain volume (nWBV) is a segment of all the voxels showcased in a tissue image, which are ordered more effectively in longitudinal MRI images. This enhances the effectiveness of the application of machine and deep learning in the overall detection process as the images are more clear and with a standardized format of NiFT1. In the cross-section dataset, the facial features were removed, and in contrast, the longitudinal OASIS dataset retains them, providing minimal impact on the segmentation algorithms. The decline in nWBV value is a key indicator of the presence of dementia. Examples of other neuroimaging datasets are Alzheimer's Disease Neuroimaging Initiative (ADNI) [16] and Clinical Record Interactive Search system (CRIS) [6].

Detection of dementia using neuroimages is a long and labor-intensive process given the magnitude of factors taken into account for the process. Specialized and sophisticated machines are required to capture the necessary details over a series of interactions. The individuals are elderly patients who need extra support and care during the diagnosis process. Since the syndrome is progressive in nature, neuroimages can be used as a final measure to detect the severity of the syndrome in addition to several other alternatives that can also capture behavioral patterns and relevant essential details.

Internet of Things (IoT) is vastly applied in the field of healthcare. It has evolved over the years where it is possible to capture essential human health information at very intricate levels. Once such a large amount of data is collected, it becomes challenging to handle the complex and unique data. The field of health care is data-intensive. Machine and deep learning algorithms offer the benefits of processing such sensory-based information in a streamlined and time-efficient manner. This progress assists various physicians, clinicians, doctors, and caregivers. Nonintrusive sensors are a preferred choice for geriatric care [17] Medical tests can now be performed at the ease of convenience of the elderly near their bedside in a safe and effective manner, which is also known as point of care (POC) diagnostics. Elderly individuals have the tendency to slow down their regular activity performances because of their age. The symptoms of dementia can be identified by monitoring their regular activities closely. Such studies use the concept of Activities of Daily Living (ADLs) as their primary input. The activities range from grooming, walking, eating, dressing, etc. This is an indication of the overall well-being of the individual, the choices they make, and the capacity for them to perform these tasks with or without assistance.

ADLs are broadly classified into,

- *BADLs*: Basic Activities of Daily Living
- *IADLs*: Instrumental Activities of Daily Living

BADLs focus on very basic, routine tasks as indicated above. IADLs focus on slightly complex tasks of managing money, shopping, cooking, housekeeping, and medication. Assessment tools are designed to process and evaluate such data. They predict the success of the living condition at the moment or identify behavioral patterns in the individuals present at the facility center. The tools are used to assess impairments for detailed diagnosis.

Patient health is monitored intricately to detect ultra-fine details using the Katz Index of Independence scale or Lawton IADL scale. Smart homes use a plethora of sensors to capture ADL data for the detection of MCI or AD in patients. One such study was performed by researchers at Washington State University. ADL data was captured to generate a dataset, Center for Advanced Studies in Adaptive System (CASAS) to understand the correlation of memory abilities with the performance of regular routine activities [7]. The smart environment was set up using motion sensors, door sensors, hot or cold water sensors, temperature sensors, and electricity-usage sensors.

Detection of dementia in the geriatric population is crucial. Videos offer the advantage of being nonintrusive while trying to monitor an individual in a smart environment. Direct installation of sensors on the body can be a hassle for elderly patients. Hence, images extracted from video feeds provide samples to understand non-stationary aspects of behavioral patterns while individuals perform regular activities. Videos are a unique form of modality explored in the field of dementia detection. The evident variations in behavioral patterns in dementia patients.

Studies have been performed to understand how agitation, sleep patterns, gait, and non-verbal communication can be used to identify specific features related to dementia.

Agitation can be used as an indicator to know how severely the patient has been impacted. A study has been conducted by researchers from Ontario [39] where they have used video surveillance for the same. In Long Term Care (LTC) homes, experts and staff can use this pertinent information to take the necessary measures for superior care of the patient that has been impacted. Deep learning models have been built to detect agitation as an anomalous behavior in individuals using unsupervised learning presented as a proof-of-concept. Spatio-temporal information is used with computer vision to provide critical details used in the detection process. The information is extracted from the videos, which is a reliable and non-invasive mechanism implemented. The overall environment is monitored and not just the individual, which provides a holistic view of the situation while diagnosing. Similar existing studies showed that convolutional LSTM autoencoders were a preferable choice against regular convolutional and deep autoencoders. DeepFall framework is an example where video data was used to extract useful spatial and thermal features.

Ambient Assisted Living (AAL) utilizes video information for critical analysis. AUXILIA [28] is a prime example that implements an interactive fall detection mechanism using videos. Good quality sleep is also used as a barometer for identifying variations in patients influenced by dementia. The REM and non-REM phases provide additional information needed for long-term analysis of the behavior. Light and deep sleep can be distinguished using machine and deep learning. The use of a contactless system is a preferable choice, and a system with smart sensors integrated with audio-visual capabilities offers a suitable solution.

A prime objective of detecting dementia is to accurately diagnose it at an early stage. This helps in slowing down the progression by taking relevant measures. Biometric recognition can be combined in the study of early detection. Human gait is an essential feature utilized. It offers the advantage of being easily measurable in varied circumstances. A study conducted by Ref. [43] geriatric care specialists in China developed a mechanism to implement the same. The use of gait analysis is a novel method used in the detection of the syndrome. An overall system is built using Kinect 2.0, a motion-sensing device to capture essential input data. Gait data is extracted visually in a detailed form. The skeleton-based gait information is applied to a CNN model that detects the presence of dementia by processing single-task and dual-task gait in gait cycles.

The use of videos in providing assistive care to advanced-stage dementia patients is explored in Ref. [32]. An individual can communicate non-verbally as well, the approach highlights the use of artificial intelligence as a medium to battle such a situation in an objective manner. Adaptive interaction is an approach where a caregiver uses repetition and imitation of body language, gestures to communicate patiently and effectively with the patient. Simple Linear Iterative Clustering (SLIC) is an algorithm applied to cluster pixels effectively, which enhances the overall image processing. The study uses videos of therapeutic sessions to detect the motion of the patients, and frame differencing technique is applied to detect such movements. A novel algorithm is proposed to showcase the estimation of the levels of patient engagements during adaptive interactions.

Audio biomarkers and memory tests are used to detect dementia. Variation in speech is a key element to detect the state of the mind and judge the proper functioning of one's cognition. Speech data can be processed using machine and deep learning techniques for the detection of MCI or Alzheimer's disease (AD). In the case of AD, loss of brain cells and connections between the neurons are evident in the initial stages while leading to the accumulation of plaques and tangles, at the later stages.

Spontaneity and fluency in speech is an important indicator of good cognition. Some of the key tests used in the detection of dementia at a granular level are Mattis Dementia Rating Scale, CDR Scale, Hachinski Ischemic Scale, Hamilton Depression Rating Scale, Blessed Dementia Scale, NYU rating scale, and MMSE. MMSE is a widely used memory test to detect dementia. Memory and thinking are evaluated using such tests also formally known as cognitive assessments. An individual loses the capability to comprehend, calculate, learn, and think as the syndrome progresses. These tests help in capturing essential details of the cognitive state of the individual. A CSF leak leads to changes in vision, cognition, and behavior.

A dementia patient exhibits variations in cognitive and behavioral patterns as well, which can be studied by neuropsychologists. Neuropsychological assessments are a barometer to test and quantify the dysfunction of the brain by analyzing and studying the complex relationship between the brain and behavior. One of the examples of this can be seen in a study done by Ref. [23] where a database such as Pitt Corpus of DementiaBank is useful in the process. Similarly, PET scans can be used with neuropsychology to detect DLB more accurately at the early stages. Neurophysiology provides additional details, which can be combined to identify sections of the brain that can showcase the variations of sensory perceptions and motor symptoms. Patients impacted by the symptom speak slowly and have disfluency.

Novel approaches are explored in the domain using voice technology. Speech detection helps in identifying the varied stages of dementia and also further supports the prediction of severity using acoustic features. Feature-level fusion and score-level fusion can be performed to evaluate the performance of the machine and deep learning models used to detect dementia. It is a non-invasive technique to diagnose the same. The status can be identified using linguistic and paralinguistic speech parameters.

Another study has been performed by Ref. [42], Framingham Heart Study (FHS) by researchers using voice recordings and deep learning for dementia detection. Responses of the individuals for verbal tests are captured meticulously. The study is able to identify and classify the individuals who had normal cognition, MCI, or dementia. An LSTM and CNN architecture was utilized to build the model for dementia screening in a streamlined and automated manner. It offers the benefit of least human intervention while processing the features directly from the audio content. Boston Process Approach is a novel technique to assess the cognition levels in-depth offering the benefit of knowing how a patient performed during the tests along with the success or failure of it. It enables the clinicians to identify specifically which portion of the brain is impacted and may be functioning improperly.

The use of multiple modalities enhances the dementia detection system as seen in the Alzheimer's Dementia Recognition through Spontaneous Speech (ADReSS) Challenge as seen in Ref. [22]. It stands for ADReSS where detection of AD is performed by extracting features from both acoustic waveforms and transcriptions. It is essential to use a standardized dataset of spontaneous speech for improving the accuracy of detection, which has been addressed by the challenge. Several systems can be built using the combined form of data to detect the stages of impact at preclinical, mild, and progression.

The characteristics of speech have unique features which when varied influence intelligibility or the capacity to be understood. Some of them include - pitch, pauses, rhythm, rate, and disfluency. Patients with dementia are characterized by having lower speaking fluency. With rhythmic patterns, the detection process is simplified as behavioral patterns can be utilized additionally. Prosody pertains to the combination of tonal, rhythmic, and intonation characteristics of speech. These features are also included in the dementia detection process. i-vector and x-vector are used in speech recognition. Features related to the speaker are captured in a compressed manner using an i-vector. There are variable-length speech segments that are mapped to embeddings using a deep neural network known as an x-vector. The input is an audio file that is represented by embeddings that are used in the classification process.

Cookie theft picture is also a common method used to detect dementia and capture essential details of the individual while assessment of the cognition level. One of the commonly used methods to extract features for an audio input is Mel frequency cepstral coefficients (MFCC) which have 39 features. Correlation-Based Feature Selection (CFS) algorithm is used for the selection of features using correlation among them. Some of the software used in the process are Kaldi Speech Recognition Toolkit, openSMILE for audio feature extraction, my-voice-analysis a python library for voice analysis, SIDEKIT a python toolkit used for speech and language research, ALIZE a C++ toolkit used for speech recognition, MSR a MATLAB-based tool used for feature extraction in speech recognition tasks, Spear-BOB a toolbox for speech recognition, SPro a toolkit to extract features of speech-related activities. Acoustic features have the extension of SPRO4, HTK, HDF5. SVM, LDA, and many more machine learning techniques were applied in several studies analyzed.

In another study, [40] dementia was detected in the preclinical stage using vocal features in daily conversations. The method was implemented to assess the cognitive functions of the individual under the standardized test of Telephone Interview for Cognitive Status (TICS-J). Machine learning models were built based on Extreme Gradient Boosting (XGBoost), Random Forest (RF), Logistic Regression (LR). Using only vocal features to detect dementia is a niche area of research. The study was performed in the Hachioji city of Tokyo where individuals above the age of 65 volunteered to participate in the program. Regular telephone conversations with an AI program were arranged to discuss the overall health of the person. The AI program used for voice recognition was developed by the collaborative efforts of Softfront Japan and McCann Health Japan. PRAAT is used to extract the vocal features from the recorded conversations.

10.3 APPLICATION OF MACHINE AND DEEP LEARNING METHODS TO DETECT DEMENTIA

Early-stage detection of dementia is sought after to assist in providing superior benefits to clinicians and individuals under observation. NLP and TL are explored in existing studies in the domain of dementia detection. Most studies begin exploration and research with the standard machine and deep learning models and slowly extend the applicabilities in novel and unique ways. Multiple modalities can be combined to detect dementia based on the requirement of the research work undertaken. The studies have shown that a combined approach is able to provide good results in dementia detection.

The standalone application of standard machine and deep learning algorithms provides useful information in the early detection of dementia. In Ref. [31], the authors have explored the vast repository of PubMed and MEDLINE to compile a survey of the most commonly used machine learning techniques implemented in the dementia detection process. The literature survey was conducted by using a combination of keywords [27]. Major categories were identified as cognitive assessment, neuroimaging, and speech analysis in the dementia detection process. The study highlighted the use of ML technologies such as SVM, RF, PCA, LDA, Naive Bayes (Bayesian network), Neural Network, Deep learning (multi-layer NNs), and DL technologies as deep NNs, autoencoders, CNNs, RNNs. The different types of modalities used to detect the presence of dementia included genetics, neuroimaging, cognitive, assessment, free texts, routine electronic health record data. Early diagnosis of dementia faces several real-time practical challenges. The use of multiple forms of high dimensional data in machine learning models is an approach explored to cause an impact on the process [26]. Brain scans, daily routine data, biological samples, and clinical data are applied to machine learning models to detect the early onset. Unsupervised forms of learning are also applied in the detection of dementia [12]. The scope of MCI to progress to dementia is a vast area of research focusing on early onset of dementia detection. Studies are performed to detect MCI which identifies the atrophies in the brain and growth of lesions. Standard machine and deep learning methods are analyzed from a pool of literature with specific keywords using Quality Assessment of studies of Diagnostic Accuracy in Systematic reviews (QUADAS) tool [13]. Some of the common deep learning architectures implemented in the detection process include CNNs, RNNs, Deep Belief Network (DBNs), Restricted Boltzmann Machines (RBMs), Deep Boltzmann Machines, and Deep Encoders. Important information is extracted from the brain using extraction tools such as Brain Extraction Tool (BET) and FFMRIB Software Library (FSL) [37].

The use of NLP and TL offer additional benefits in the detection process. Linguistics is the study of language. Language is the capacity to generate and apprehend spoken and written words. Phonemes, morphemes, lexemes, syntax, and context are the five major constituents of a language. Dementia patients can be identified with changes in language usage. Aphasia is a disorder that is generated in any individual when they are unable to communicate, where specific portions of the brain are impacted related to language processing. In geriatric individuals, the language skills decline and showcase themselves in the form of such changes. Basic abilities to read, write, speak or understand a language cause a hindrance in the individual affected.

There are various biomarkers used to detect dementia traditionally, the use of language impairment is a unique and novel approach explored. DementiaBank offers relevant resources. Narrative samples extracted from the description of a picture are used essentially in the detection process. Linguistic and acoustic features are extracted from audio files for additional processing. Linguistic features and characteristics vary based on the task. If the translation is involved, it is different. In the case of dementia detection, it can be related to transcribing. The objective of such studies largely pertains to developing state-of-the-art methods to detect dementia using language impairment.

Linguistic alterations are used to detect dementia in patients. Very minor changes can be key indicators in identifying different cognitive symptoms which are processed using NLP. Patients can experience disarray while communicating or processing linguistic information. Such disorders are also used as an indication to understand how it impacts dementia and its growth in the individual.

Studies have been performed using spontaneous speech for the early diagnosis of dementia. Language-related features are extracted from speech samples using CLAN which processes transcriptions for further analysis. SVM classifier is applied for the overall detection process.

In Ref. [11], biosensors are used to compile essential patient information providing assistance to medical caregivers in inpatient care. Studies have shown that control patients and patients diagnosed with dementia can be uniquely identified by the use of an additional variable of language samples. Deep learning models using CNN, LSTM-RNNs are used to detect and classify patients by analyzing relevant linguistic features. Novel techniques are also explored and implemented in the overall detection process such as activation clustering and first-derivative saliency.

Human speech can be categorized as unstructured data. NLP offers the benefit of processing such data by converting the voice or text into strings. Processing pipeline is a process with multiple steps that use trained models to generate an output considering the tone of the voice, or length of the sentence. To predict, decode and assimilate human language NLP uses Language Processing Pipelines. There are sub-processes involved which essentially reduces the input data into small forms to further undergo reconstruction before generating the relevant output. The steps involved are namely

- Sentence segmentation
- Word tokenization
- Text lemmatization
- Predicting parts of speech for each token
- Text lemmatization
- Identifying stop words
- Dependency parsing

In a collaborative study performed [36], NLP was used to develop a pipeline to identify the presence of dementia by detecting motor signs in a group of patients. Rigidity, freezing or tremor are some examples of motor signs. This information assists clinicians in the screening process. The study was performed using a platform Clinical Record Interactive Search System (CRIS) using an NLP algorithm and specialized software, General Architecture for Text Engineering (GATE). It is an open-source software used exclusively for text analysis. ADEPt is a pipeline implemented in the study as well. This is also an example where NLP has been applied in clinical gerontology, which constitutes the treatment, care, and diagnosis of the elderly.

Handcrafted features are used to build classification or regression models to detect dementia. They require the support of expert knowledge in the automation process. With the rapid progress being made in the field of artificial intelligence, machine and deep learning are applied to ease the work process of experts in the field of health and patient care. Specialized features can be explored using TL as it is able is share knowledge learned from a large dataset focusing on a simple task to a smaller dataset needed for a unique task. It expands the utility of pre-trained models to provide for innovative solutions. The similarity factors are transferred as much as possible to provide a feasible model for detection. Selection of the pre-trained model is also an important step in the overall process. Customization of the model to suit the needs and requirements of dementia research is equally challenging.

Speech and cognition are correlated. They are used to detect dementia in spite of having limited availability of baseline data. The address challenge provides a potential solution in such situations. Data is carefully curated by researchers with details of patients based on their age, gender, and cognitive status. The use of multiple modalities offers a vast array of features that can be used to detect dementia using TL. The use of images, speech, audio, and language are widely explored in several studies applying machine and deep learning. TL permits the use of existing knowledge learned from larger and relevant datasets, offering a wider range of applicability in the field of healthcare and patient care.

The application of TL requires the utility of standardized models. MobileNet is an example model that trains on images to detect patterns for further analysis. In the case of a textual input, BERT is used as a standard model for training. Audio samples are trained on a specialized base model such as YAMNet. Patients interact with caretakers to share their thoughts, where their speech is transcribed and also used in the dementia detection process. To train such unique data, the Mockingjay model is preferred.

When TL is applied, various modalities can be tested extensively for the task of dementia detection and a comparison can be drawn accordingly. Concepts of multitask learning can also be explored to identify inconsistencies and regions of improvement in the studies performed. The use of pre-trained models as stated offers computational benefits, leading to cost-effective solutions being implemented in the field.

In various studies [44] performed using TL for detection of the syndrome, the chosen pre-trained model addresses overfitting using fine-tuning. The last few layers of the deep learning model are replaced with suitable layers to perform the classification task in an effective manner. A combination of acoustic, linguistic, and handcrafted features is used in the detection of AD or MCI with deep learning. CNN, RNN, and LSTM architectures can be applied. Multimodal and multitask TL techniques are also explored to provide a competitive cost-effective solution. Multiple inputs can be combined to understand the influence of different feature sets. The Dual-BERT model is used for this purpose where TL is applied to a combination of speech and audio input. Different tasks share commonalities and differences, they can be used as well to improve the efficiency of the dementia detection model. PyTorch and Tensorflow are vastly used in the overall implementation process. Standard evaluation metrics are applied in the study performed.

Geriatric care is expensive and requires specialized attention from caregivers. Dementia care uses novel methods to further expand the implementation of TL. In another study [30], an ensemble model is generated constituting of linguistic, acoustic, and cognitive features. The severity of dementia is detected with ANNs using specialized temporal characteristics.

The use of attention-based TL in multi-class classification tasks can also be explored and seen in studies [38]. The source of input is derived from ADNI where MRI images are processed to provide an output in 4 categories. Boosting techniques are applied for varying the hyperparameters and optimizing the parameters.

With the advent in technology, there is scope for improvement in building innovative solutions by combining several inputs and building multimodal frameworks for dementia detection. Various researchers are now able to explore and extend the standard applications of machine and deep learning for early-stage dementia detection in novel and effective ways. Several frameworks are explored by experts analyzing a wide variety of medical data. In Ref. [25], EEG recordings are provided as input for dementia classification in an automated fashion. CWT and Bis features are extracted to process the EEG data. The model proposed is compared with AE, MLP, LR, and SVM-based multimodal classification models.

Deep learning models utilize multitask learning to detect Alzheimer's [24]. The detection process relies on time series data as the primary input. MRI and PET images are combined with cognitive scores, neuropathology, and cognitive performance data. The authors developed a framework to classify dementia at an early stage into MCI, AD, and CN stages. Ensemble learning is explored in the dimension of deep learning where the model proposed uses CNN and BiLSTM architectures for the task of classification using multiple modalities.

A combination of cross-sectional, longitudinal, and cognitive performance biomarkers was integrated to build a novel framework. The proposed system implemented a multimodal recurrent neural network and GRU-based model for Alzheimer's detection [18]. ADNI is a database that provides longitudinal data along with several types of biomarker data that include cross-sectional neuroimaging, longitudinal fluid, cognitive performance information. Disease classification is performed into MCI-C, MCI-NI, CN, and AD using three representations of 'baseline', 'single modal', and 'proposed'. 'Baseline' represents the scenario where features related to multimodal data are extracted. The extraction and use of longitudinal data are applicable to the 'single modal' scenario. The proposed model uses a combination of features extracted from both longitudinal and multimodal data.

The utility of multiple forms of input provides a holistic approach in understanding the various clinical stages. Clinical data correlates to geographical, cognition-based tests, biomarkers, imaging summary score information. MRI data provides critical information from cross-sectional images used for diagnosis. Genetic data is used in the process of detection by applying whole-genome sequencing information. Feature extraction is performed using autoencoders. Clustering and perturbation analysis further assist in the feature learning process. Shallow and deep models built with the multimodality approach [41].

Dementia detection at an early stage is performed using novel techniques while applying standard machine and deep learning methods. The studies have thrown light on the task of combining different types of relevant inputs for better performing models, improvements in the classification of dementia and its stages at the early onset are showcased experimentally.

10.4 CONCLUSION

Dementia is on the steady rise enabling medical researchers and AI community to work in tandem to develop innovative solutions for the early detection process and prevent progression. Individuals are impacted by slower cognitive abilities and motor skills when showcasing symptoms of dementia. Most studies indicate the use of neuroimages for the prediction of the onset largely. Less complex and cost-effective alternatives are also explored in the field of research of AI and healthcare. Sensors are used in a smart environment that captures binary values as ADL data to identify the symptoms. Video samples provide an overview of the movements of the individual under supervision and care, images are a powerful measure of the overall scenario involved. In the case of audio, speech, and text data linguistic features are extracted and transcribed, which can highlight the changes in the speaking patterns, thus knowing more about the cognitive effects. The different feature sets and their combinations enhance the study of dementia prediction in a non-invasive manner. Machine and deep learning approaches provide several useful advantages to handle data-intensive approaches. NLP and TL offer key advantages while tackling the varied forms of data in an effective and useful manner. The objective of the study focuses on and highlights the use of the multimodality approach in dementia detection. Caretakers, medical experts, and clinician benefit from better approaches in the fight for the prevention of dementia globally.

REFERENCES

[1] Ferrari, E., Cravello, L., Bonacina, M., Salmoiraghi, F., and Magri, F. Chapter 3.8: Stress and dementia. In: T. Steckler, N. Kalin, and J. Reul (Eds), *Handbook of Stress and the Brain*, volume 15 of *Techniques in the Behavioral and Neural Sciences*, pp. 357–370. Elsevier, 2005. DOI: 10.1016/S0921-0709(05)80064-1.

[2] Marcus, D. S., Fotenos, A. F., Csernansky, J. G., Morris, J. C., and Buckner, R. L. Open access series of imaging studies: Longitudinal mri data in nondemented and demented older adults. *Journal of Cognitive Neuroscience*, 22(12):2677–2684, 2010.

[3] National Health Portal. 2015. https://www.nhp.gov.in/disease/neurological/dementia
[4] Doody, R. Dementia- an overview, 2015. https://www.sciencedirect.com/science/article/abs/pii/S0921070905800641
[5] Clinical Dementia Rating, 2016. https://www.sciencedirect.com/topics/neuroscience/clinical-dementia-rating
[6] Alzheimer's Disease Neuroimaging Initiative, 2017. https://adni.loni.usc.edu/
[7] Casas Dataset, 2017. http://casas.wsu.edu/datasets/
[8] Gamir-Morralla, A., López-Menéndez, C., Medina, M., and Iglesias, T. Chapter 7: A novel neuroprotection target with distinct regulation in stroke and alzheimer's disease. In: I. Gozes (Ed.), *Neuroprotection in Alzheimer's Disease*, pp. 123–147. Academic Press: Cambridge, MA, 2017. ISBN 978-0-12-803690-7, DOI: 10.1016/B978-0-12-803690-7.00007-7.
[9] Mini-Mental State Examination, 2018. https://www.sciencedirect.com/topics/medicine-and-dentistry/mini-mental-state-examination
[10] Rapidly Progressive Dementias, 2018. https://memory.ucsf.edu/dementia/rapidly-progressive-dementias
[11] Karlekar, S., Niu, T., and Bansal, M. Detecting linguistic characteristics of alzheimer's dementia by interpreting neural models. In *Proceedings of the 2018 Conference of the North American Chapter of the Association for Computational Linguistics: Human Language Technologies, Volume 2 (Short Papers)*, pp. 701–707, New Orleans, LA. Association for Computational Linguistics, 2018.
[12] Cleret de Langavant, L., Bayen, E., and Yaffe, K. Unsupervised machine learning to identify high likelihood of dementia in population-based surveys: Development and validation study. *Journal of Medical Internet Research*, 20(7):e10493, 2018. ISSN 1438-8871. DOI: 10.2196/10493.
[13] Pellegrini, E., Ballerini, L., del C. Valdes Hernandez, M., Chappell, F. M., González-Castro, V., Anblagan, D., Danso, S., Muñoz-Maniega, S., Job, D., Pernet, C., Mair, G., MacGillivray, T. J., Trucco, E., and Wardlaw, J. M. Machine learning of neuroimaging for assisted diagnosis of cognitive impairment and dementia: A systematic review. *Alzheimer's & Dementia: Diagnosis, Assessment & Disease Monitoring*, 10:519–535, 2018. ISSN 2352-8729. DOI: https://doi.org/10.1016/j.dadm.2018.07.004.
[14] Centers for Disease Control and Prevention, 2019. https://www.cdc.gov/aging/dementia/index.html
[15] Dementia, 2019. https://pubmed.ncbi.nlm.nih.gov/30561351/
[16] Maudsley Biomedical Research Centre, 2019. https://www.maudsleybrc.nihr.ac.uk/facilities/centre-for-neuroimaging-sciences/
[17] Choudhuri, A., Chatterjee, J. M., and Garg, S. Chapter 6: Internet of things in healthcare: A brief overview. In: V. E. Balas, L. H. Son, S. Jha, M. Khari, and R. Kumar (Eds.), *Internet of Things in Biomedical Engineering*, pp. 131–160. Academic Press, 2019. ISBN 978-0-12-817356-5. DOI: 10.1016/B978-0-12-817356-5.00008-5.
[18] Lee, G., et al., Predicting alzheimer's disease progression using multi-modal deep learning approach. *Scientific Reports*, 9(1):1952, 2019. ISSN 2045-2322. DOI: 10.1038/s41598-018-37769-z.
[19] Dementia Australia, 2020. https://www.dementia.org.au/about-dementia/what-is-dementia

[20] Types of Dementia, 2020. https://www.hopkinsmedicine.org/health/conditions-and-diseases/dementia
[21] National Health Service, 2020. https://www.nhs.uk/conditions/dementia/about/
[22] Campbell, E. L., Docío-Fernández, L., Raboso, J. J., and García-Mateo, C. Alzheimer's dementia detection from audio and text modalities. 2020.
[23] Chakraborty, R., Pandharipande, M., Bhat, C., and Kopparapu, S. K. Identification of dementia using audio biomarkers. 2020.
[24] El-Sappagh, S., Abuhmed, T., Riazul Islam, S., and Kwak, K. S. Multimodal multitask deep learning model for alzheimer's disease progression detection based on time series data. *Neurocomputing*, 412:197–215, 2020. ISSN 0925-2312. DOI: 10.1016/j.neucom.2020.05.087.
[25] Ieracitano, C., Mammone, N., Hussain, A., and Morabito, F. C. A novel multimodal machine learning based approach for automatic classification of eeg recordings in dementia. *Neural Networks*, 123:176–190, 2020. ISSN 0893-6080. DOI: 10.1016/j.neunet.2019.12.006.
[26] Myszczynska, M. A., Ojamies, P. N., Lacoste, A. M. B., Neil, D., Saffari, A., Mead, R., Hautbergue, G. M., Holbrook, J. D., and Ferraiuolo, L. Applications of machine learning to diagnosis and treatment of neurodegenerative diseases. *Nature Reviews Neurology*, 16(8):440–456, 2020. ISSN 1759-4766. DOI: 10.1038/s41582-020-0377-8.
[27] Rawat, R. M., et al. Dementia detection using machine learning by stacking models. In *2020 5th International Conference on Communication and Electronics Systems (ICCES)*, pp. 849–854, Coimbatore, India. IEEE, 2020.
[28] Roman Siedel, T. S., et al., Contactless interactive fall detection and sleep quality estimation for supporting elderly with incipient dementia. *Current Directions in Biomedical Engineering*, 6(3):388–391, 2020. DOI: 10.1515/cdbme-2020-3100.
[29] Ryu, S.-E., Shin, D.-H., and Chung, K. Prediction model of dementia risk based on xgboost using derived variable extraction and hyper parameter optimization. *IEEE Access*, 8:177708–177720, 2020.
[30] Sarawgi, U., Zulfikar, W., Soliman, N., and Maes, P. Multimodal inductive transfer learning for detection of alzheimer's dementia and its severity, 2020.
[31] Tsang, G., Xie, X., and Zhou, S.-M. Harnessing the power of machine learning in dementia informatics research: Issues, opportunities, and challenges. *IEEE Reviews in Biomedical Engineering*, 13:113–129, 2020. DOI: 10.1109/RBME.2019.2904488.
[32] Zhang L, O. A., et al., Quantification of advanced dementia patients' engagement in therapeutic sessions: An automatic video based approach using computer vision and machine learning. In *Annual International Conference of the IEEE Engineering in Medicine and Biology*. 2020. DOI: 10.1109/EMBC44109.2020.9176632.
[33] Dementia Friendly Wyoming, 2021. https://www.dfwsheridan.org/types-dementia
[34] National Institute of Aging, 2021. https://www.nia.nih.gov/health/what-is-dementia
[35] World Health Organisation (2021) Dementia, 2021. https://www.who.int/news-room/fact-sheets/detail/dementia

[36] Al-Harrasi, E. I., et al., Motor signs in alzheimer's disease and vascular dementia: Detection through natural language processing, co-morbid features and relationship to adverse outcomes. *Experimental Gerontology*, 146:111223, 2021.

[37] Bansal, D., Khanna, K., Chhikara, R., Dua, R. K., and Malhotra, R. A systematic literature review of deep learning for detecting dementia. In: D. Goyal, A. K. Gupta, V. Piuri, M. Ganzha, and M. Paprzycki, (Eds.), *Proceedings of the Second International Conference on Information Management and Machine Intelligence*, pp. 61–68. Springer: Singapore, 2021. ISBN 978-981-15-9689-6.

[38] Guram, M. H. et al. Improved demntia images detection and classification using transfer learning base convulation mapping with attention layer and xgboost classifier. *Turkish Journal of Computer and Mathematics Education (TURCOMAT)*, 12(6):217–224, 2021.

[39] Khan, S., et al., Unsupervised deep learning to detect agitation from videos in people with dementia. *IEEE Access*, 2021. DOI: 10.13140/RG.2.2.33167.51361.

[40] Shimoda, A., Li, Y., Hayashi, H., and Kondo, N. Dementia risks identified by vocal features via telephone conversations: A novel machine learning prediction model. *PLoS One*, 16(7):e0253988, 2021.

[41] Venugopalan, J., Tong, L., Hassanzadeh, H. R., and Wang, M. D. Multimodal deep learning models for early detection of alzheimer's disease stage. *Scientific Reports*, 11(1):3254, 2021. ISSN 2045-2322. DOI: 10.1038/s41598-020-74399-w.

[42] Xue, C., Karjadi, C., Paschalidis, I. C., Au, R., and Kolachalama, V. B. Detection of dementia on raw voice recordings using deep learning: A framingham heart study. *Alzheimer's Research & Therapy*, 13(1):146, 2021.

[43] Zhang, Z., et al., Deep learning based gait analysis for contactless dementia detection system from video camera. In *2021 IEEE International Symposium on Circuits and Systems (ISCAS)*, pp. 1–5. 2021. DOI: 10.1109/ISCAS51556.2021.9401596.

[44] Zhu, Y., Liang, X., Batsis, J. A., and Roth, R. M. Exploring deep transfer learning techniques for alzheimer's dementia detection. *Frontiers in Computer Science*, 3:22, 2021. ISSN 2624-9898. DOI: 10.3389/fcomp.2021.624683.

Chapter 11

Heart attack analysis and prediction system

Ashish Kumar Das, Ravi Vishwakarma, Adarsh Kumar Bharti, and Jyoti Singh Kirar
DST-CIMS, Banaras Hindu University

CONTENTS

11.1 INTRODUCTION

The heart is considered an important organ to a human. If a heart doesn't perform its operation properly, it will affect various organs of the human-like brain, lungs, etc. According to the UN, the one-third population worldwide died from heart condition and cardiovascular diseases. Heart disease and attacks are found to be one of the reasons for

DOI: 10.1201/9781003368342-11

deaths in developing and developed countries. The heart circulates blood throughout the blood vessels present in the heart system. Blood provides the body with vitamins and nutrients, further aiding in the removal of metabolic wastes, and if blood within the body is inadequate, then several organs like neural structure and vital organs fail and lead to the death of the patient.

Heart disease factor include:

- High cholesterol
- High blood pressure
- Diabetics
- Smoking and consuming alcohol
- Being obese
- Family history of coronary illness

Symptoms of heart attack:

- Shortness of breath
- Pain and discomfort in chest
- Pain travels to left or right arm or to neck, back or stomach, etc
- Fatigue and Cold sweat and unsteadiness
- Rapid or irregular heartbeat

The effective prevention of heart attack is also a target of the research. The rest of this paper describes the data mining process. The survey is briefly discussed and problems are identified. In this chapter, methodology is discussed, and results are given in sections. This chapter finally gives conclusion and future work.

11.1.1 Literature survey and comparative analysis

This chapter predicts the heart attack in both males and females. It only contains dataset of those individuals who are above 25 years i.e., teenagers are not included. Detailed information, such as risk factors, about heart attack has been explained in this chapter in a concise manner. The data mining and machine learning algorithm is used to predict the heart attack within individual.

Sushmita Manikandan [1] built a model for predicting the heart attack in patient using classifier, i.e., Naïve Bayes algorithm. The data set was taken from the UCI machine learning repository containing 14 features including a target feature. She aims to predict whether the individuals are prone to heart attack or not based on the risk factors. The accuracy score of 81.25 is obtained by using Naïve Bayes Algorithm.

Nida Khateeb and Usman Muhammad [2] Proposed various models for heart attack prediction using a classifier algorithm i.e., K-Nearest Neighbor. The dataset was taken from UCI Machine Learning repository containing 13 features and a target feature of records of 303 patients. Various machine learning and data mining techniques were used such as Naïve Bayes, K-Nearest Neighbor, and Bagging Technique were used here for experimentation. The accuracies of models were calculated without feature reduction. The results were NB, KNN, DT, and Bagging with accuracies of 58.74%, 52.8%, 54.78%, and 59.73%, respectively. This system can be reliable as its accuracy using NB, KNN, and DT classifiers has been tested using dataset 14 features. These results are reliable as it has been tested using all the features mentioned.

Radhimeenakshi [3] Proposed a system for predicting and classifying the heart disease and heart attack using techniques like Support Vector Machine and Artificial Neural Network techniques. The dataset was taken from the UCI machine learning repository. It has 303 records and 14 features in all including a target feature. The target feature was to predict whether patient is prone to heart disease or not. Support Vector Machine models were used to predict the trained and tested dataset and delivered an accuracy score of 84.7% and with a precision of 85.6% whereas Artificial Neural Network showed an accuracy of 81.8 and precision score of 83.3. It is clearly seen that Support Vector Machine performed better than Artificial Neural Network in terms of accuracy and precision. The advantage of ANN is that it performs better in terms of specificity and adaptability to extensive training because of its tendency to classify non-linear data and the handling of multiple features effectively.

11.2 GOALS

The main aim is to predict and detect heart attack in patient or individual at an early stage.

- Through this, the present research work aims to administrate proper treatment to patient.

- The present work also aims to reduce high death rate occurred due to heart attacks.
- This has been achieved by building solution using machine learning and data mining techniques like logistic regression and decision tree algorithm.
- The present research work aims to build a high-accuracy model and models that take less time to predict the output with decent accuracy in case of emergency for which important selection of features are required.
- The present work contains medical history or patient's record. The data is stored in the system and after pre-processing, it is split into train and test dataset and then fed to the machine learning models to learn from the train dataset and test model's accuracy by predicting the patients with heart-related problem by comparing with known class variable.
- Also, to identify hidden patterns from the dataset that were previously unknown and also to find a significant pattern from the dataset through visualization and model building. The system accepts new patient data and process it to predict the probability of the patient suffering from heart attack.

11.3 DESIGN

11.3.1 Data collection

The dataset [4] is collected from Heart Disease Dataset in the UCI machine learning repository. UCI is a collection of databases that are used for the implementation of machine learning algorithm. The dataset used here consists of 303 data and 14 features including a target feature. Here the present research work predicts the target feature, i.e., whether an individual is prone to heart attack or not based on these 13 features.

11.3.1.1 Feature information

The dataset which the present research work considered consists of 13 features (risk factors) such as age of the patient (age), gender of the patient (sex), chest pain type (cp), resting blood pressure (trtbps), cholesterol in mg/dL (chol), fasting blood sugar (fbs > 120 mg/dL), resting electrocardiographic results (restecg), maximum heart rate (thalachh), exercise included angina (exng), and previous peak (old peak), slope of the peak exercise ST segment (slp), number of major vessels (caa), and thal rate (thall).

Few of the features are discussed below.

1. *High blood pressure (trtbps):* High blood pressure puts extra stress on the heart and other organs. Checking our blood pressure value regularly is critical in order to avoid long-term complications such as heart disease, heart failure, stroke, impaired vision, kidney disease, etc.
2. *Chest pain type (cp):* Chest pain is the major cause of heart-related problems, and in most of the cases, it is life-threatening. Whether the chest pain is actually severe or not can only be diagnosed by doctors. Patients feel chest pain descending from the neck to the upper abdomen. Causes of chest pain include:

   Sharp sensation, burning, squeezing, or crushing sensation, coronary artery disease (CAD), and myocardial infarction (heart attack).
3. *Cholesterol (chol):* Cholesterol is a wax-like substance found in the blood and arteries. Human body cells need cholesterol to build healthy cells, but excess of cholesterol can lead to the risk of heart-related disease. With cholesterol increment, the body generates fatty deposits in the blood vessels and arteries. Eventually, fatty deposits grow and make blood difficult to flow through the arteries leading to cardiovascular disease and heart attack. If the cholesterol level is more than 200 mg/dL there is a possibility that the patient might suffer from heart disease.
4. *Fasting blood sugar (fbs):* A blood sample is taken from an overnight fasting, and if the blood sugar level is more than 110 mg/dL, then the individual is highly prone to diabetic. Diabetic is a chronic problem, and if it remains for prolonged time, then it will result in heart disease and heart attacks. This could also result in high blood pressure leading to deteriorate the health condition of the heart.
5. *Electrocardiographic results (restecg):* An electrocardiogram captures the electric signals of the heart to investigate the health of the heart. It is a test to detect heart-related issues and associated disease. The doctor uses an electrocardiogram to detect: Abnormal heart

rhythm (arrhythmias) detects whether you have had any previous heart attack. The graph will show whether the individual is having a chance of heart attack or not.

6. *Exercise-induced angina (exng):* Angina is a symptom caused when blood flow in the heart tissue reduces leading to a pain in the chest. If angina pain is felt in the chest due to performing exercise, then this might result in heart diseases and attacks.

   If symptoms like shortness of breath or chest pain occur while performing any kind of physical activity for some minutes or more, then that individual may be at risk of heart attack.
7. *Coronary artery (caa):* Another important feature is coronary artery-related disease. Coronary artery provides oxygen, nutrients, and blood to the heart. The disease arises when major vessels related to the heart get damaged or diseased, resulting in CAD. It also occurs when coronary arteries become narrow or blocked. There are three types of CAD, which include:
   - *Obstructive:* Blood vessels have narrowed or blocked.
   - *Non-obstructive:* Blood vessels are narrower because of branching or heart muscle squeezing tightly on the vessels.
   - *SCAD:* Spontaneous coronary artery dissection (SCAD) refers to the blood vessels tearing in the heart.

All these three types are responsible for knowing the degree of heart attack of an individual of any age or gender.

11.3.2 Data pre-processing

The raw data is transformed into an understandable format and stored in the form of comma-separated values (CSV). The collected data had some missing and duplicated values, which have been taken care of properly and accurately. The dataset was analyzed, and normalization was performed too to improve integrity. Data visualization is performed to understand the feature relation with each other and drawing insights that were previously unknown. After that, it was split into training and testing dataset for model building. Various classification models were implemented and tried to find a model that worked efficiently with the dataset by comparing it with other models (Figure 11.1).

11.3.3 Architecture diagram

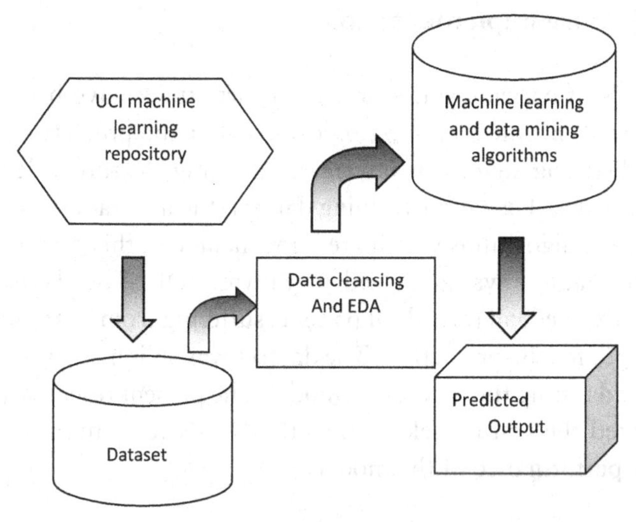

Figure 11.1 Architecture diagram of our prediction process.

11.3.4 Machine learning approach

The present research work implemented various machine learning models to predict heart attacks in patients based on feature values. Since the aim of the present work is to predict heart attack in patients, supervised machine leaning algorithms like classification models were used as the class variable is binary in the dataset. Here supervised machine learning algorithms are used to predict heart attack.

1. Logistic Regression
2. Decision Tree Classification Algorithm
3. Random Forest Classifier
4. Support Vector Machine
5. K-Nearest Neighbor
6. Naive Bayes Algorithm

11.3.5 Hardware and software

The present research work used a device with specifications of 4 GB of RAM size, Windows 7, a 2.1 GHz CPU, and a tool like Python programming language.

11.4 IMPLEMENTATION

11.4.1 Feature implementation

The records of patients suffering from heart attack have been collected from the UCI machine learning repository. For the prediction, different machine learning algorithms were used. After feature selection and training the model using the training dataset, the accuracy was compared with different algorithms which are implemented in this present research work. The dataset was analyzed in Jupyter IDE. The dataset, which contained the medical records of patients suffering from heart attack, was used as input for the prediction. The dataset was split into two subsets for training and testing the prediction model. The present research work also implemented the feature selection methods to select important features for better performance of the models.

11.4.2 Data visualization

Here the graphical representation of information, patterns, and trends are explained in a well-defined manner. Below are some of the visualizations of some risk factors of heart attack in the dataset used in this present research work.

Figure 11.2 explains the results of the patients' (male and female) diagnosis of heart attack gotten from the risk variable, which is the "output variable" of the dataset used. The "output variable" shows whether a patient is susceptible to heart attack or not. The blue color of the bar chart represents the patients with lesser chances of having heart attack, while the orange color represents patients with a high chance of having heart attack. It showed that 92 male patients and 72 female patients have suffered from heart attack, whereas 114 male patients and 24 female patients have not suffered from heart attack according to the dataset used (Figure 11.3).

In this bar chart, the blue color shows the number of patients having a lower chance of having heart attack due to exercise-induced angina (exng), whereas the orange color shows the numbers of patients having a higher chance of having heart attack due to exercise-induced angina, regardless of gender and age. Here, the binary number 0 indicates that the patients have symptoms of exercise-induced angina, and the binary number 1 indicates that the patients do not have symptoms of exercise-

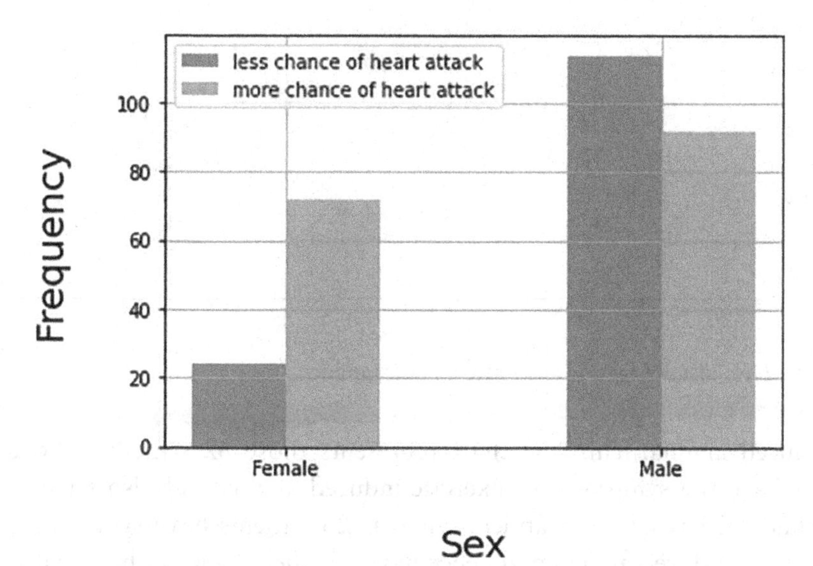

Figure 11.2 Chances of different levels of heart attack for different genders.

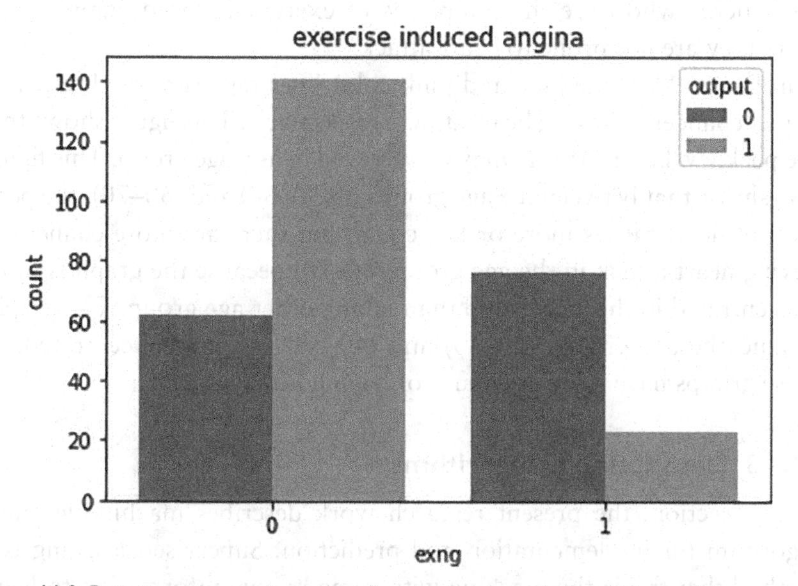

Figure 11.3 Patients with exercise-induced angina (exercise-induced chest pain).

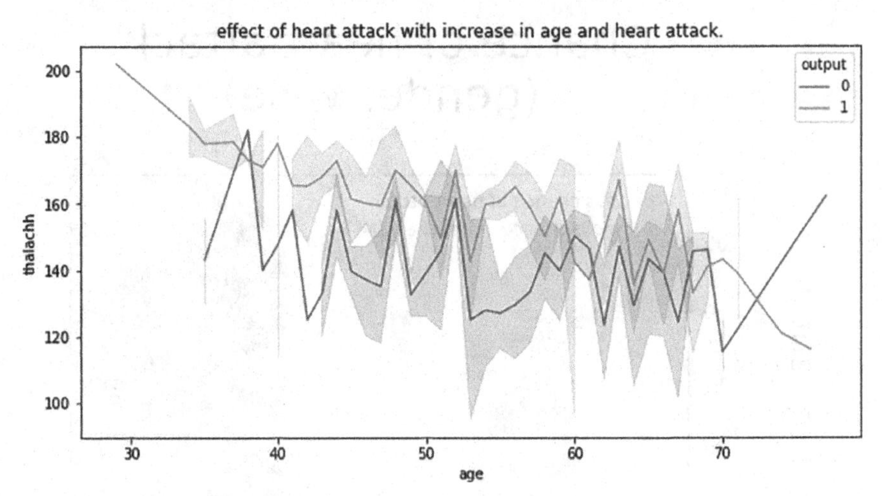

Figure 11.4 Effect of age and heart rate on heart attack.

induced angina. This bar chart represents those 62 patients who do not have the symptoms of exercise-induced angina and also have less chance of having heart attack, whereas 23 patients have symptoms of exercise-induced angina and hence have a higher chance of having heart attack. But there are 141 patients who do not have symptoms of exercise-induced angina; even then, they are prone to heart attack, and there are 76 patients who have the symptoms of exercise-induced angina; even then, they are not prone to heart attack.

In Figure 11.4, the blue and pink color lines represent the lower and higher chances of having heart attack, respectively. This figure shows that the peak level of heart rate may be achieved in any age group. This figure also shows that between the age groups of (50–60) and (60–70), the peak level of heart rate is more or less equal, but there are more chances of having heart attack in the age group (60–70) because the graph is more concentrated in this age group than in any other age group. The graphs around the age groups (30–40) and (40–50) are less concentrated, so these groups have a lower chance of having heart attack.

11.4.3 Description of algorithms

In this section, the present research work describes machine learning algorithm for implementation and prediction. Supervised learning is a method that trains the machine with some known information to learn from data and draw insights that will help in building the model for the prediction of heart attack in patient.

The present research work used six algorithms to predict heart attack in individuals.

- Logistic Regression [5]
- Decision Tree Classification Algorithm [6]
- Random Forest Classifier [7]
- Support Vector Machine [8–10]
- K-Nearest Neighbor [11]
- Naive Bayes Algorithm [12]

11.4.4 Training and testing dataset

Training and testing of the data are very important concepts when it comes to model building. In machine learning, the algorithm learns from the datasets. They tried to find relationship between the data points and analyze patterns to make a decision. The better the training, the better the result. After training the data, the present research work tries to access the performance of the model that is built. To do that, a test dataset is fitted to the model by providing the test data to it and trying to predict the target feature. Here, the present research work splits the dataset into two parts: one part of the data that contains 80% of the dataset is used for training the model, and the rest of the 20% is used for testing the model. The present research work can perform testing and training of the data by importing the package train_test_split from sklearn.

11.4.5 Algorithm accuracy

During implementation, the present research work uses different algorithms, which are described above, while considering a different number of feature sizes or Chi-scores. The present research work found that the more useful the features for prediction, the higher the score. After implementation, the present research work found that logistic regression classifier performs better for prediction with ten best features. The following accuracies are obtained by using K-fold cross-validation to remove over- and under-fitting in our dataset. The accuracies mentioned are basically average accuracies obtained by taking different K-folds.

The highest accuracy of logistic regression is 0.96. The present research work also tried obtaining accuracies with different features using these algorithms, but only with ten features did logistic regression have highest average accuracy of 85.09%.

11.4.6 Quantitative analysis

The present research work tried to compare the results with the rest of the classification models. In the previous studies mentioned [1–3], model the systems with algorithms such as Logistic Regression, Random Forest, Decision Tree, Naïve Bayes, and K-Nearest Neighbor and obtain accuracies with different features. The comparison with other studies that were mentioned earlier is mentioned in these tables (Table 11.1).

The Random Forest accuracy of our model is comparatively high when taken with ten features. The accuracy is the average accuracy obtained by K-fold cross-validation technique, with highest accuracy of 85.2% and lowest accuracy of 75.34%.

Below Table 11.2 compare with other study.

The Decision Tree average accuracy of our model is not performing well with ten features (Table 11.3).

Tables 11.4 and 11.5 show the accuracies of KNN and SVM with other studies.

Table 11.1 Model accuracy

Model	*Accuracy (%)*	*Time (seconds)*
Logistic regression	85.09	0.04514
Decision tree	73.83	0.02977
Random forest	83.42	0.51574
SVM	79.44	0.03066
KNN	77.79	0.02958
Naïve Bayes	75.44	0.02199

Table 11.2 Naïve Bayes algorithm accuracy comparison

Research study	*Features*	*Accuracy (%)*
Manikandan [1]	13	81.25
Khateeb and Muhammad [2]	13	58.74
Our model	10	75.44

Table 11.3 Decision tree accuracy comparison

Research study	*Features*	*Accuracy (%)*
Khateeb and Muhammad [2]	14	84.26
Our Model	10	73.83

Table 11.4 KNN algorithm accuracy comparison

Research study	*Features*	*Accuracy (%)*
Khateeb and Muhammad [2]	13	52.80
Our model	10	77.79

Table 11.5 SVM algorithm accuracy comparison

Research study	*Features*	*Accuracy (%)*
Radhimeenakshi [3]	13	84.7
Our model	10	79.44

11.5 EXPERIMENTS

In this section, the evaluation of our implemented model is conducted and explained. The present research work tries to analyze the complexity of the model and resolve the issue. In the present research work, we have analyzed the model accuracy algorithms to acquire knowledge about our proposed model.

The present research work has also analyzed the models to justify their effectiveness by performing some experiments with the test dataset. In addition to that, the performance of the algorithms used in our prediction with different sizes of datasets with different algorithms and with different feature selection methods particularly. Some of them are described below.

11.5.1 Forward feature selection

Forward Feature Selection is a method [13] of selecting best features out of number of features. Table 11.6 shows the algorithm's accuracy with best ten features and time taken by them. Here, it is seen the logistic regression performs better, and SVM and KNN found to be close

Table 11.6 Model accuracy

Model	*Accuracy (%)*	*Time (seconds)*
Logistic regression	84.96	0.05179
Decision tree	76.14	0.02567
Random forest	82.09	0.52828
SVM	84.43	0.05382
K-Nearest Neighbor	83.43	0.03217
Naive Bayes	78.12	0.02203

Table 11.7 Model accuracy

Model	*Accuracy (%)*	*Time (seconds)*
Logistic regression	84.40	0.02747
Decision tree	73.83	0.01702
Random forest	80.47	0.57965
SVM	81.10	0.01444
KNN	78.46	0.01734
Naive Bayes	77.77	0.00973

competitors to it, and it is observed that it was not performing well as compared to Table 11.1 feature selection methodology.

11.5.2 Linear discriminant analysis (LDA)

It [14] is a dimensionality reduction technique in which a dataset of high dimensional space is present research worked into a dataset of lower dimensional space. It helps to find the area that maximizes the separation between multiple classes and helps in classification. The present research work has reduced our dataset to a single dimensional dataset, trained and tested our dataset, and tabled the accuracy. Logistic regression performs better here, with accuracy of 84.40%. If time is taken into consideration, then Naive Bayes will perform better in medical emergency. Still, it doesn't improve the model's performance, and hence the chi-square feature selection technique is still dominating, as mentioned in Table 11.1 (Table 11.7).

11.5.3 Results

As seen in the Experiment section, models were performing well with different feature selection methodologies, but they lagged behind those in Table 11.1. The present research work compares logistic regression to some well-known classifiers and finds that logistic regression outperforms the other models with an accuracy score of 85.09. When compared with different authors, as mentioned earlier, our model's timely performance and accuracy were better under the circumstances.

11.6 CONCLUSION AND FUTURE WORKS

This research work presents a model that has been built using existing machine learning techniques to predict heart attacks in patients using the dataset from UCI machine learning depository. The removal of duplicates from the data for checking outliers and null values to prediction is done. The over-fitting problem was prevented by using cross-validation. During cross-validation, the dataset was partitioned into *k*-subsets called folds. Then, iterating with *k*–1 folds to train and the remaining to test which allows test set of data to be unseen for selecting the final model's. The present research work tried building algorithm for comparative purposes such as Random Forest, SVM, KNN, Decision Tree, and Naive Bayes classifiers used for model building with the same dataset. It has been found that logistic regression works better than any other algorithms after chi-squared forward feature selection method is implemented in our dataset with best ten features. New patterns were discovered after feature selection, such as the priority order of risk factors in the prediction of heart attacks in patients.

There can be many other techniques of data mining algorithms, such as neural network and deep learning algorithms, that can be used to get better models and higher accuracy than this, but this one does not need them because the number of study variable is less.

As a part of the future scope of this system, newly introduced classification algorithms can be used in order to improve the accuracy.

This present research work could assist medical professionals in predicting the heart attack in new patients by entering the required parameters into the model and obtaining the output based on the input. Early detection and prediction of heart attacks in patients will reduce the mortality rate due to heart attack.

REFERENCES

[1] S. Manikandan, Heart attack prediction system. *2017 International Conference on Energy, Communication, Data Analytics and Soft Computing (ICECDS)*, Chennai, 2017, p. 817820.

[2] N. Khateeb, U. Muhammad, Efficient heart disease prediction system using K-Nearest Neighbor classification Technique. *Proceedings of the International Conference on Big Data and Internet of Things*, London, United Kingdom, December 20–22, 2017.

[3] S. Radhimeenakshi, Classification and prediction of heart disease risk using data mining techniques of Support Vector Machine and Artificial Neural Network. *2016 3rd International Conference on Computing for Sustainable Global Development (INDIACom)*, New Delhi, 2016, pp. 3107–3111.

[4] kaggle, Heart Attack Analysis and Prediction Dataset, Available at https://www.kaggle.com/rashikrahmanpritom/heart-attack-analysis-prediction-dataset.

[5] S.B. Kotsiantis, I. Zaharakis, P. Pintelas, Supervised machine learning: A review of classification techniques. *Emerging Artificial Intelligence Applications in Computer Engineering*, 2007, 160(1): 3–24.

[6] Y. Yan-Song, *Decision Tree Methods: Applications for Classification and Prediction*. Shanghai Municipal Bureau of Publishing: Shanghai, 2015. ncbi.nlm.nih.gov.

[7] A. Liaw, M. Wiener, Classification and regression by random Forest. *R News*, 2002, 2(3): 18–22.

[8] M.E. Mavroforakis, S. Theodoridis, A geometric approach to support vector machine (SVM) classification. *IEEE Transactions on Neural Networks*, 2006, 17(3): 671–682.

[9] J.S. Kirar, R.K. Agrawal, Relevant frequency band selection using sequential forward feature selection for motor imagery brain computer interfaces. *2018 IEEE Symposium Series on Computational Intelligence (SSCI)*, pp. 52–59, 2018. doi: 10.1109/SSCI.2018.8628719.

[10] J.S. Kirar, R.K. Agrawal. Composite kernel support vector machine based performance enhancement of brain computer interface in conjunction with spatial filter. *Biomedical Signal Processing and Control*, 2017, 33: 151–160.

[11] Z. Deng, et al., Efficient kNN classification algorithm for big data. *Neurocomputing*, 2016, 195: 143–148.

[12] K. Dnuggets, Naive Bayes Algorithm: Everything you need to know, Available at https://www.kdnuggets.com/2020/06/naive-bayes-algorithm-everything.html.

[13] T. Hastie et al., *The Elements of Statistical Learning*. Springer: Berlin, Germany.

[14] G. Banu, Predicting thyroid disease using linear discriminant analysis (LDA) data mining technique. *Communications on Applied Electronics*, 2016, 4: 4–6. doi: 10.5120/cae2016651990.

Chapter 12

Utility of exploratory data analysis for improved diabetes prediction

Udita Goswami, Yashaswa Verma, Anwesha Kar, and Jyoti Singh Kirar
Banaras Hindu University

CONTENTS

DOI: 10.1201/9781003368342-12

12.1 INTRODUCTION

Diabetes is an intimately acquainted word in the current world and a pivotal challenge in both developed and developing nations. The pancreas secretes insulin, a chemical in the body that allows glucose to pass from food into the circulatory system. The absence of this chemical due to malfunctioning of the pancreas forms diabetes, which can bring about coma, renal/retinal failure, pathological destruction of pancreatic beta cells, cardiovascular dysfunction, cerebral vascular dysfunction, peripheral vascular diseases, sexual dysfunction, joint failure, weight loss, ulcer and pathogenic effects on immunity. As per World Health Organization (WHO), research on diabetes patients shows that diabetes among grown-ups (more than 18 years of age) has ascended from 4.7% to 8.5% from 1980 to 2014, respectively, and is rapidly growing up in second and third world countries. A portion of the measurable discoveries in 2017 showed that around 451 million individuals were living with diabetes around the world; further, this toll will increase to 693 million by 2045. One such study shows that the severity of diabetes is such that a large portion of a billion groups will have diabetes worldwide, and this number will increase from 25% to 51% in 2030 and 2045, respectively. The pervasiveness of diabetes is significantly found among different nations such as Canada, China, USA, India, and so forth, which makes diabetes a significant reason for death on the planet. The construction and deployment of an early predictive method in order to seclude such illnesses can save a huge number of human lives. In any case, there is no drawn-out remedy for diabetes, but it can be controlled and prevented if an early prediction is possible. The prediction is a challenging task, as the distribution of classes for all attributes is not linearly separable. However, different classification procedures of supervised machine learning can do this forecast; still, picking the best technique is extreme. Consequently, for this reason, we have applied here a portion of the famous classification and ensemble methods such as Decision Trees, K-Nearest Neighbour, Logistic Regression, Random Forest Classifier and Support Vector Classifier on the dataset and built the best model for diabetes prediction.

12.2 LITERATURE REVIEW

- Mitushi Soni, Dr. Varma and others presented their Diabetes Prediction Model in 2020, in which they used machine learning techniques such as Support Vector Machine (SVM), K-Nearest Neighbour (KNN), Decision Trees, Logistic Regression, Random Forest and Gradient Boosting.
- Aishwariya Mujumdar, Dr. Vaidehi and others proposed a prediction model in 2019 where they implemented Support Vector Classifier, Random Forest Classifier, Decision Tree Classifier, Extra Tree Classifier, Ada Boost, Linear Discriminant Analysis (LDA) and several other classifiers.
- Dr. Kayal Vizhi and Aman Dash presented a robust framework for diabetes prediction in 2020 where they implemented major steps of machine learning using classifiers such as KNN, Logistic Regression, SVM, Decision Trees and Artificial Neural Network (ANN).
- In 2016, M.S. Barale, D.T. Shirke and others presented a hybrid prediction model, which includes a Simple K-means clustering algorithm, integrated by the application of classification algorithm.
- Md. Kamrul Hasan, Md. Ashraful Alam and others presented an article on the prediction of diabetes using machine learning algorithms in health care in 2020 where they applied seven different machine learning algorithms and compared their performances.

12.3 PROPOSED SYSTEM

Machine learning is actually a subfield of Artificial Intelligence that enables machines to improve a given task with its experience. It is crucial to note that all machine learning techniques are classified as Artificial Intelligence. However, the corollary is not true since some basic rule-based engines could be classified as AI, but they do not learn from experience. These techniques provide us with efficient results, which are achieved by collecting knowledge and building various classification and ensemble models from the collected dataset. These techniques are as supervised learning, unsupervised learning, semi-supervised learning and reinforcement learning.

In our project, we have used supervised machine learning. Here the algorithms are designed in such a manner that they can learn from the examples, and the processes are carried out under surveillance. In general, just as a teacher teaches the activities to be carried out in a class, these algorithms also work in the same way. During the process of training in this algorithm, we always focus on finding and recognizing the patterns in the data such that it can correlate with our desires in the form of outputs. Post-training, we feed in new, unseen inputs and determine under which labels the new inputs will be classified, based on prior training data.

Now we construct our proposed system for the experiment, here we start from:

i. Collection of the data.
ii. Data cleansing.
iii. Exploratory data analysis (EDA) is carried out to get initial intuitions about the dataset and to pictorially depict them.
iv. Based on insights using EDA, the outliers are identified and dealt with.
v. Then on filtered data, we perform feature selection.
vi. We perform data standardization prior to feeding the data into suitable models.
vii. Next, we move on to model building.
viii. During training, a classification algorithm is fed with data points with an assigned category. The task expectation of a classification algorithm is to take an input value, and based on the training data provided, assign it a class or category that it fits into. In our dataset, we have two classes: Class with Diabetes and the other without Diabetes, so now this problem can further be simply seen as a Binary Classification problem. The algorithm is given training data with population that is both diabetic and non-diabetic, based on this prior data our model will map and find the features within the data that correlate to either of the classes. Here the mapping function is of the form: $-y = f(x)$. Then, when provided with an unknown observation, the model will use this function to determine whether the observation is diabetic.
ix. Classification problems can be solved with a number of algorithms, which are further discussed in this report.
x. Post this; we measure the performance of each ML technique using K-fold cross-validation, ROC and hyperparametric tuning.
xi. At last, we make a comparative analysis of our proposed method with other project works on the same dataset.

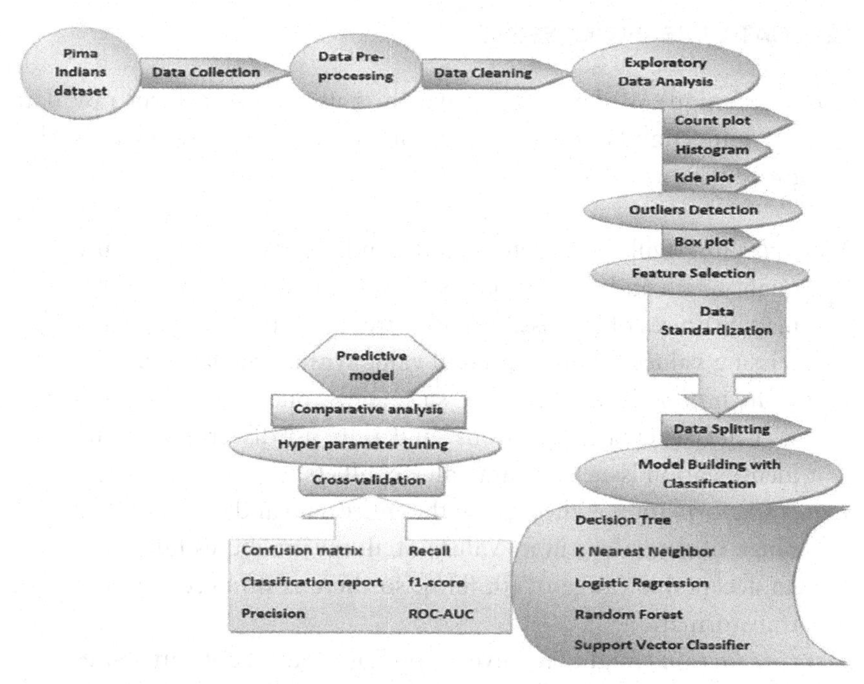

Figure 12.1 Flow – diagram of the proposed architecture.

Here, Figure 12.1 gives a well-executed flow diagram of our proposed framework for diabetes prediction.

12.4 DATA COLLECTION

Our source data for diabetes prediction is publicly available at UCI ML repository and Kaggle as –PIMA Indians Dataset. There are eight numerical variables, zero categorical variables and one target variable in this dataset. Since the data contains only numerical features, we have checked whether any of them are stored as text and found out that there are no features that are stored as text, so we can proceed safely. The dataset also has 500 non-diabetic patients and 268 diabetic ones (represented as Outcome 0 and 1, respectively).

12.5 DATA PRE-PROCESSING

It is a technique of data mining which is used to transform raw data into an understandable piece of information. This process is further categorized as–

Data cleaning will filter, detect, and handle dirty data to ensure quality data and quality analysis results. In this scenario, there may be noises of impossible and extreme values or outliers and missing values. There is no null value within the dataset.

Data integration is not needed, since only one dataset is used with no schema integrations, and thus no discernible entity identification issues or data value conflicts.

Data transformation is checked on the entire data and on the overall range of the values in it. Values of all the attributes fall under an acceptable range of [0, 846], so there is no need for data transformation.

Data reduction might involve dropping redundant attributes through attribute dimensionality reduction but there are no related cases detected.

12.5.1 Exploratory data analysis

EDA aims to perform initial investigations on the data before formal modelling by using graphical representations or visualizations. The summarized information on main characteristics and hidden trends in data can help the doctor to identify concerned areas and problems.

Outcome labels and count plot: Taking a closer look at the outcome labels, there are two classes of diabetes outcome with quantitative discrete binary data values, where 1 has 268 instances, and 0 has 500 as clearly depicted in Figure 12.2.

Histogram: It is used in order to display the shape and spread of the continuous sample data.

From Figure 12.3, we can see that the attributes are more or less positively skewed.

Outliers detection using box plots: While dealing with the outliers we have used box plots that depict a method of graphically illustrating groups of arithmetic data via their quartiles. In

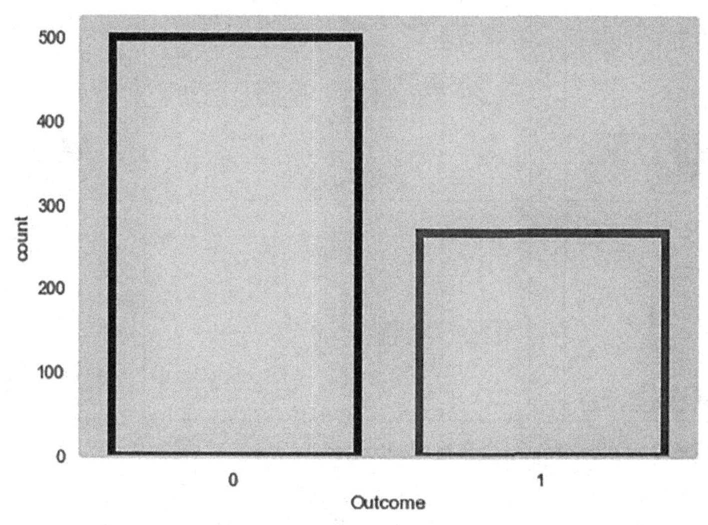

Figure 12.2 Histogram depicting the count of Non-Diabetic (0) i.e. 500 persons and Diabetic (12.1) i.e. 268 persons of the population.

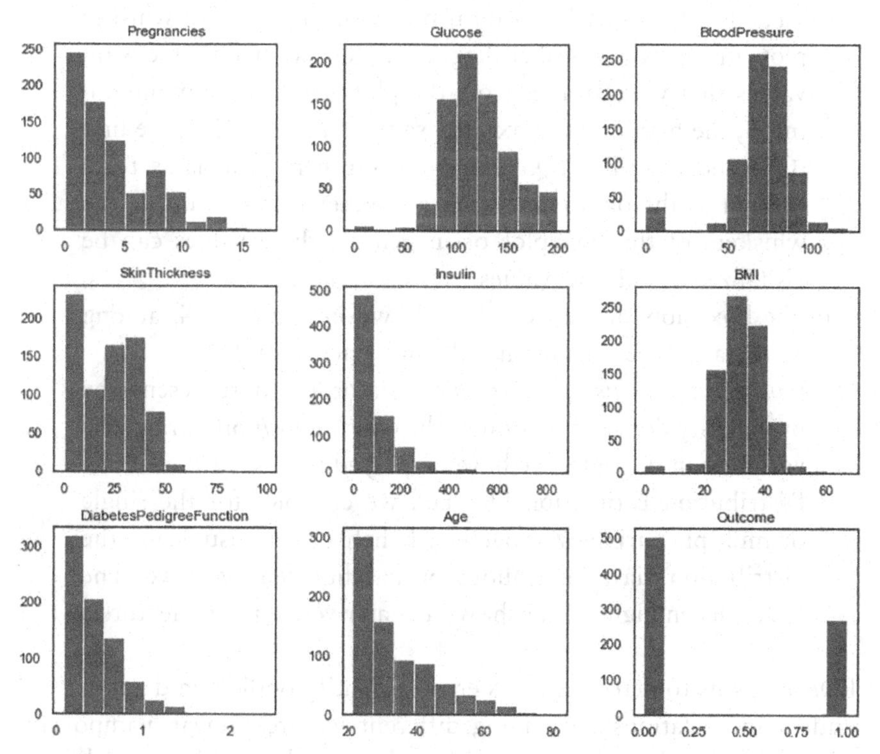

Figure 12.3 Histogram of various attributes in dataset.

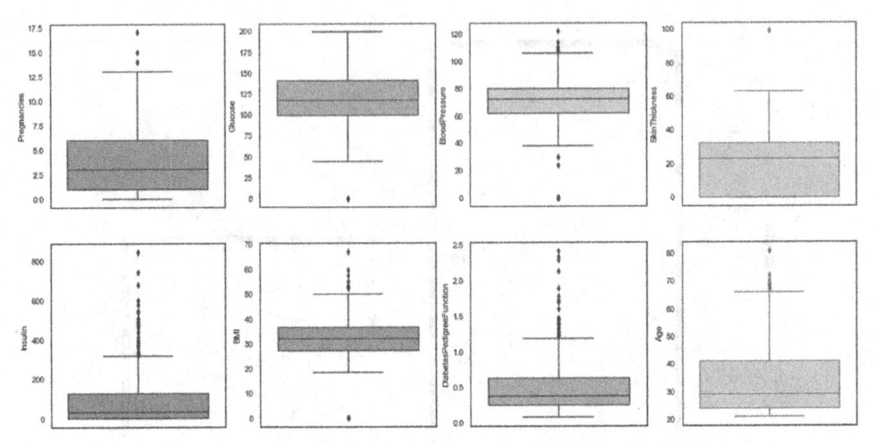

Figure 12.4 Box plot of attributes in the dataset.

these plots, there are lines extending from the boxes, termed as whiskers that present variability outside the upper and lower quartiles. Hence, we can term box plots as box-and-whisker plots or box-and-whisker diagrams. Here we mainly focus on values that we can infer from the plot, such as the minimum (min), the maximum (max), the sample median (Q2), the first (Q1) and the third (Q3) quartiles. Outliers in a dataset are defined as the data points that are either located outside the whiskers of the box plot or in general these values can be visualized as extreme values.

In the box plots of diabetes data shown in Figure 12.4, among all the attributes, insulin has the most no. of outliers.

Data visualization using KDE plot: In order to represent the probability density function of the continuous/non-parametric variables in the data, we have employed the use of the Kernel Distribution Estimation Plot i.e., we can plot for the single or multiple variables altogether. It helps us in visualizing the distribution via a continuous probability density curve. The KDE plot in Figure 12.5 shows a neater version of all features.

EDA helps us to detect obvious errors, identify outliers in datasets, and understand relationships among different features, unearth important factors, find hidden patterns within data, and provide us with new insights.

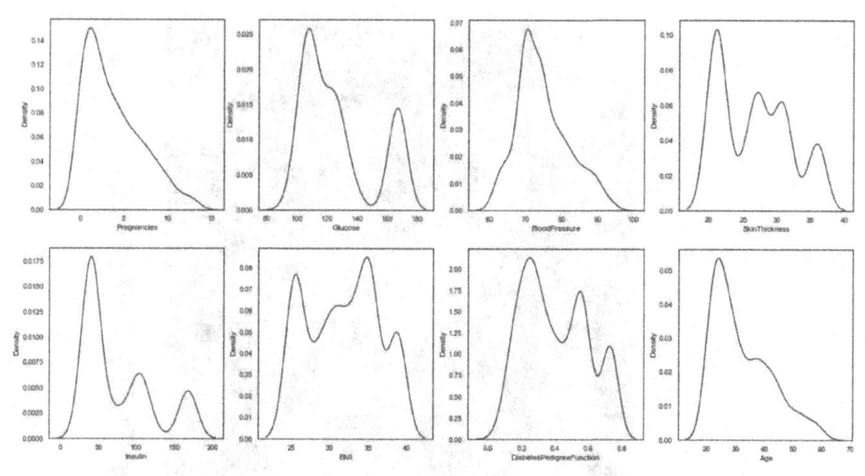

Figure 12.5 KDE plot for attributes without outliers.

12.5.2 Feature selection

After we are done with the visualizations, we have gone for feature selection of the attributes. This method of machine learning helps us to get the best set of features, which are useful in building a good model. We have intensively used the method of correlation matrix using heat map in this regard.

Correlation matrix using heat map: Heat Maps are the methods of graphically depicting the data. Here the correlation between the data values is represented via colours and numeric values. As per the statistical definition of correlation, it's a measure of the degree of linear relationship between two variables and more. One intuition of using this is that variables that are highly correlated with the target variables have a higher numeric value or a darker colour tone here and are termed as good variables for modelling. From the heat map shown in Figure 12.6, we can see that almost all predictor variables were weakly correlated among themselves. Using these intuitions, we shall let go of the variables having a lower value of the coefficient in accordance with the target variable. We will now set an absolute value; let's assume 0.3 to be the threshold for the selection of our variables.

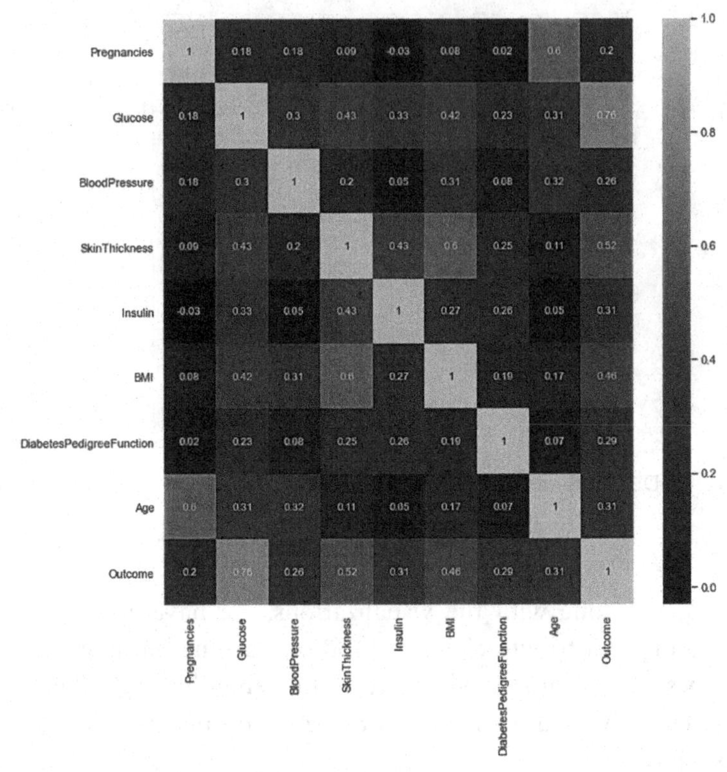

Figure 12.6 Correlation matrix of the attributes.

Based on these criteria, we have considered Glucose, Skin Thickness, Insulin, BMI and Age for final model building.

12.6 DATA STANDARDIZATION

After feature selection, we have constructed a standardized version of the data. Since all the selected features are at different scales, we have transformed the data into a common scale. As part of the Data Preparation field, it deals with the transformation of datasets after the data is pulled from source systems and before it's loaded into target systems. In our dataset, we have done scaling of the data set using Sklearn's *StandardScaler()*. This is the technique to rescale the attributes for achieving standard Gaussian distribution with parameters as 0 and 1 i.e. Mean = 0 and variance = 1. This further helps to deal with the skewness in the data by reducing it.

12.6.1 Data splitting

Under this, the dataset will be split into two groups namely the training group and the testing one. Now we had employed the train_test_split() function of Sklearn for this purpose. The attributes in both of the sets are similar but the point of difference is the attribute values. The training and construction of the classification models are done using the training group values. Prior to evaluating the model performance based on the performance metrics, the test group is used to predict the classifications of the new unbiased data that were not used to train the model.

12.7 MODEL BUILDING

The dataset will now be inserted into several classification models. We have used numerous classification techniques to predict the output variable, in this case, the diabetic and non-diabetic patients. The motto is to evaluate their performance. To name a few methodologies used here are as follows.

12.7.1 Decision trees

Let the training vectors be denoted as $x_i \in R^n, i = 1, \ldots, l$ along with a label vector as $y \in R^l$. The motto here is to do a partition in such a manner that the samples from the feature space with the same labels/same target values should get grouped together.

Let the data at node m be represented by S_m with N_m samples. Let the candidate split $\theta = (j, t_m)$ consist of a feature j and threshold t_m, such that we partition the data into and subsets.

$$S_m^{\text{right}}(\theta)\, S_m^{\text{left}}(\theta) = \{(x,\ y)\,|x_j \le t_m\} \tag{12.1}$$

$$S_m^{\text{right}}(\theta) = \frac{S_m}{S_m^{\text{left}}(\theta)} \tag{12.2}$$

Now we will compute the impurity function or the loss function which is denoted here by $H()$, so as to evaluate the quality of our candidate split of node,

$$G(S_m,\ \theta) = \frac{N_m^{\text{left}}}{N_m} H\left(S_m^{\text{left}}(\theta)\right) + \frac{N_m^{\text{right}}}{N_m} H\left(S_m^{\text{right}}(\theta)\right) \tag{12.3}$$

Now, the aim is to pick those bunches of parameters that are minimizing the impurity.

$$\theta^* = \underset{\theta}{\arg\min}\ G(S_m, \theta) \tag{12.4}$$

We will now recourse for the subsets $S_m^{\text{left}}(\theta)$ and $S_m^{\text{right}}(\theta)$ till we have attained the maximum allowable depth, i.e. $N_m <$ min.samples or $N_m = 1$.

12.7.1.1 Classification criteria

Here our target variable is an outcome of classification, which in turn is taking on the values $0, 1, 2, \ldots, K-1$, for the node m, let p_{mk}

$$p_{mk} = \frac{1}{N_m \sum_{y \in S_m} I(y=k)} \tag{12.5}$$

be the proportion of class k observations in node m. If m is a terminal node, *predict_proba* for this region is set to p_{mk}. Common measures of impurity are the following.

$$\text{Gini :} \quad H(S_m) = \sum_k p_{mk}(1 - p_{mk}) \tag{12.6}$$

$$\text{Entropy :} \quad H(S_m) = -\sum_k p_{mk} \log\ p_{mk} \tag{12.7}$$

$$\text{Misclassification :} \quad H(S_m) = 1 - \max_k\ p_{mk} \tag{12.8}$$

12.7.2 K-nearest neighbor

It is used to identify and cluster the data points into multiple classes or groups so that we can use this for the prediction of an upcoming new sample point. It is a non-parametric, lazy learning algorithm. It classifies new cases based on a similarity measure (i.e., distance functions).

12.7.2.1 Distance-weighted k-NN

First, we replace

$$f(q) = \underset{v \in V}{\text{argmax}} \sum_{i=1}^{k} \delta(v, f(x_i)) \text{ by}$$

$$f(q) = \underset{v \in V}{\text{argmax}} \sum_{i=1}^{k} \frac{1}{(x_i, x_q)} \delta(v, f(x_i)) \tag{12.9}$$

We can also consider here general kernel functions like Parzen Windows may be, instead of inverse distance.

12.7.2.2 Predicting continuous values

We replace

$$f(q) = \underset{v \in V}{\operatorname{argmax}} \sum_{i=1}^{k} w_i \delta(v,\ f(x_i)) \quad \text{by :}$$

Now we'll have, $w_i = 1$ for all

$$f(q) = \frac{\sum_{i=1}^{k} w_i f(x_i)}{\sum_{i=1}^{k} w_i} \tag{12.10}$$

12.7.3 Logistic regression

It is a method that is used intensively in regression, predictive analysis as well as for classification purposes. Here the motto is to conduct an analysis in such was that the dependent variable gets classified in binary classes. Its equation is obtained as

$$y = b_1 x_1 + b_2 x_2 + b_3 x_3 + \cdots + b_n x_n \tag{12.11}$$

Further, as an addition to this, we evaluate logit or the sigmoid.

12.7.4 Random forest

It is based on the concept of multiple decision trees and some of its benefits of over tree algorithm is that it doesn't overfit. Further, the motto here is to calculate the Gini importance by assuming that we have two child nodes as it's done in binary trees:

$$ni_j = w_j C_j - w_{\text{left}}(j)\, C_{\text{left}}(j) - w_{\text{right}}(j)\, C_{\text{right}}(j) \tag{12.12}$$

where,

ni is denoted as the importance of node j
w_j is indicated as weighted number of samples reaching node j
C_j is denoted as impurity value of node j
left (j) is denoted as child node from the left split on node j
right (j) is denoted as child node from the right split on node j

Now, we shall evaluate the importance of each feature in that of the decision tree as

$$fi_i = \frac{\sum_{j:\text{ node } j \text{ splits on feature } i} i_j}{\sum_{k\in \text{ all nodes}} ni_k} \tag{12.13}$$

here, fi_i = importance of feature

The values will be normalized now using:

$$\text{Norm } fi_i = \frac{fi_i}{\sum_{j\in\text{all features}} fi_j} \tag{12.14}$$

At the Random Forest level, the final feature importance is given as the average of all the trees.

$$\text{RF } fi_i = \frac{\sum_{j\in \text{ all trees}} \text{norm } fi_j}{T} \tag{12.15}$$

here,

RF fi_i is denoted as the importance of feature i calculated from all trees

norm fi_j is denoted as the normalized feature importance for feature i in tree j

T = total number of trees

12.7.5 Support vector classifier

SVC is used for both regression and classification. The concept on which we make separating plane or decision boundary is based on equation which is of the form

$$y = m\,x + c \tag{12.16}$$

Let us consider the mathematical equation:

$$g(x) = w^T x + b \tag{12.17}$$

$$\begin{aligned} \text{Maximize } k \text{ such that}: \quad & -w^T x + b \geq k \quad \text{for } d_i = 1 \\ & -w^T x + b \leq k \quad \text{for } d_i = -1 \end{aligned}$$

Value of (x) depends upon $\|w\|$, so we have to keep a look at the following:

1. Keep $\|w\|$ = 1 and maximize (x)
2. Keep $(x) \geq 1$ and minimize $\|w\|$

12.8 EXPERIMENTAL RESULTS

12.8.1 Classification model performance

Now, we will evaluate the model performance using various metrics such as Confusion matrix, Classification report, Area Under the curve (AUC) and Receiver Operator Curve (ROC).

12.8.1.1 Confusion matrix

This is a tabular representation for evaluating the performance of the classification models. From the set of test data for which the true values are known, we apply these methods and compare their metrics. It has four different combinations of predicted and actual values in the case for a binary classifier (Table 12.1).

In this Figure 12.7,

TP = True Positive
FP = False Positive
FN = False Negative
FP = True Negative

The confusion matrix of Random Forest Classifier is the best as it is correctly able to predict the occurrence of Diabetes in 110 patients and the non-occurrence of Diabetes in 46 patients, followed by the confusion matrix of Decision Trees which is correctly able to predict the occurrence of Diabetes in 110 patients and the non-occurrence of Diabetes in 45 patients, then comes the confusion matrix of KNN which is correctly able to predict the occurrence of diabetes in 110 patients and the non-occurrence of Diabetes in 45 patients, after this the confusion matrix of Support Vector Classifier comes, which is correctly able to predict the occurrence of Diabetes in 100 patients and the non-occurrence of

Table 12.1 Confusion matrix

Predicted values		*Actual values*	
		Positive (1)	*Negative (0)*
	Positive (1)	TP	FP
	Negative (0)	FN	TN

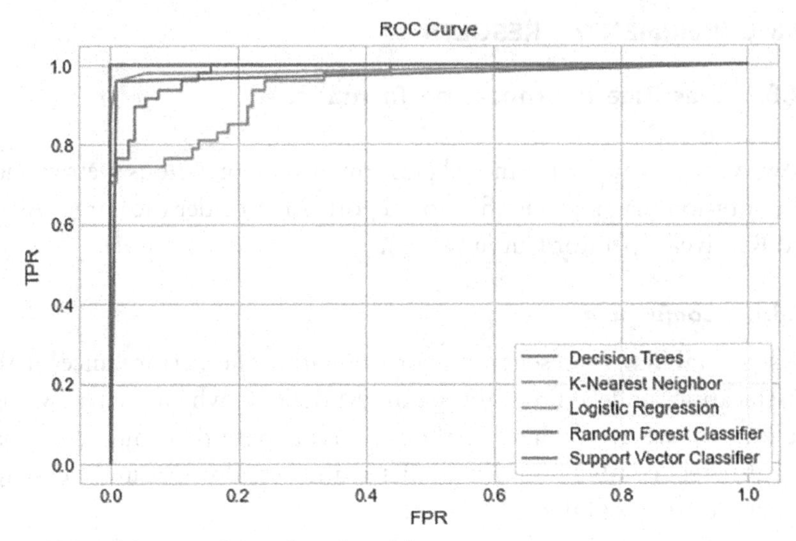

Figure 12.7 ROC curve of the selected models.

Diabetes in 36 patients and finally it is the confusion matrix of Logistic Regression, which is correctly able to predict the occurrence of Diabetes in 98 patients and the non-occurrence of Diabetes in 35 patients.

12.8.1.2 Classification report

This is a summary or brief detail which compares several metrics of classification.

a. *Accuracy*: It is defined as the number of values that our model has been able to predict rightly. Accuracy alone cannot tell the full story when working with a class-imbalanced dataset in which there is a significant disparity between the number of positive labels and negative labels. The formula for accuracy is given by

$$\text{Accuracy} = \frac{\text{TP} + \text{TN}}{\text{TP} + \text{TN} + \text{FP} + \text{FN}}$$

b. *Precision*: Out of all the classes, precision is how much we have predicted correctly. Precision should be as high as possible. The formula for Precision is given by

$$\text{Precision} = \frac{\text{TP}}{\text{TP} + \text{FP}}$$

c. *Recall*: It's the number of responses that we have evaluated correctly among the group of positive classes. It should be as high as possible. The formula for Recall is given by

$$\text{Recall} = \frac{\text{TP}}{\text{TP} + \text{FN}}$$

d. *f1-score*: It's the method employed when we need to compare two classifiers and formulated as the inverse of the arithmetic mean of inverse of precision and recall. As a result, the classifier will only get a high F-1 score if both recall and precision are high. The formula for f1-score is given by

$$f1\text{–score} = \frac{2 \times \text{Recall} \times \text{Precision}}{\text{Recall} + \text{Precision}}$$

12.8.1.3 Area under the curve

It's a 2-D area under the ROC curve and ranges from 0 to 1. For an ML technique that classifies the data or predicts it 100% wrong, has an AUC of 0 and the ML technique that classifies the data 100% correct, has an AUC of 1.

12.8.1.4 Receiver operator curve

It is used to pictorially represent the performance of the model and its thresholds. This curve plots two parameters:

- True Positive Rate (TPR)
- False Positive Rate (FPR)

The formulae for TPR & FPR are given as follows-

$$\text{TPR} = \frac{\text{TP}}{\text{TP} + \text{FN}}$$

$$\text{FPR} = \frac{\text{FP}}{\text{TN} + \text{FP}}$$

An ROC curve plots TPR vs. FPR at different classification thresholds. From Figure 12.7, we can clearly see that the ROC curve of Random Forest Classifier is the best as its AUC score is 1.0.

12.8.2 K-fold cross-validation

It is a procedure used to estimate the skill of the model on the dataset and to avoid overfitting or underfitting. In general, the K-fold cross-validation is conducted where the value for k is chosen such that each of the train set or test set is large enough to be statistically representative of the broader dataset. We have chosen the value of k as 10.

In Table 12.2, we have summarized the performance of the selected ML techniques based on various attributes like Train accuracy, Test accuracy, Precision, Recall, f1-score, AUC and K-fold cross-validation score. From this table we can infer that the test accuracy is the highest for Random Forest Classifier (99.35%), the AUC value is the greatest for Random Forest (1.00) and its K-fold Cross-validation score is 98.3%, which implies that the classifier is 98.3% accurate in fitting the model on the data and more competent in avoiding overfitting. So, it is now clear that this classifier will give the best prediction.

12.8.3 Hyperparameter tuning

These are the parameters that govern the entire training process and directly control the behaviour of the training algorithm. They have a crucial impact on the potential of the model that is being trained. Now in order to have the best hyperparameters for our model we now employ the following methods as – *Grid Search* and *Random Search*.

a. *Grid search*: Here a search is carried out among the set of hyperparameters and further it helps to find the optimal combinations. The main demerit of this process is that it can be time-consuming and computationally expensive.
b. *Random search*: Here, we use this procedure which searches within the specified subset of hyperparameters randomly unlike Grid Search. In our project, we used Grid Search on KNN and Logistic Regression models and Random Search on Support Vector Classifier model, among them K-Nearest Neighbour gives the best score with the best parameter 'n-Neighbours = 5'. Its major advantage is that it has a low processing time.

Table 12.2 Summary table for selected ML techniques

Models	*Train accuracy*	*Test accuracy*	*Precision (%)*	*Recall (%)*	*f1-score*	*AUC*	*K-fold cross-validation score*
Decision tree	1.000	0.980	98	99	0.99	0.974	0.968
Random forest	1.000	0.993	100	100	1.00	1.000	0.983
K-nearest neighbours	0.961	0.980	98	99	0.99	0.986	0.929
Logistic regression	0.902	0.893	89	92	0.90	0.944	0.894
Support vector machine	0.946	0.919	90	97	0.94	0.983	0.920

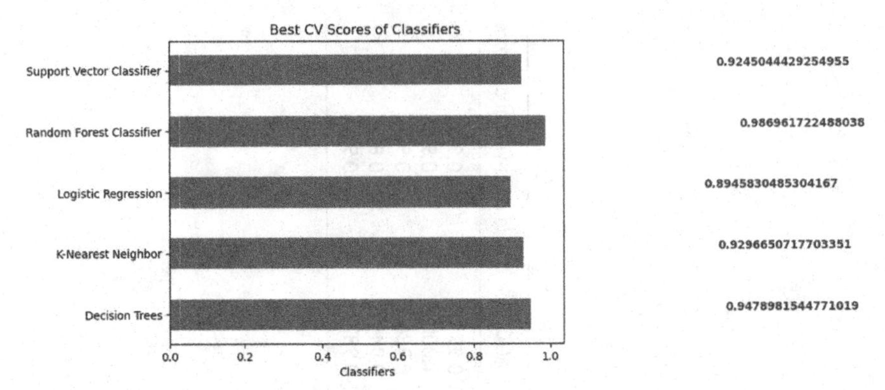

Figure 12.8 Cross-validation scores of the different ML methods using hyperparameter tuning.

As per the plot given in Figure 12.8, it is evident that Random Forest Classifier has performed better than the other classifiers. Hence, we shall save our predictive model with this classifier.

12.9 COMPARATIVE ANALYSIS

In Table 12.3, we have done a comparative analysis of our proposed framework against state-of-the-art works. Here, the overall comparison is made on the project description, and outcomes of the respective projects, followed by gaps in research methodologies and finally contrasting changes that we have incorporated in our proposed framework to make it more refined and user-friendly.

In Table 12.4, we have made a comparison of our proposed framework against the state-of-the-art works based on the accuracies of our selected ML techniques like Decision Trees, KNN, Logistic Regression, Random Forest Classifier and Support Vector Classifier.

CONCLUSION

The main motto behind selecting this topic for the project work is the early prediction of Diabetes in the human body by using various Classification techniques of supervised machine learning so that the common people can get the essence of Artificial Intelligence at an affordable cost in lesser time. KNN, Logistic Regression, Support Vector Machine, Decision Tree and Random Forest are the classification algorithms, which

Table 12.3 Comparative analysis of our proposed framework against the state-of-the-art works

Author's name	*Description*	*Outcomes*	*Research gap*	*Contrast*
Mitushi Soni and Sunita Varma (2020)	In this project work, Classification and Ensemble techniques like K-Nearest Neighbour (KNN), Logistic Regression (LR), Decision Tree (DT), Support Vector Classifier (SVM/SVC), Gradient Boosting (GB) and Random Forest (RF) were used to predict diabetes. The accuracy is different for every model when compared to other models	Random forest classifier has given the maximum accuracy of 77.17%, followed by logistic regression 75.2%, SVM 71.13% and KNN 68.9%	The model can be improved to increase the precision and recall value and can be tested on real-time data	Feature selection and K – fold cross-validation technique has resulted in an increase in the precision and recall values. Random Forest stands out with maximum precision (1.00) and recall (1.00)
Aishwariya Mujumdar and Vaidehi (2019)	Big data analytics and machine learning classification techniques were widely used in this prediction model in order to cope up with large volumes of databases in the healthcare sectors and also to discover hidden patterns from the data	Here KNN and SVM have given accuracies of 90% and 70% respectively. These are compared on the basis of their performance in diabetes forecasting	The prediction model can be further improved to increase the accuracy	Using data pre-processing and standardization procedures, we were able to improve the model and attain significantly better results
Kayal Vizhi, Aman and Dash (2020)	Their entire procedure was based on a machine learning workflow. They had undergone many steps such as data exploration, feature engineering, advanced feature selections, model building and hyperparameter tuning	Here the classifier LR has achieved the highest accuracy of 77.64% followed by RFC (74.75%), KNN (71.15%), decision trees (68.55%) and SVM (65.61%)	The accuracy of the model is low which can be increased	Hyperparameter tuning was implemented to get better accuracy with LR, DT, KNN, SVM and RFC

(Continued)

Table 12.3 (Continued) Comparative analysis of our proposed framework against the state-of-the-art works

Author's name	*Description*	*Outcomes*	*Research gap*	*Contrast*
M.S. Barale and D.T. Shirke (2016)	In this paper, the classifiers like LR, ANN, SVM and DT were used for the classification of the dataset. After k -means clustering, the author had acted upon by removal of the mislabelled instances from the database. Further, the remaining instances were used as input to the classifiers ANN, LR and DT	The developed models cascaded k-means combined with logistic regression and k-means combined with artificial neural network gave accuracy above 98% while k-means combined with SVM achieved the accuracy of 95.31%. The processed data was also analysed using ANN, SVM and LR yielding accuracies of 75.10%, 79.32% and 76.10%, respectively	The performance of reported classifiers can be improved by using ensemble methods	K-fold cross-validation optimized the model accuracies to a larger extent
Kamrul Hasan et al. (2020)	In this paper, a robust framework was proposed for diabetes prediction where outlier rejection, data standardization, feature selection and K-fold cross-validation were employed along with different ML classifiers	The results had established the efficacy of the recommended model in the early detection of diabetes	A large number of features were extracted which increased the execution time	Through data filtration and outlier detection, we have sorted out the valuable features from the dataset thereby decreasing the runtime of the model

Table 12.4 Comparative performance of our proposed framework against the state-of-the-art works

Classifiers	*Accuracy (in %)*					
	Our project	*Mitushi Soni and Sunita Varma (2020)*	*Aishwariya Mujumdar and Vaidehi (2019)*	*Kayal Vizhi, Aman and Dash (2020)*	*M.S. Barale and D.T. Shirke (2016)*	*Kamrul Hasan et al. (2020)*
DT	98.00	76.81	95.42	68.55	78.93	93.45
KNN	98.00	68.9	90	71.15	74.30	92.6
RFC	99.30	77.17	96.32	74.75	81.61	96.56
LR	89.30	75.20	82.36	77.64	76.10	88.56
SVC	91.90	71.13	70.00	65.61	79.32	89.10

are used on the dataset to build the best predictive model with the highest accuracy among all. Here, EDA & Feature selection have played a crucial role in robust and precise prediction. Hyperparameters tuning also increased the learning capability of the classifiers. The grid search cross-validation score of Random Forest is the best i.e. 98.69%, which made it the most preferred classifier among all. The proposed model can be applied to many medical contexts and research fields to verify their generality and versatility in the prediction of the disease.

REFERENCES

Aishwariya Mujumdar, Vaidehi, "Diabetes Prediction using Machine Learning Techniques", *International Conference on Recent Trends in Advanced Computing*, 2019.

Kamrul Hasan, AshrafulAlam, Dola Das, Eklas Hossain, Mahmudul Hasan, "Diabetes Prediction Using Ensembling of Different Machine Learning Classifiers", *IEEE Access*, 2020. DOI: 10.1109/ACCESS.2020.2989857.

Kayal Vizhi, Aman Dash, "Diabetes Prediction Using Machine Learning", *International Journal of Advanced Science and Technology*, 29(6), 2020, 2842–2852.

M.S. Barale, D.T. Shirke, "Cascaded Modelling for PIMA Indian Diabetes Data", *International Journal of Computer Applications*, 39(11), (2016), 0975–8887.

Mitushi Soni, Sunita Varma, "Diabetes Prediction using Machine Learning Techniques", *International Journal of Engineering Research & Technology (IJERT)*, 9(9), 2020, 921–925.

Chapter 13

Fundus image classification for diabetic retinopathy using deep learning

Monika Mokan, Soharab Hossain Shaikh, and Devanjali Relan
BML Munjal University

Goldie Gabrani
VIPS-TC College of Engineering

CONTENTS

13.1 INTRODUCTION

The complication in diabetic retinopathy (DR) occurs due to elevated blood sugar levels, and it damages the retinal blood vessels. It also results in swelling and leaking [30]. In an advanced stage of DR, it may cause blindness which is quite common in developed nations [34]. It has a significant financial impact on society, particularly on healthcare systems [6, 15, 19]. It is thus always advisable that frequent retinal screening for diabetic patients is carried out to discover DR early and manage its progression. This can prevent blindness for approximately 90% of cases

DOI: 10.1201/9781003368342-13

of visual loss. As a result, it's critical to categorise and stage the severity of DR in order to find the right treatment.

Retinopathy is a type of retinal degeneration that happens regularly in the eye as a result of a systemic condition such as diabetes or hypertension. Microaneurysms (MA) (small dots in a fundus camera image), Haemorrhages (HR) (blood deposits on the retina caused by a microaneurysm), Cotton Wool Spots (CWS) (round or oval white fluffy lesions), Hard Exudates (HE) (lipoprotein deposits caused by abnormal vascular leakage and appear as white or yellowish-white), Druse (small round or oval) (Figure 13.1).

Ophthalmologists' physical diagnosis of DR is time-consuming and labour-intensive, and it is prone to disease misdiagnosis. As a result, employing a computer-aided diagnosis system can help diagnose while also saving money, time, and effort. Deep learning (DL) has arisen

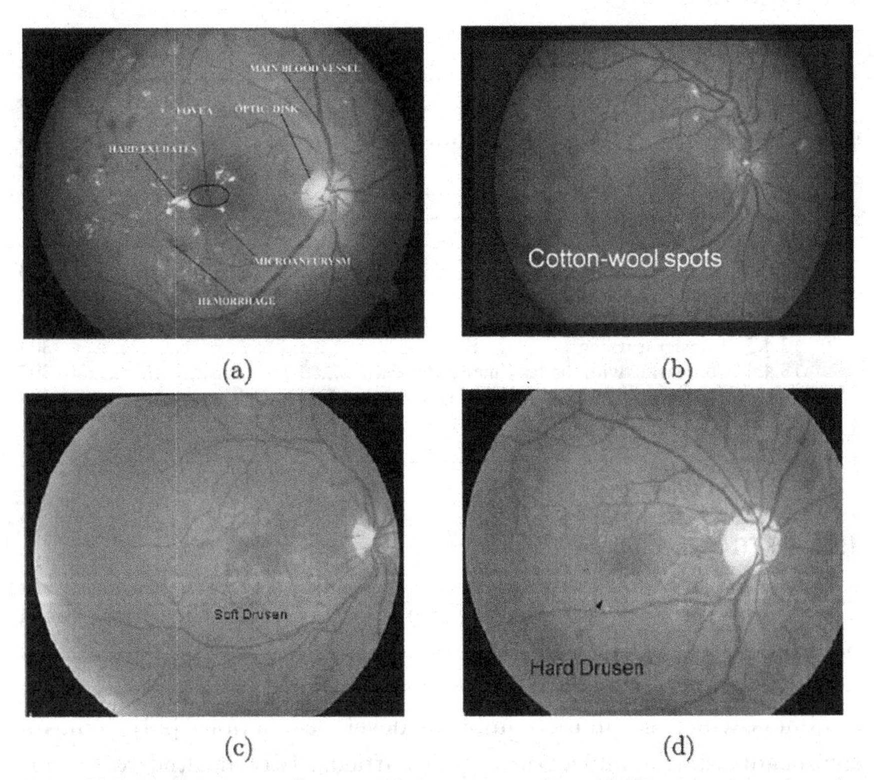

Figure 13.1 Examples image showing different retinopathies. (a) Microaneurysms haemorrhages and hard exudates, (b) cotton-wool spot, (c) soft drusen, and (d) hard rusen.

and gained recognition in various sectors during the previous decade, including medical picture analysis. DL approaches do not necessitate the extraction of hand-crafted features, but they still necessitate a large amount of data for training. Machine learning, on the other hand, necessitates the extraction of handcrafted features but does not require a significant amount of data to train.

Numerous attempts have been made to design a system that can automatically perform DR classification using DL to aid ophthalmologists in the early detection of the condition. However, the majority of this research focused solely on detecting DR rather than detecting different stages of DR. Furthermore, there have been few attempts to identify and locate all types of DR lesions as these lesions to assess the severity of DR and track its course. Several attempts have been made to use DL to automate the classification of DR images in order to aid ophthalmologists in the early detection of the ailment. However, the majority of this research focused solely on detecting DR rather than detecting different stages of DR. In a few proposed systems, it has been attempted to identify various DR stages to assess the severity of DR and track its course.

We try to classify the DR images based on their severity in the current work. The following is the format of this chapter: Section 13.2 provides the relevant literature while Section 13.3 gives the detailed methodology. The experiments and findings are described in Section 13.4. Section 13.5 contains the discussion and conclusion.

13.2 RELATED WORK

Many automated systems to classify diabetic retinopathy (DR) stages and lesion classification have been developed in the past [2, 9, 12, 16, 17, 21, 22, 24–26, 35]. Literature shows that for DR classification and localisation of retinal fundus images CNN has been used widely. The DR detection has been performed by many researchers either in the form of binary DR classification [9, 12, 17, 21, 22, 25] or in the form of multi-level DR classification [5, 10, 13, 18, 20, 31–33]. Binary classification has a basic flaw in that it simply categorises the DR images into two groups, ignoring the five main DR stages. The precise DR stages must be identified to select an appropriate treatment strategy and avoid retinal degeneration.

The authors in Ref. [4] provide an extensive survey on DL-based computer-based diagnostic systems for diabetic retinopathy. The chapter provided a comprehensive view of different diabetic retinopathy biomarkers and lesions. The research on disease detection and its progression using fundus imaging in its early stages aid ophthalmologists to save a lot of time and effort.

In Ref. [36] the author proposed a diabetic retinopathy recognition and classification system that used a combination of ensemble models. Various attempts were in binary and multi-class classification, and some of the state-of-the-art research is mentioned in Table 13.1. The table shows the various approaches used by different authors.

13.3 METHODOLOGY

We solve a multi-class image classification problem to identify diabetic retinopathy severity levels. We first pre-process the images as stated below. The rationale behind this step is also highlighted in the following subsection. Subsequently, a baseline-convolutional neural network (CNN) is trained on the training set and tested on the test set. Next, we carried out several experiments with transfer learning using some popular pre-trained CNN models. Finally, we used one such transfer learning model as a feature extractor, trained several machine learning classifiers, and compared their performances. The details have been mentioned in the following subsections.

13.3.1 Material

On a scale of 0–4, the suggested approach leverages images from Kaggle [1] to determine the presence of diabetic retinopathy in each image (0 being the No sign of DR and 4 being Proliferative DR. There is a considerable class imbalance present in the data. The number of images with a label 0 (representing there is no DR or not diseased) is manyfold compared to the nearest next majority class. The total number of samples in the dataset is 35, 108 acquired from a different camera system and under various imaging conditions. The number of samples with no DR (label 0) is 25,802. In contrast, the number of samples of the other diabetic severity classes with labels 1 (Mild), 2 (Moderate, 3 (Severe), 4 (Proliferative) DR are 2,438, 5,288, 872 and 708, respectively.

Table 13.1 State of art method using deep learning model for diabetic retinopathy grading

Author and reference	*Objective*	*Method*	*Accuracy/results*	*Pros or cons*
Alyoubi et al. [3]	Classifies DR images into 5 stages	Deep Learning Model: CNN512 and YOLOv3.	86% and 89%	Localisation of lesions can be improved by adding more layers to the CNN512.
Jiang et al. [16]	DR classification and lesion detection	Deep learning-based multi-label classification model with Gradient-weighted Class Activation Mapping (Grad-CAM)	94.4%	Strength: Grad-CAM model which automatically outlined the specific region of each lesion. But the Upsampling to coarse heatmap results in artefacts and loss in signal
Qureshi et al. [26]	Automatic recognition of the DR stage	Multi-layer architecture of active deep learning (ADL)	98%	ADL requires very large amount of data to perform better
Wang et al. [31]	DR severity level prediction	Composite deep neural network model	Sensitivity: 92.59% and specificity: 96.20%	L requires very large amount of data
Zhang et al. [36]	Automated DR identification and grading system	Neural Networks (NN) based on mixture of CNN and customised standard Deep NN	Sensitivity: 98.1% and a specificity:98.9%.	Study was conducted by using different combinations of classifiers to create optimal model but how these classifiers are chosen not explained.

(Continued)

Table 13.1 (Continued) State of art method using deep learning model for diabetic retinopathy grading

Author and reference	*Objective*	*Method*	*Accuracy/results*	*Pros or cons*
Gayathri et al. [11]	Binary and multi-class classification of DR	CNN model architecture with J48 classifier	Accuracy-99.89% (binary classification) 99.59% (multi-class classification)	J48 classifiers are unstable, which means that a slight change in the data can result in a significant change in the structure of the best decision tree.
Yash Choudhary et al. [7]	Autonomous DR detection	Google EfficientNet model with some modification	Precision: 81% , recall: 80% , F1 score: 80% and quadratic weighted kappa: 91.25%	EfficientNet model gives high accuracy but the effectiveness of model scaling also relies heavily on the baseline network

Due to this heavily imbalanced dataset, building a multi-class-classifier model that produces a high accuracy without learning anything meaningful pattern from the sample images is not easy. There are many techniques to deal with class imbalance (sampling-based techniques like SMOTE or data augmentation-based techniques etc.). However, in this chapter, we like to explore the first-hand results obtained from different transfer learning models and compare the results with a convolutional baseline model. Therefore, we sub-sampled the images from all five categories taking only 708 samples from each class category forming a dataset of 3,540 samples to work with.

13.3.2 Image pre-processing

The fundus images were gathered from a variety of sources using a variety of imaging techniques. The colour tone, brightness and illuminations are not uniform across all the images. This imposes a great challenge on the performance of the classifier model. Suitable image pre-processing and transformation needs to be carried out. Figure 13.2 shows three images. The first image is the original sample (three-channel RBG image), whereas the second image is the greyscale. Images can be processed in grayscale to make the classifier colour-invariant. However, the colour could be an important feature, especially for identifying the proliferative class. Many sample images contain bloody retinal images showing a high severity level diabetic retinal condition.

The last image is obtained after suitable image transformation. Clearly, the transformed image has better contrast, and the veins on the retina are shown distinctively. These features could be useful for downstream tasks. It is important to note that the original images are of very high resolution and contain a black background along the border. This black background

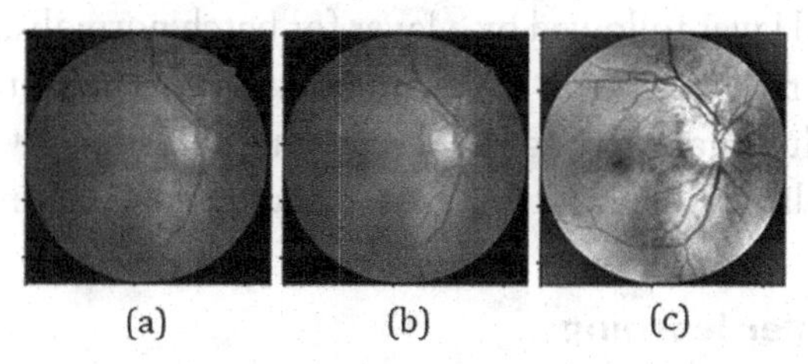

Figure 13.2 Figure showing (a) original three-channel RBG image, (b) gray-scale and (c) transformed image.

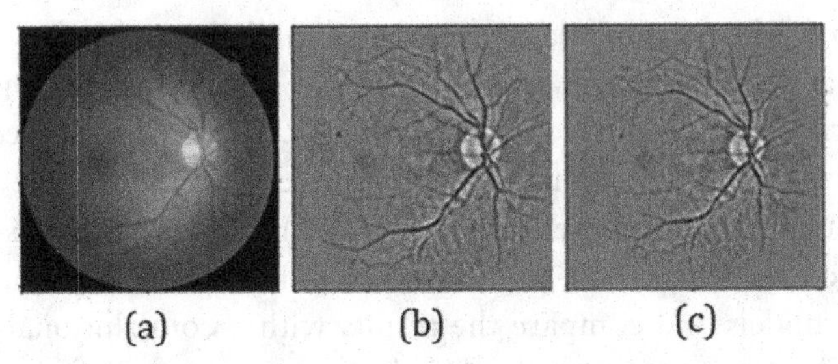

Figure 13.3 Figure showing (a) original three-channel RBG image, (b) transformed image with cropping to the approximate radius, and (c) image transformed image without applying the cropping.

does not provide any distinctive feature to the classifier. Therefore, the images are cropped to reduce the spatial dimensions.

Image transformation has been applied to convert the original fundus image into a more desired colour-invariant representation. The images are cropped to the centres to hold the circular shapes of the retina after applying an adaptive local intensity subtraction to supplement the large change in illumination (brightness). Figure 13.3 shows an original fundus image along with the transformed image in the middle, which is cropped to the approximate radius of the circular retina. The third image is obtained when we just apply the image transformation without applying the cropping with respect to the radius. These images could be further experimented with to understand whether the rounded shape of the retina could be a useful feature in discriminating between different DR categories.

13.3.3 Baseline-CNN model

We built a CNN to classify the fundus images. The model contains four CNN blocks cascaded in a series. Each block is a combination of a Convolutional layer followed by a layer for batch normalisation followed by dimension reduction with a max-pooling layer. The features extracted by the convolutional layers are subsequently classified by feed-forward layers (Multi-layered Perceptron) at the end of the CNN network.

13.3.4 Transfer learning

For the purposes of this research, some well-known pre-trained convolutional models were used. Models being used are the famous VGG-16 network [27], ResNet-50 [14], Inception-V3 [28] and Efficient-Net [29]. Transfer learning has been applied in two different configurations.

- *Configuration-1: Use model as a feature extractor*: The original models were loaded with pre-trained weights trained on the ImageNet dataset. It was repurposed to suit the current five-class classification problem by discarding the top layers and adding two feed-forward dense layers on top of the model. In this configuration, the newly added head acted as a classifier. The earlier layers of the original network were frozen to make them non-trainable. The learning rate parameter was set to be relatively large. The model was then trained on the training dataset for 25 epochs. During training, after every epoch, the performance was evaluated on a validation set.
- *Configuration-2: Fine Tuning*: In this configuration, the earlier model was taken with the already-trained head. Some of the deeper convolutional layers were unfrozen to further train them. A relatively smaller learning rate was chosen. Then the network was again trained on the training dataset for 20 epochs.

13.4 RESULTS

This section summarises the findings from the experiments.

13.4.1 Evaluation metrics

We have used the kappa score and AUC as the evaluation metrics. The following is the justification for adopting these evaluation metrics: Cohen's weighted kappa is a widely used measure of agreement between observed raters in cross-classification. It is used to calculate a statistic that measures inter-rater and intra-rater reliability for qualitative and categorical questions [23]. It is often thought to be a more reliable statistic than a simple percentage agreement estimate since it considers the possibility of the agreement occurring by chance. The fundus images have been manually labelled by the medical professionals. There are disagreements among those human ratings (e.g., one image has been rated by two human raters as belonging to two different severity labels).

Cohen's kappa [8] is a statistic that measures inter-annotator agreement. This score indicates how well two annotators agree on a classification task and is given by,

$$\kappa = \frac{(p_o - p_e)}{(1 - p_e)} \tag{13.1}$$

where pe is the expected agreement when both annotators give labels randomly, and po is the empirical probability of agreement on the label assigned to any sample (the observed agreement ratio).

We choose AUC as another metric (even though this metric is generally used in a binary-classification setting). AUC is a composite measure of performance that takes into account all possible categorisation levels. Because different raters' labels differ, it's more crucial to keep track of how well forecasts are ranked rather than their absolute values. AUC seems to be a suitable metric for this purpose.

13.4.2 Baseline-CNN model

The model was trained for 20 epochs. The loss on the training set drops slowly. However, there is a sudden surge observed in the validation loss after 15th epoch. The accuracy, on the other hand, increases slowly. As an alternative, the model could be trained for a few more epochs. This is shown in Figure 13.4.

However, as the loss and accuracy plots for training and validation data show a little divergence from each other, we stop training after $20th$ epoch and save the model from running into an over-fitted stage.

13.4.3 Transfer learning

Figure 13.5 shows the metrics (loss, AUC on training set) for Efficient-Net, VGG-16, Resnet-50 and Inception-V3 models when trained in feature extraction mode (configuration 1). As shown in the plot, we observe a steady fall in the loss till the 13th epoch. Afterwards, the loss flattens slowly. On the other side, the increase in AUC score is rather less-steep. The Inception-V3 model fails to match the scores of the other models.

Figure 13.6 shows the metrics (loss, AUC on validation set) for Efficient-Net, VGG-16, Resnet-50 and Inception-V3 models when trained in feature extraction mode (configuration 1). We observe a steady

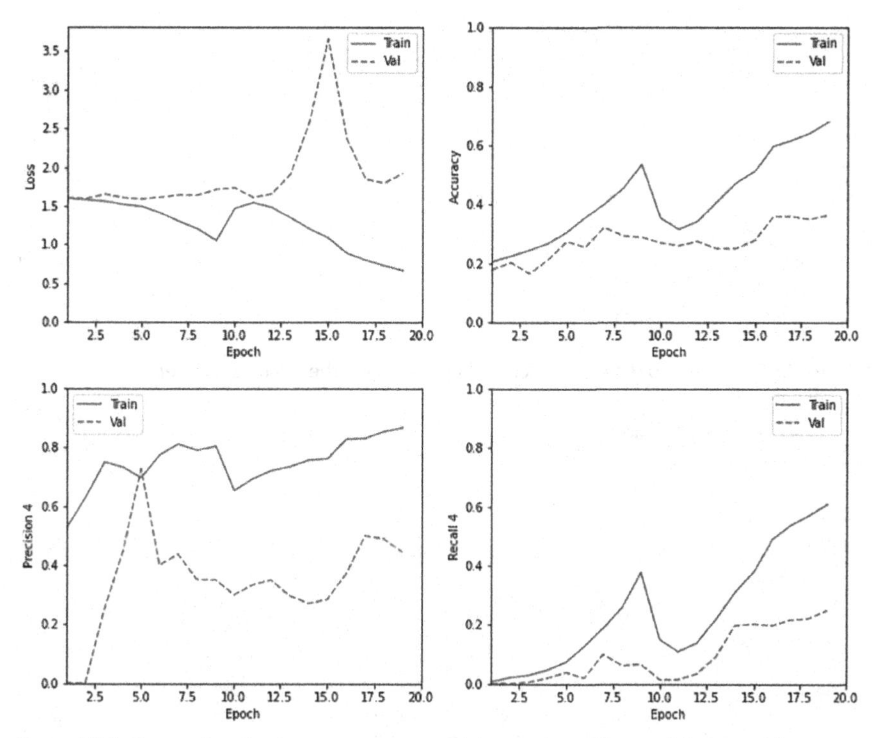

Figure 13.4 Figure showing loss, accuracy, precision and recall on validation and training set.

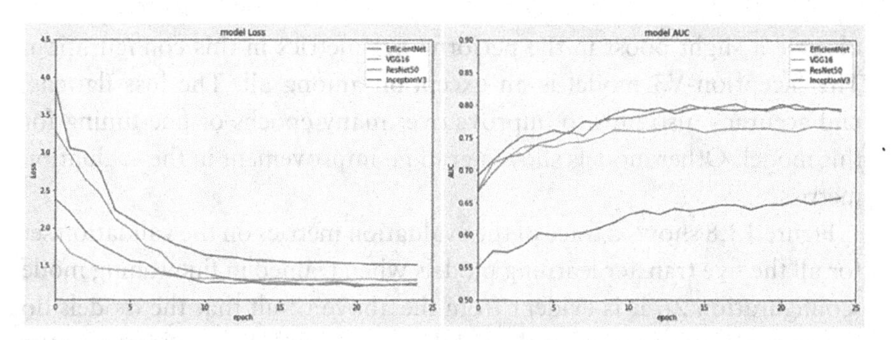

Figure 13.5 Figure showing the loss and AUC plots on the training dataset.

fall in the loss. However, the trajectory looks much noisier. A similar but complementary plot has been observed for the AUC metric.

Figure 13.7 shows a trace of the evaluation metrics (loss, AUC on training set) for all the five transfer learning models when trained in fine-tuning mode (configuration 2). Compared to configuration 1, we

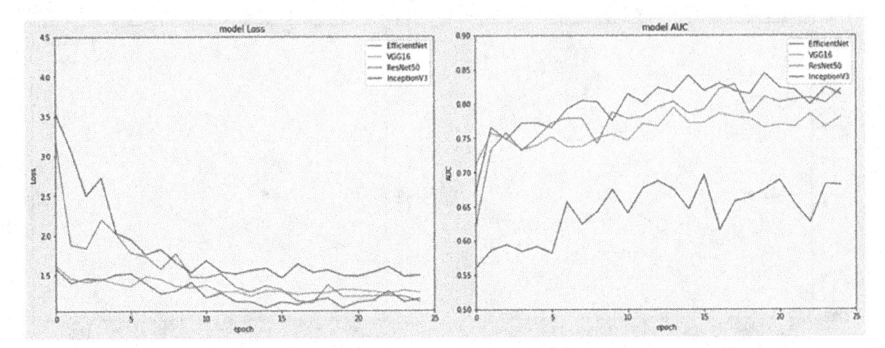

Figure 13.6 Figure showing the loss and AUC plots on the training dataset.

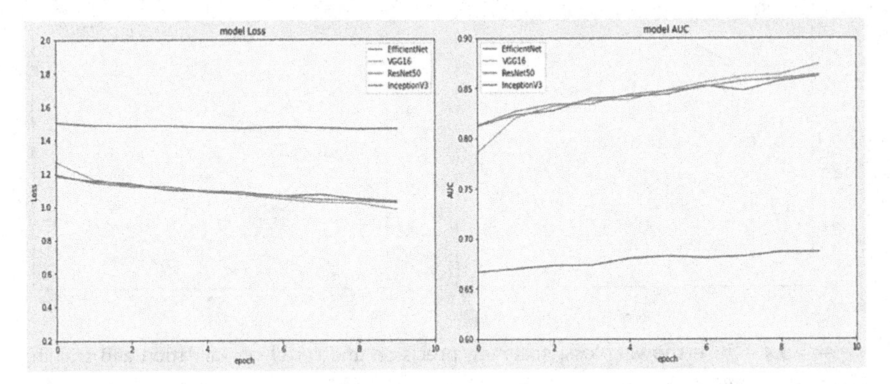

Figure 13.7 Figure showing the loss and AUC plots on the training dataset.

observe a slight boost in the performance metrics in this configuration. The Inception-V3 model is an exception among all. The loss flattens, and accuracy also fails to improve over many epochs of fine-tuning for this model. Other models show a gradual improvement in the evaluation metrics.

Figure 13.8 shows a trace of the evaluation metrics on the validation set for all the five transfer learning models when trained in fine-tuning mode (configuration 2). It is evident from the above result that the models do not improve the metrics on the validation set, and there is a jitter in the plot for the VGG-16 model. This suggests that further training the model in fine-tuning mode will overfit the model, and the model will not benefit in generalising the unseen data.

Table 13.2 summarises the performance comparisons of the four transfer learning models with respect to the AUC and the kappa metrics on the test dataset for both configurations. It is evident from the results that fine-tuning surely boosted the performance of the model. The pre-

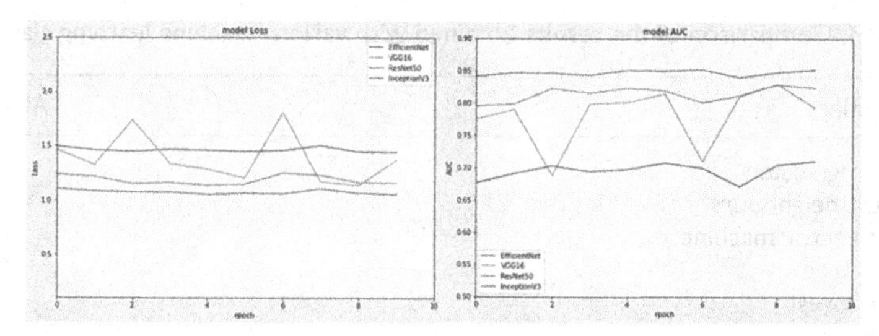

Figure 13.8 Figure showing the loss and AUC plots on the training dataset.

Table 13.2 Summarises the performance comparisons of the four transfer learning models with respect to the AUC and the kappa metrics

Transfer learning mode	Custom new FFN (top head - configuration-1		Fine-tuning (selected top layers – configuration-2	
	AUC	Weighted Kappa	AUC	Weighted Kappa
Efficient-Net	0.73	0.59	0.77	0.68
VGG-16	0.74	0.56	0.78	0.67
ResNet-50	0.75	0.59	0.80	0.65
Inception-V3	0.64	0.31	0.66	0.41

training of the model in the feature extraction model was useful for this classification task.

13.4.4 Comparing with the baseline-CNN

The performance of the baseline-CNN model has been compared with the pre-trained model based on the selected metrics in Table 13.3. In terms of both the metrics, all other pre-trained CNNs performed better than the baseline-CNN.

Table 13.3 Performance of the baseline-CNN model has been compared with the pre-trained model

Transfer learning models fine-tuning (selected top layers – configuration-2)	Custom new FFN (top head - configuration-1	
	AUC	Weighted Kappa
Efficient-Net	0.77	0.68
VGG-16	0.78	0.67
ResNet-50	0.80	0.65
Inception-V3	0.66	0.41
Baseline CNN	0.62	0.29

Table 13.4 Comparison of the results obtained with various machine learning classifiers

ML classifiers	AUC score
Logistic regression	0.70
K-nearest neighbours	0.62
Support vector machine	0.73
Decision tree	0.63
Random forest	0.70
AdaBoost	0.67

13.4.5 Comparison between different machine learning models

We have used VGG16 as a feature extractor and trained several machine learning classifiers on the feature vectors extracted from the training dataset. We have carefully chosen the machine learning classifiers to have a good balance between the different ways a typical machine learning model learns the decision boundaries for a given set of feature points. We have selected a distance-based classifier like K-nearest-Neighbour; a probabilistic model like Logistic Regression; an entropy-based model like Decision Tree and two ensemble-based learners – Random Forest and AdaBoost classifiers. We have also chosen a Support Vector classifier for comparing the results. The results on the test set are summarised in Table 13.4.

The K-nearest-neighbours classifier was trained with $k = 5$ as this is a five-class classification problem. The decision tree classifier was trained with a depth-cutoff regularisation of 5. The random forest classifier model was created for a forest containing 100 decision trees. The number of estimators for the AdaBoost algorithm has been set to 50. The Support Vector classifier performs the best, followed by Logistic Regression and Random Forest.

13.5 CONCLUSION

Deep learning-based techniques can work as a great assistive technology for countrywide DR screening from retinopathy images. Using a convolutional neural network, we discussed multiple strategies for identifying DR severity levels from fundus images in this chapter (CNN). There are several methods proposed by many researchers to deal with the DR images. However, our primary focus is to study the effectiveness of

CNN-based models using transfer learning for DR severity classification. In this study, we have analysed the results obtained from various pre-trained CNN models using transfer learning and compared the results with a custom baseline-convolutional network. We have initially applied image pre-processing to reduce the variations of colour tone, brightness and illuminations present in the input fundus photographs. Multiple experiments have been conducted utilising many pre-trained CNN models, including VGG-16, ResNet-50, Inception-V3, and Efficient-Net. Transfer learning was used in two distinct settings (model that has been pre-trained as a feature extractor and is in the fine-tuning setting), and the outcomes were quantified using two evaluation metrics. We observed a small gain in the performance metrics during fine-tuning mode compared to the initial setup. On the specified metrics, the baseline-CNN model's performance was compared to that of the other pre-trained models. All other pre-trained CNNs outperformed the baseline-CNN on both evaluation metrics AUC and Kappa. Among all the pre-trained models with fine-tuning, ResNet-50 gave the highest AUC score of 80%. In addition, we have compared the performance of several conventional machine learning algorithms – support vector machine, K-nearest-neighbours classifier, decision tree and ensemble techniques – random forest and AdaBoost. Support Vector Machine produced the highest accuracy. The convolutional features extracted from the fundus images seem to be useful in solving the classification task. There could be many alternative ways to approach this DR classification problem, e.g., using hybrid architectures like a multi-head model, combining images from both left and right eyes, etc.

REFERENCES

[1] Diabetic Retinopathy Detection, https://www.kaggle.com/c/diabetic-retinopathy-detection/data?select=sample.zip.

[2] Qaisar Abbas, Imran Qureshi, and Mostafa EA Ibrahim. An automatic detection and classification system of five stages for hypertensive retinopathy using semantic and instance segmentation in densenet architecture. *Sensors*, 21(20):6936, 2021.

[3] Wejdan L Alyoubi, Maysoon F Abulkhair, and Wafaa M Shalash. Diabetic retinopathy fundus image classification and lesions localization system using deep learning. *Sensors*, 21(11):3704, 2021.

[4] Norah Asiri, Muhammad Hussain, Fadwa Al Adel, and Nazih Alzaidi. Deep learning based computer-aided diagnosis systems for diabetic retinopathy: A survey. *Artificial Intelligence in Medicine*, 99:101701, 2019.

[5] Jyostna Devi Bodapati, Nagur Shareef Shaik, and Veeranjaneyulu Naralasetti. Composite deep neural network with gated-attention mechanism for diabetic retinopathy severity classification. *Journal of Ambient Intelligence and Humanized Computing*, 12, 9825–9839, 2021.

[6] Melissa M Brown, Gary C Brown, Sanjay Sharma, and Gaurav Shah. Utility values and diabetic retinopathy. *American Journal of Ophthalmology*, 128(3):324–330, 1999.

[7] Yash Choudhary, M Eliazer, and Aditya Jain. Automated detection and grading of diabetic retinopathy using cnn. *Turkish Journal of Physiotherapy and Rehabilitation*, 32:3, 2021.

[8] J. Cohen. A coefficient of agreement for nominal scales. *Educational and Psychological Measurement*, 20:37–46, 1960.

[9] Sraddha Das, Krity Kharbanda, M Suchetha, Rajiv Raman, and Edwin Dhas. Deep learning architecture based on segmented fundus image features for classification of diabetic retinopathy. *Biomedical Signal Processing and Control*, 68:102600, 2021.

[10] Omar Dekhil, Ahmed Naglah, Mohamed Shaban, Mohammed Ghazal, Fatma Taher, and Ayman Elbaz. Deep learning based method for computer aided diagnosis of diabetic retinopathy. In *2019 IEEE International Conference on Imaging Systems and Techniques (IST)*, pp. 1–4. Abu Dhabi, United Arab Emirates, IEEE, 2019.

[11] S Gayathri, Varun P Gopi, and Ponnusamy Palanisamy. A lightweight cnn for diabetic retinopathy classification from fundus images. *Biomedical Signal Processing and Control*, 62:102115, 2020.

[12] Waleed M Gondal, Jan M Köhler, René Grzeszick, Gernot A Fink, and Michael Hirsch. Weakly-supervised localization of diabetic retinopathy lesions in retinal fundus images. In *2017 IEEE International Conference on Image Processing (ICIP)*, pp. 2069–2073. National Convention Center in Beijing, China. IEEE, 2017.

[13] Along He, Tao Li, Ning Li, Kai Wang, and Huazhu Fu. Cabnet: Category attention block for imbalanced diabetic retinopathy grading. *IEEE Transactions on Medical Imaging*, 40(1):143–153, 2020.

[14] Kaiming He, Xiangyu Zhang, Shaoqing Ren, and Jian Sun. Deep residual learning for image recognition. In *Proceedings of the IEEE Conference on Computer Vision and Pattern Recognition*, pp. 770–778, Las Vegas, NV, USA. 2016.

[15] Jonathan C Javitt, Lloyd Paul Aiello, Yenpin Chiang, Frederick L Ferris, Joseph K Canner, and Sheldon Greenfield. Preventive eye care in people with diabetes is cost-saving to the federal government: implications for health-care reform. *Diabetes Care*, 17(8):909–917, 1994.

[16] Hongyang Jiang, Jie Xu, Rongjie Shi, Kang Yang, Dongdong Zhang, Mengdi Gao, He Ma, and Wei Qian. A multi-label deep learning model with interpretable grad-cam for diabetic retinopathy classification. In *2020 42nd Annual International Conference of the IEEE Engineering in Medicine & Biology Society (EMBC)*, pp. 1560–1563. Montreal, QC, Canada. IEEE, 2020.

[17] Hongyang Jiang, Kang Yang, Mengdi Gao, Dongdong Zhang, He Ma, and Wei Qian. An interpretable ensemble deep learning model for diabetic retinopathy disease classification. In *2019 41st Annual International Conference of the IEEE Engineering in Medicine and Biology Society (EMBC)*, pp. 2045–2048. Berlin, Germany, July 23–27, 2019. IEEE, 2019.

[18] Sara Hosseinzadeh Kassani, Peyman Hosseinzadeh Kassani, Reza Khazaeinezhad, Michal J Wesolowski, Kevin A Schneider, and Ralph Deters. Diabetic retinopathy classification using a modified xception architecture. In *2019 IEEE International Symposium on Signal Processing and Information Technology (ISSPIT)*, pp. 1–6. IEEE, 2019.

[19] Mark Lambert. Cost-effectiveness of detecting and treating diabetic retinopathy. *Annals of Internal Medicine*, 125(11):939, 1996.

[20] Xiaomeng Li, Xiaowei Hu, Lequan Yu, Lei Zhu, Chi-Wing Fu, and Pheng-Ann Heng. Canet: cross-disease attention network for joint diabetic retinopathy and diabetic macular edema grading. *IEEE Transactions on Medical Imaging*, 39(5):1483–1493, 2019.

[21] Yi-Peng Liu, Zhanqing Li, Cong Xu, Jing Li, and Ronghua Liang. Referable diabetic retinopathy identification from eye fundus images with weighted path for convolutional neural network. *Artificial Intelligence in Medicine*, 99:101694, 2019.

[22] Muhammad Mateen, Junhao Wen, Sun Song, Zhouping Huang, et al. Fundus image classification using vgg-19 architecture with pca and svd. *Symmetry*, 11(1):1, 2019.

[23] Mary L McHugh. Interrater reliability: The kappa statistic. *Biochemia Medica*, 22(3):276–282, 2012.

[24] Samuel Ofosu Mensah, Bubacarr Bah, and Willie Brink. Towards the localisation of lesions in diabetic retinopathy. In: Kohei Arai (Ed.), *Intelligent Computing*, pp. 100–107. Springer: Berlin/Heidelberg, Germany, 2021.

[25] Ramon Pires, Sandra Avila, Jacques Wainer, Eduardo Valle, Michael D Abramoff, and Anderson Rocha. A data-driven approach to referable diabetic retinopathy detection. *Artificial Intelligence in Medicine*, 96:93–106, 2019.

[26] Imran Qureshi, Jun Ma, and Qaisar Abbas. Diabetic retinopathy detection and stage classification in eye fundus images using active deep learning. *Multimedia Tools and Applications*, 80(8):11691–11721, 2021.

[27] Karen Simonyan and Andrew Zisserman. Very deep convolutional networks for large-scale image recognition. arXiv preprint arXiv:1409.1556, 2014.

[28] Christian Szegedy, Vincent Vanhoucke, Sergey Ioffe, Jon Shlens, and Zbigniew Wojna. Rethinking the inception architecture for computer vision. In *Proceedings of the IEEE Conference on Computer Vision and Pattern Recognition*, pp. 2818–2826, Las Vegas, NV, USA. 2016.

[29] Mingxing Tan and Quoc Le. Efficientnet: Rethinking model scaling for convolutional neural networks. In *International Conference on Machine Learning*, pp. 6105–6114. PMLR, Long Beach, California, USA. 2019.

[30] G Thomas, Y Harold Robinson, E Golden Julie, Vimal Shanmuganathan, Seungmin Rho, and Yunyoung Nam. Intelligent prediction approach for diabetic retinopathy using deep learning based convolutional neural networks algorithm by means of retina photographs. *Computers, Materials & Continua*, 66(2):1613–1629, 2021.

[31] Shaohua Wan, Yan Liang, and Yin Zhang. Deep convolutional neural networks for diabetic retinopathy detection by image classification. *Computers & Electrical Engineering*, 72:274–282, 2018.

[32] Jialiang Wang, Jianxu Luo, Bin Liu, Rui Feng, Lina Lu, and Haidong Zou. Automated diabetic retinopathy grading and lesion detection based on the modified r-fcn object-detection algorithm. *IET Computer Vision*, 14(1):1–8, 2020.

[33] Xiaoliang Wang, Yongjin Lu, Yujuan Wang, and Wei-Bang Chen. Diabetic retinopathy stage classification using convolutional neural networks. In *2018 IEEE International Conference on Information Reuse and Integration (IRI)*, pp. 465–471. Salt Lake City, UT, USA. IEEE, 2018.

[34] Rhys Williams, M Airey, H Baxter, J Forrester, T Kennedy-Martin, and A Girach. Epidemiology of diabetic retinopathy and macular oedema: A systematic review. *Eye*, 18(10):963–983, 2004.

[35] Gabriel Tozatto Zago, Rodrigo Varejão Andreão, Bernadette Dorizzi, and Evandro Ottoni Teatini Salles. Diabetic retinopathy detection using red lesion localization and convolutional neural networks. *Computers in Biology and Medicine*, 116:103537, 2020.

[36] Wei Zhang, Jie Zhong, Shijun Yang, Zhentao Gao, Junjie Hu, Yuanyuan Chen, and Zhang Yi. Automated identification and grading system of diabetic retinopathy using deep neural networks. *Knowledge-Based Systems*, 175:12–25, 2019.

Chapter 14

Emerging role of artificial intelligence in precision oncology

Vinod Kumar Singh
Jawaharlal Nehru University

14.1 INTRODUCTION

A cell is the fundamental structural and functional unit of life. The biological processes such as cell division, DNA replication, transcription, etc. are vital for a cell to live and respond to the environment. A biological process involves a series of biochemical reactions and is regulated by many other biological processes; examples include gene expression, protein–protein/substrate interaction, protein modification, etc. All the information regarding order, timing, and location of biological processes are encoded in the cellular genome. Hence, genome is a complete set of genetic instructions and is made up of deoxyribonucleic acid (DNA) (Alberts et al., 2002; Lewin, 2000).

A genome includes both coding regions known as genes and non-coding DNA. Where genes are the functional units of inheritance that control the transmission and expression of certain traits. Most of the

DOI: 10.1201/9781003368342-14

genes achieve their effect by directing the synthesis of proteins that carry out a variety of functions. A wide variety of genes in a cell are regulated by epigenome (made up of chemical compounds and proteins) that can attach to the DNA and gives a cell a different gene expression profile to dictate its role in the tissue. Thus, epigenome changes the way cells use genetic instructions without changing the sequence of the DNA (Lewin, 2000).

In the life journey of a body cell, somatic mutations continue to occur due to multiple intrinsic and extrinsic mutational processes, each of which generates a unique combination of mutation types known as "mutational signatures" in the genome (Alexandrov et al., 2013a; Helleday et al., 2014). Hence, the cells within the same tissue may have a distinct set of somatic mutations. A large chunk of these mutations does not impact any biological process and are known as passive mutations. Only a small fraction of these mutations, known as driver mutations, alters the expression of genes involved in cell division or cell death and cell movement (Figure 14.1). Few genes can become activated in such a way that enhances cell division or prevent cell death such genes are known as oncogenes. Alternatively, some genes known as tumor-suppressor genes (TSG) become inactivated and are not available to apply checks or brakes to these processes. The activation of oncogenes or inactivation TSGs can take place in three ways: (i) through mutations that cause amplification or deduction of gene expression; (ii) copy number gain or complete deletion of the gene; and (iii) epigenetic expression or silencing of gene (Baylin and Jones, 2016). Hence, any change in the genome sequence can be deleterious or advantageous to the cell (King and Robins, 2006). If the rapidly dividing cells have a selective advantage over the normal cells, the tumor grows, infiltrates surrounding tissues, and can spread to other parts of the body. This abnormal growth of

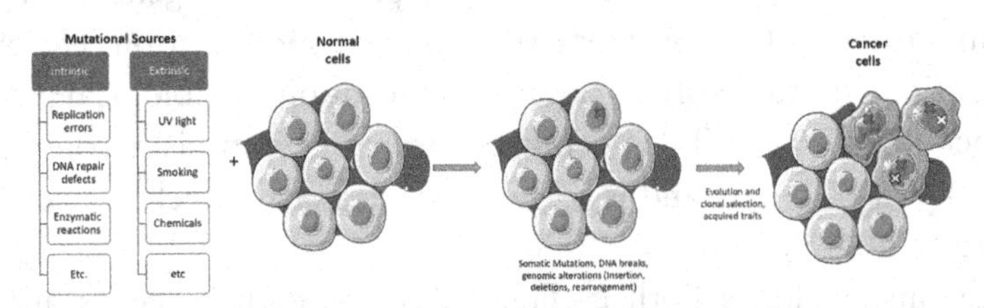

Figure 14.1 Development of cancer: Extrinsic and intrinsic mutational sources damages driver genes in normal cells followed by evolution and clonal selection of cancer hallmarks. (Parts of figure are taken from SMART, smart.servier.com.)

cells interferes with the digestive, nervous, circulatory system, and other body functions (King and Robins, 2006; Tokheim et al., 2016). Most cancers evolve from a single cell by acquiring stochastic and sequential, genetic and epigenetic changes over time, which leads to heterogeneity among cancer cells and is visible in the form of subclones. This evolutionary dynamics of sub-clonal cells create difficulties in characterizing cancer (Chowell et al., 2018). A normal cell doesn't become cancer cell suddenly; it has to acquire six major hallmarks (acquired traits) during the multistep tumor development that provide diversification among the sub-clonal population (Alkhazraji et al., 2019). These traits include sustaining growth signaling, insensitive to anti-growth signaling, evading cell death, sustaining limitless replicative potential, inducing angiogenesis, and activating tissue invasion and metastasis (Hanahan, 2022; Hanahan and Weinberg, 2011).

Cancers can originate from various body organs and have phenotypic diversity such as cell surface receptors, mutations, growth rate, and cell death depending on the blood supply and tumor microenvironment. Cancer development and progression mechanism also depend on diverse factors like genetics to epigenetics. Inter-tumor heterogeneity (among different patients) and intra-tumor heterogeneity (within the same tumor) impose challenges in early detection, diagnosis, and treatment response. Certain cancers, such as gastric and pancreatic cancers, can only be diagnosed at their advanced stage (Patel et al., 2020).

After decades of research, many measurable characteristics (known as biomarkers) exclusive to cancer cells have been identified. Recent developments in next-generation sequencing (NGS), bioinformatics, and computational analysis techniques added new biomarkers and enhanced our understanding of cancer development and progression. Ongoing global cancer projects have created a massive amount of multi-omics data (genomics, proteomics, metabolomics, and epi-genomics) and non-omics data (pathological imaging, clinical data, treatment response, and demography) (Campbell et al., 2020; Goyal, 2019). This multimodal data has provided a unique opportunity to re-examine the cancer development process. The use of artificial intelligence (AI) based models, specifically machine learning (ML) models, has shown the capacity to integrate this data in a nonlinear fashion to learn and discover potential cancer biomarkers or biomarker patterns. Identified biomarkers have shown encouraging outcomes in the early detection of cancer and individual treatment guidance. These developments have shifted the focus of treatment from nonspecific cytotoxic therapy to more precise treatment based on the patient's clinical and molecular profile (Chaudhary et al., 2018; Chowell et al., 2021; Jiao et al., 2020; Lapuente-Santana et al., 2021; Patel et al., 2020; Tran et al., 2021; Zhang et al., 2018). Thus, the tailor-made cancer treatment approach, known as "precision oncology," plays a crucial role in clinical decision-making while reducing exposure to ineffective or unnecessary therapies. However, the effectiveness and efficiency of AI/ML-based models primarily depend on the effectiveness of biomarkers, training sample size, and data characteristics. Hence, understanding the dataset can be a critical factor while selecting a suitable AI model.

This chapter discusses the emerging role of diverse molecular and clinical data obtained from advanced experimental techniques such as sequencing to profile cancer patients and discover cancer-associated biomarkers. This chapter also highlights some ongoing major cancer projects and the limitations of the generated dataset. We examined some studies where AI-based approaches are successfully used to discover biomarkers, driver genes, and relationships between genotypes and phenotypes by integrating diverse molecular data. In the end, we discuss the current challenges faced by oncologists in the AI-assisted precision treatment of cancer patients.

14.2 PROFILING OF CANCER PATIENTS USING ADVANCED EXPERIMENTAL TECHNIQUES

Advances in experimental technologies ranging from NGS to mass spectrometry have generated a plethora of multidimensional molecular data, also known as "omics" data. Application of AI-based methods has integrated a diverse range of omics data such as genomics, epigenomics, transcriptomics, metabolomics, and proteomics, responsible for tumorigenesis ((Bailey et al., 2018; Baylin and Jones, 2016); (Poirion et al., 2021; Porta Siegel et al., 2018)). Moreover, the non-omics data, such as clinical, demographical, and epidemiological also associated with tumor development and prognosis. Non-omics data is mainly obtained through a pre-elaborated process done either by the patient about their lifestyle habits or symptoms or by the physician/pathologists about the characterization of the tumor such as tumor stage, tumor size, cell surface receptors, etc. Despite large availability, non-omics data lacks a standardization process in recording, which impacts data quality and comparability that ultimately influences the outcome. Although to understand cancer progression and development, it is important to consider interactions between all properties of the data, irrespective of their type or source (de Maturana et al., 2019). However, current cancer patients' precise treatment approach in clinical practice is largely based on a few genomics features, e.g., mutations and genomic alterations (Herbst et al., 2018). The depth and duration of treatment response also vary widely among cancer patients (Jänne et al., 2015) and the biological explanation for the underlying differences is not fully understood. Therefore, the current research is focused on integrating multi-omics data and finding complex interactions between them to make precise treatment effective in cancer patients (de Maturana et al., 2019). Therefore, decreasing costs and turnaround time of sequencing, and the improvements in bioinformatics analysis is enhancing the clinical interpretation of genomic results. These developments have encouraged the scientific community for comprehensive profiling of patients in precision medicine.

14.3 MAJOR ONGOING PROJECTS AND RESOURCES AVAILABLE FOR CANCER RESEARCH

Considering the role of cancer data in understanding cancer progression and development, leading research institutes around the globe had initiated various cancer projects for data collection and sharing. To facilitate integrated analysis, data of thousands of patients is made available on multiple online platforms and some of them are tabulated (Table 14.1) below. Since data is associated to human subject, all the data-sharing platforms follow good privacy protection guidelines.

In recent years, the volume and complexity of scientific and clinical data in oncology have grown rapidly and are available at shared data storage platforms. The Cancer Genome Atlas (TCGA) (Collins and Barker, 2007; Garber, 2005) project alone brings together researchers from diverse backgrounds and multiple institutes to molecularly characterize over 20,000 primary and corresponding normal samples from 33 types of cancer. This project has gathered petabytes of genomic, epigenomic, transcriptomic and proteomic data, which has been used to enhance cancer diagnosis, treatment, and prevention. The number of

Table 14.1 Resources for visualizing and exploring cancer genomes.

Resource	*Weblink*	*Description*
The Cancer Genome Atlas (TCGA) (Collins and Barker, 2007; Garber, 2005)	https://www.cancer.gov/	Genomic, proteomic, epigenomic, and transcriptomic dataset integrated with exploration and analysis tools. It supports several cancer genome programs
International Cancer Genome Consortium (ICGC) (Zhang et al., 2019)	https://dcc.icgc.org/	Genomic, epigenomic, and transcriptomic dataset integrated with exploration and analysis tools
The American Association for Cancer Research's (AACR) Project Genomics, Evidence, Neoplasia, Information, Exchange (GENIE) (Sweeney et al., 2017)	https://www.aacr.org/professionals/research/aacr-project-genie/aacr-project-genie-data/	Facilitate sharing of integrated genomics and clinical datasets across multiple institutions worldwide
GenomePaint (Zhou et al., 2021)	https://genomepaint.stjude.cloud/	Visualizes somatic coding and non-coding alterations in pediatric cancer dataset
Therapeutically Applicable Research to Generate Effective Treatments (TARGET)	https://ocg.cancer.gov/programs/target	Project aimed at comprehensive molecular characterization to determine the genetic changes that drive the initiation and progression of childhood cancer
cBioPortal ((Cerami et al., 2012; Gao et al., 2013))	https://www.cbioportal.org/	Provides visualization, analysis, and download of large-scale cancer genomics data set
Interactive genome viewer (IGV) (Robinson et al., 2011)	https://software.broadinstitute.org/software/igv/	A high-performance visualization tool for the interactive exploration of genomic data
Oncology Precision Network (OPeN) (Nadauld et al., 2017)	https://syapse.com/	The oncology precision network data-sharing consortium
COSMIC, the Catalogue of Somatic Mutations in Cancer	https://cancer.sanger.ac.uk/cosmic	To study the impact of somatic mutations in human cancer

samples and data in the ongoing projects is increasing every year. Hence, data-driven approaches are becoming popular in cancer treatment.

14.4 FRAMEWORK FOR PRECISION ONCOLOGY

Continuous expansion in data opens the gateway for a deeper understanding of cancer progression and, accordingly, more precise, and effective treatment. The availability of enormous and heterogeneous data has enhanced the performance of AI-based models in multiple applications related to precision oncology such as diagnosis, predicting drug-response or clinical outcome, etc. (Luchini et al., 2021; Tran et al., 2021). AI-based precision oncology is still in the development phase and is not widely adopted by oncologists due to lack of consensus about the treatment (Chae et al., 2017; Murali et al., 2020). However, a typical framework for precision oncology is described in Figure 14.2.

In a typical precision oncology framework, the genomic and clinical medical records data of cancer patients is used to build the AI-based model for cancer treatment. To achieve best treatment outcomes, these

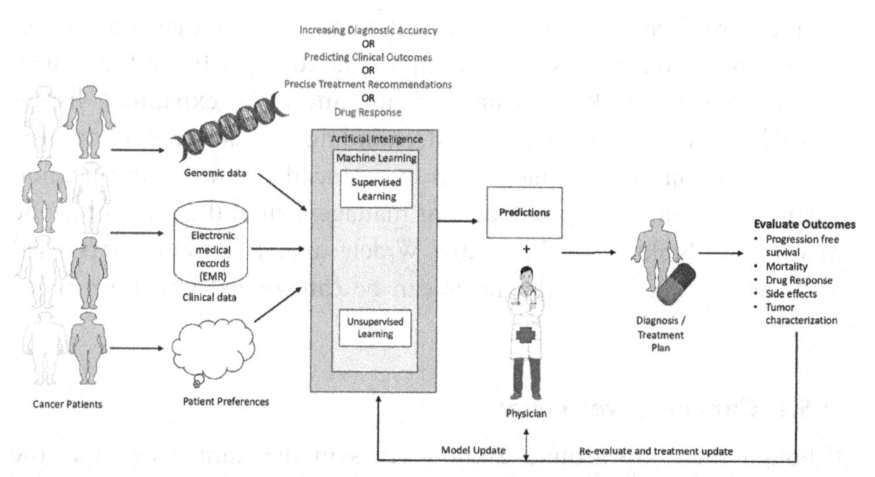

Figure 14.2 A typical outline of precision oncology. Genomics and clinical data are collected with patient's consent and preferences. Data profile of the patient is used for machine learning-based personalized treatment recommendations, which are further evaluated by a team of expert physicians. After the treatment, the outcomes are evaluated, and treatment and ML model are also updated if required. (Parts of figure are taken from SMART, smart.servier.com.)

models are updated continuously on the availability of new patients' data and evaluation of treatment outcomes by a team of experts.

14.5 WIDELY USED BIOMARKERS AND THEIR APPLICATIONS IN AI-BASED PRECISION ONCOLOGY

A biomarker is a measured characteristic that describes normal or abnormal cells by analyzing biomolecules such as DNA, RNA, proteins, and chemical modifications on biomolecules. Cancer biomarkers are used to measure the risk of cancer development/progression or potential response to therapy and are an important part of clinical decision-making (Goossens et al., 2015). There are two categories of cancer biomarkers based on their usage: (i) predictive biomarkers predict the response to specific treatment such as the presence of activating mutations in KRAS gene, an oncogene, are indicative of patient's insensitivity to EGFR inhibitor drugs (Van Cutsem et al., 2009) and (ii) prognostic biomarkers are used to indicate how a clinical situation such as cancer reoccurrence and progression, is likely to turn out in future after the treatment (Goossens et al., 2015).

Cancer, by large, is a genome-based disease rather than only gene-based. Therefore, efforts have been made to identify and use new genome-wide biomarkers to understand cancer. An expanding list of biomarkers not only helped in understanding the cancer development and progression but also facilitated the clinically relevant stratification of cancer patients to improve patient management and treatment at the early phase (Sinkala et al., 2020). Widely available biomarkers used in cancer treatment and diagnosis can be categorized into four major categories.

14.5.1 Cancer driver genes

Although there are around 20,000 genes in the human genome, the abnormal expression of only a tiny fraction of genes helps characterize and understand tumors. In general, these genes are mutated abnormally at a high frequency across tumors, and their expression decides the fate of cancer origin. Therefore, they are the most valuable biomarkers. Numerous methods have been developed to identify driver genes, where most methods basically depend on occurrence-based and positive selection criteria (Arnedo-Pac et al., 2019; Martínez-Jiménez et al., 2020). However for driver discovery, it is important to consider the local mutation rate to avoid the detection of false-positive drivers and to identify those with low mutation recurrence. Many complex statistical models have been proposed to estimate of local mutation rate by integrating diverse types of genomic context data, (Bailey et al., 2018; Dietlein et al., 2020; Weghorn and Sunyaev, 2017). At the same time, deep learning (DL) models can simultaneously fuse the mutation rate, functional the impact of mutations, and similar gene expression patterns to predict driver genes with high accuracy (Luo et al., 2019).

14.5.2 Driver mutations

Most of the initial studies were focused on driver mutations in protein-coding genes. However, the developments in whole-genome sequencing (WGS) made it possible to examine driver events in non-coding regions such as promoter and enhancer regions. In general, a driver mutation occurs more frequently than expected and is highly likely to be selected during tumor development. Finding the expected mutations in a region is a real challenge due to extensive variability in mutation rate across the cancer genome, which depends on the chromatin states or accessibility and replication timing. Hence, identification driver events in the non-coding regions are highly impacted by inaccurate local mutation rate estimation and incomplete annotation of regulatory regions (Rheinbay et al., 2020). Both coding and non-coding driver events impact the expression of many cancer driver genes and are considered important biomarkers.

The limitation with non-coding driver events is that their true labels on the pathogenicity are not available that can be used for training. Hence to develop a pathogenicity prediction model of these driver events, it is important to transform the problem into multiple-instance learning problem (MIL), where driver-gene pairs are considered as bag and regulatory elements as instances. MIL maps the bags in a new feature space where negative and positive bags can be separated by a normal classification model ((Chen et al., 2006; Nieboer and de Ridder, 2020; Nieboer et al., 2021)). This approach is quite effective in detecting pathogenic non-coding drivers and has applications in many other oncology treatments (Xiong et al., 2021).

14.5.3 Cancer-associated fibroblasts

Cancer-associated fibroblasts (CAFs) are used to capture the tumor microenvironment, which is crucial for characterizing cancer. Studies have shown that functional differences among CAF play a significant role in diverse treatment responses and considering CAF heterogeneity into account can influence the cancer treatment response (Junttila and De Sauvage, 2013). A recent study on lung cancer, have captured the functional difference among CAF by clustering them based on three biomarker genes expression i.e., HGP, FGF7 and phospo-SMAD2, involved in signaling of proliferation and growth. These clustered subtypes show diverse degree of clinical response to the treatment and are associated to tumor immune microenvironment (Hu et al., 2021).

14.5.4 Mutational signatures

WGS has revealed thousands of mutations present in a cancer patient due to multiple mutational sources that were active at some time point in a cancer cell. Each mutational source generates a characteristic mutational signature. Thus, a cancer genome may have multiple mutational signatures. Mutational signatures are represented by the contribution of six base substitution mutations (C > A, C > G, C > T, T > A, T > C, and T > G) in the cancer genome. The probability of a mutation depends on the genomic context. Therefore, to increase the resolution among signatures, immediate base context information of each base substitution mutation is also added (Nik-Zainal et al., 2012). Since there are four bases, a mutational signature is described by $4 \times 6 \times 4 = 96$ mutation types described in Figure 14.3.

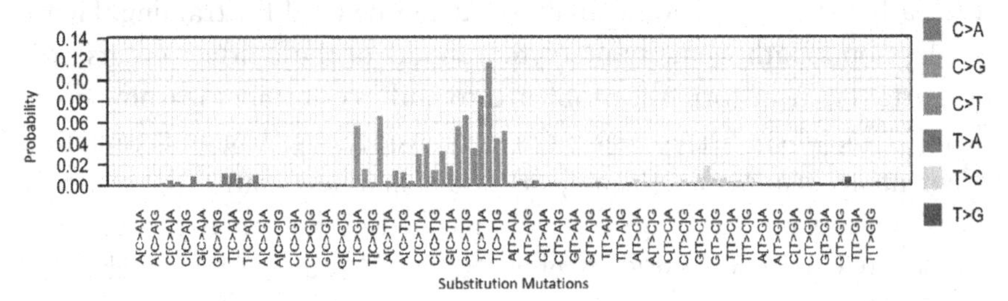

Figure 14.3 A mutational signature representation. Six substitution mutations (represented in different colors) along with immediate context based on the x-axis and y-axis represent their contribution to the cancer genome. Figure is generated using "deconstructSigs" an R-package.

Mutational signature modeling can be understood by the topic modeling problem of text mining, where a document is a mutational catalogue of a cancer patient and mutation types are the words of a document. Topic modeling aims to represent a document by a non-negative linear combination of different topics, where each topic has a unique frequency spectrum of words. Whereas, mutation signature modeling is used to represent the mutational profile of a cancer genome by a non-negative linear combination of "mutational signatures", where each mutational signature is a unique frequency spectrum of mutation types. The non-negative matrix factorization (NMF) technique had been widely used for topic modeling. However, in 2013, Alexandrov utilised the NMF on mutation data from thousands of cancer patients for mutational signature modeling. (Alexandrov et al., 2013a,b; Campbell et al., 2020; Carbonetto et al., 2021; Xu et al., 2003).

A study on cancer patients used a supervised lasso logistic regression model and identified a subset six mutational signatures that were able to predict tumors with nonfunctional BRCA1/BRCA2 gene. This subset of signatures was associated with the homologous recombination pathway abrogation in cancer cells (Davies et al., 2017). Mutational signatures also have the ability to unveil mismatch repair deficient cancers, which show response to Immune Checkpoint Blockage (ICB) treatment ((Koh et al., 2021; Ma et al., 2018; Schrock et al., 2019)). Thus, mutational signatures are the secondary biomarkers derived from the mutations with numerous possibilities to subtype cancers by estimating the active mutational sources. Analysis of mutational signatures is gaining popularity in cancer genetics, with emerging implications for cancer evolution, prognosis, clinical decision-making, and tumor classification.

Genomic profiling of cancers provides valuable information about the (epi)genetic alterations. However, using only genetic driver events as biomarkers for clinical decision-making is insufficient in some cancer types, such as some pediatric and prostate cancers with very few or no recurrent mutations (Gröbner et al., 2018; Vogelstein et al., 2013). In addition, genomic profiling to find variation in oncogenes or TSG doesn't provide enough information about the corresponding pathway activation i.e., the presence of mutations doesn't guarantee the activation of cancer driver pathways (Chen et al., 2014). The most comprehensive approach to overcome these challenges is to do an integrated analysis of omics (genomic, epigenomic, proteomic, transcriptomic, and metabolomic) data of tumor and their surrounding stroma and the non-omics (clinical, demographical, etc) of cancer patients (Senft et al., 2017).

14.6 MAIN CHALLENGES FOR AI IN PRECISION ONCOLOGY

Even after the successful application of AI in many cancer treatments and diagnosis studies, we are still at a bottleneck of the data-driven possibilities in precision oncology that are limited due to the following reasons.

14.6.1 Data integration

Most precision oncology ML models rely only on a subset of input data, i.e., gene expression data, single-nucleotide mutation/variants data (SNV), copy-number alterations (CNA), proteomics, epigenetics data and image data. This limits the success of ML algorithms. Moreover, data from different information resources, known as multimodal data, have distinct statistical properties that pose a challenge in data integration, which gets further complicated due to missing modalities in the data. Traditional ML techniques such as Support vector machines (SVM), Random-forest (RF), K-nearest neighbor (KNN), etc., need features to be identified by a domain expert. These algorithms can't benefit beyond a limit even after the availability of "Big Data" in cancer genomics. Fortunately, DL methods have shown the ability to outperform traditional ML methods in a wide range of real-life applications when it comes to integrating and utilizing large data (Patel et al., 2020). They can discover the relationship between different modalities and devise the best way to represent them jointly. Their multimodal learning capability can also estimate a missing modality from the observed one (Audebert et al., 2019; Ma et al., 2021; Summaira et al., 2021). They automatically extract high-level features from the data and draw complex nonlinear relationships among them. DL models can attain unprecedented generalizability from the exponentially growing data and computational power (Duda et al., 2001); (L'Heureux et al., 2017). Although DL models perform well on large data sets due to complex nature, they are not human-interpretable.

14.6.2 Heterogeneity of the cancer

Heterogeneity creates difficulty in the assessment of drug sensitivity, which has importance in therapeutic development and patient care and has applications in precision oncology, drug repurposing, and new drug development (Zhu et al., 2020). The classification algorithms used in many oncology problems, such as drug sensitivity prediction, have a few samples (s) with many biomarkers (n) (molecular features) that make them susceptible to overfitting on the test data. In multiple myeloma patients (target task), where the number of samples was low with a high number of biomarkers ($s \ll n$), this problem is addressed by transfer learning (TrLe). TrLe improves the solution by transferring the patterns learned from sensitivity prediction in other cancer types (related task) (Turki et al., 2017). Transfer learning is also used in DL models for other oncology problems, i.e., cancer-type classification, drug-response prediction, metastasis prediction, etc. ((Alawad et al., 2019; Kim et al., 2020; Sevakula et al., 2019; Zhu et al., 2020)). Datasets with $s \ll n$ property are extensively used to train ensemble-based learning models in many healthcare domains and some precision oncology applications. This approach trains thousands of models simultaneously on different learning feature subsets, and the final prediction is an ensemble of all models (Brunese et al., 2020; Gupta et al., 2020; Singh et al., 2018).

Highly heterogeneous tumors such as pancreatic cancer are difficult to treat and only a few effective treatment options are available with low success rate. Attempts have been made to classify tumors into clinically distinct subtypes by integrating diverse molecular biomarker data. However, the complexities in data integration have limited clinical outcomes (Raphael et al., 2017). To mitigate this problem, a multi-platform interactive clustering approach named as similarity network fusion (SNF) is used to segregate pancreatic tumors into two subtypes. SNF constructed the similarity network of samples for each molecular data and then fused them into one cluster network based on all underlying molecular data types. Intestinally, the SNF clustered tumor subtypes were associated with different clinical outcomes, and tumors of each subtype also had a difference in a signaling pathway, which can be useful information for potential drug target (Sinkala et al., 2020).

14.6.3 Data privacy and sharing

Many factors such as the restrictive language of patient consent forms, government regulations across countries, and incomplete annotation of data create data access and utilization problems. Research organizations are making efforts for improved data-sharing guidelines and the development of cloud-based infrastructure to store and analyze shared data ((Molnár-Gábor et al., 2017; Saunders et al., 2019)).

Besides all the above-mentioned challenges, the final performance of ML models is highly dependent on the quality and quantity of the training data (Duda et al., 2001). In case of too many features, a substantial amount of training data might be required for better generalization, which can be difficult for the human subject.

14.7 LIMITATIONS OF TARGETED THERAPIES AND PRECISION ONCOLOGY TRIALS

The objective of precision oncology is to match cancer patients to targeted therapies. Our discussion clearly shows a major hurdle to its evidence-based execution is the overwhelming heterogeneity in the genetic landscape of tumors and the distinctive evolutionary track of each cancer type and patient (Campbell et al., 2020). Although precise cancer treatment therapies are evolving into achievable standards, still there are significant concerns described below.

1. Only a few treatment strategies have reliable predictive biomarkers and evidence of their clinical benefits found for a few genomic alterations in limited number of cancer types. Furthermore, the use of rare biomarkers for trial-based studies during cancer patient selection may cause high screening failure rates and only one or a few patients may have an exceptional response. Hence, intense efforts are being taken by National Cancer Institute (NCI) to molecularly characterize the tumors of exceptional responder (https://www.ctsu.org).
2. The development of targeted therapy needs strong evidence of genetic alterations in tumor behavior. Furthermore, it is also important to important to address the function of these alterations with a treatment therapy or a targeted agent on tumor progression (Conley, 2015; Meric-Bernstam et al., 2015).

3. ML-assisted decision-making raises the questions of responsibility of errors. Due to complexity involved, it would be unclear what proportion of legal or moral responsibility lies with medical professionals, programmers in hospital, model developers, etc.

Despite all these challenges, NGS-based genetic screening methods can effectively discover genetic variants that may be linked to a higher risk of cancer development. But of course, after getting clinically relevant biomarkers from the genomic data require data of tens of thousands of patients with comprehensive clinical characterization. In a well-documented case, patients with *BRCA1/2* mutations and specific genetic variants have quantifiable effects on breast cancer development (Easton et al., 2015).

14.8 CONCLUDING REMARKS AND FUTURE OUTLOOK

This chapter has discussed the emerging role of AI in cancer diagnosis, guiding treatment, and prognosis. The application of molecular biomarkers for the diagnosis and precise treatment of cancer represents an attractive possibility in oncology. In the last decade, developments in sequencing technologies and sophisticated computational algorithms have generated a tremendous amount of omics data that has been used to discover a wide variety of biomarkers. As DNA sequencing is now a common practice among oncologists, the amount of data generated by cancer research institutes will continue to increase. AI-based methods have shown promising results in many precision oncology applications by effectively consolidating and integrating enormous data, as discussed in this chapter. The volume and quality of omics and non-omics data is increasing rapidly, which may open the way for DL based AI methods to get exciting new insights for the precise treatment of cancer patients. Currently we are only at the bottleneck of the possibilities that can open if we overcome a few challenges discussed in the chapter.

New emerging sequencing technologies, such as long-read technologies, have substantially reduced the cost and sequencing errors; single-cell DNA sequencing technologies are enhancing our understanding of tumor heterogeneity and clonal evolution. Uncovering new applications of AI in precision oncology will require the integration of many data storage and management tools with new innovative cloud-based bioinformatics tools for visualization and interpretation of the data. This creates a hope that ongoing and future precision oncology trials will continue to add more valuable biomarkers. Their integrated study may further enhance our understanding of tumor progression, diagnosis, prognosis, and treatment.

REFERENCES

Alawad, M. et al. (2019) Deep transfer learning across cancer registries for information extraction from pathology reports. 2019 IEEE EMBS International Conference on Biomedical & Health Informatics (BHI 2019). IEEE.

Alberts, B. et al. (2002) Molecular Biology of the Cell. W. W. Norton & Co: New York.

Alexandrov, L.B. et al. (2013a) Signatures of mutational processes in human cancer. Nature, 500, 415–421.

Alexandrov, L.B. et al. (2013b) Deciphering signatures of mutational processes operative in human cancer. Cell Rep., 3, 246–259.

Alkhazraji, A. et al. (2019) All cancer hallmarks lead to diversity. Int. J. Clin. Exp. Med. 12(??), 132–157.

Arnedo-Pac, C. et al. (2019) OncodriveCLUSTL: A sequence-based clustering method to identify cancer drivers. Bioinformatics, 35, 4788–4790.

Audebert, N. et al. (2019) Multimodal deep networks for text and image-based document classification. Commun. Comput. Inf. Sci., 1167 CCIS, 427–443.

Bailey, M.H. et al. (2018) Comprehensive characterization of cancer driver genes and mutations. Cell, 173, 371–385.e18.

Baylin, S.B. and Jones, P.A. (2016) Epigenetic determinants of cancer. Cold Spring Harb. Perspect. Biol., 8, 1–35.

Brunese, L. et al. (2020) An ensemble learning approach for brain cancer detection exploiting radiomic features. Comput. Methods Programs Biomed., 185, 105134.

Campbell, P.J. et al. (2020) Pan-cancer analysis of whole genomes. Nature, 578, 82–93.

Carbonetto, P. et al. (2021) Non-negative matrix factorization algorithms greatly improve topic model fits. https://arxiv.org/abs/2105.13440.

Cerami, E. et al. (2012) The cBio cancer genomics portal: An open platform for exploring multidimensional cancer genomics data. Cancer Discov., 2, 401–404.

Chae, Y.K. et al. (2017) Path toward precision oncology: Review of targeted therapy studies and tools to aid in defining 'actionability' of a molecular lesion and patient management support. Mol. Cancer Ther., 16, 2645–2655.

Chaudhary, K. et al. (2018) Deep learning–based multi-omics integration robustly predicts survival in liver cancer. Clin. Cancer Res., 24, 1248–1259.

Chen, J.C. et al. (2014) Identification of causal genetic drivers of human disease through systems-level analysis of regulatory networks. Cell, 159, 402–414.

Chen, Y. et al. (2006) MILES: Multiple-instance learning via embedded instance selection. IEEE Trans. Pattern Anal. Mach. Intell., 28, 1931–1947.

Chowell, D. et al. (2018) Modeling the subclonal evolution of cancer cell populations. Cancer Res., 78, 830.

Chowell, D. et al. (2021) Improved prediction of immune checkpoint blockade efficacy across multiple cancer types. Nat. Biotechnol., 40(4), 499–506.

Collins, F.S. and Barker, A.D. (2007) Mapping the cancer genome. Sci. Am., 296, 50–57.

Conley, B.A. (2015) Genomically guided cancer treatments: From "promising" to "clinically useful". JNCI J. Natl. Cancer Inst., 107, 168.

Davies, H. et al. (2017) HRDetect is a predictor of BRCA1 and BRCA2 deficiency based on mutational-signatures. Nat. Med., 23, 517.

de Maturana, E.L. et al. (2019) Challenges in the integration of omics and non-omics data. Genes, 10, 238.

Dietlein, F. et al. (2020) Identification of cancer driver genes based on nucleotide context. Nat. Genet., 52, 208–218.

Duda, R.O. et al. (2001) Pattern Classification. Wiley: Hoboken, NJ.

Easton, D.F. et al. (2015) Gene-panel sequencing and the prediction of breast-cancer risk. N. Engl. J. Med., 372, 2243–2257.

Gao, J. et al. (2013) Integrative analysis of complex cancer genomics and clinical profiles using the cBioPortal. Sci. Signal., 6, l1.

Garber, K. (2005) Human cancer genome project moving forward despite some doubts in community. J. Natl. Cancer Inst., 97, 1322–1324.

Goossens, N. et al. (2015) Cancer biomarker discovery and validation. Transl. Cancer Res., 4, 256.

Goyal, M. (2019) Genome databases and browsers for cancer. Encycl. Bioinforma. Comput. Biol. ABC Bioinforma., 1–3, 1077–1082.

Gröbner, S.N. et al. (2018) The landscape of genomic alterations across childhood cancers. Nature, 555, 321–327.

Gupta, A. et al. (2020) A novel approach for classification of mental tasks using multiview ensemble learning (MEL). Neurocomputing, 417, 558–584.

Hanahan, D. (2022) Hallmarks of cancer: New dimensions. Cancer Discov., 12, 31–46.

Hanahan, D. and Weinberg, R.A. (2011) Hallmarks of cancer: The next generation. Cell, 144, 646–674.

Helleday, T. et al. (2014) Mechanisms underlying mutational signatures in human cancers. Nat. Rev. Genet., 15, 585–598.

Herbst, R.S. et al. (2018) The biology and management of non-small cell lung cancer. Nature, 553, 446–454.

Hu, H. et al. (2021) Three subtypes of lung cancer fibroblasts define distinct therapeutic paradigms. Cancer Cell, 39, 1531–1547.e10.

Jänne, P.A. et al. (2015) AZD9291 in EGFR inhibitor–resistant non–small-cell lung cancer. N. Engl. J. Med., 372, 1689–1699.

Jiao, W. et al. (2020) A deep learning system accurately classifies primary and metastatic cancers using passenger mutation patterns. Nat. Commun., 11, 728.

Junttila, M.R. and De Sauvage, F.J. (2013) Influence of tumour micro-environment heterogeneity on therapeutic response. Nature, 501, 346–354.

Kim, Y.G. et al. (2020) Effectiveness of transfer learning for enhancing tumor classification with a convolutional neural network on frozen sections. Sci. Rep., 10, 1–9.

King, R.J.B. and Robins, M.W. (2006) Cancer Biology, Third Edition, pp. 1–311. Oxford University Press: Oxford.
Koh, G. et al. (2021) Mutational signatures: Emerging concepts, caveats and clinical applications. Nat. Rev. Cancer, 21, 619–637.
L'Heureux, A. et al. (2017) Machine learning with big data: Challenges and approaches. IEEE Access, 5, 7776–7797.
Lapuente-Santana, Ó. et al. (2021) Interpretable systems biomarkers predict response to immune-checkpoint inhibitors. Patterns, 2, 100293.
Lewin, B. (2000) Genes VII. Oxford University Press: Oxford.
Luchini, C. et al. (2021) Artificial intelligence in oncology: Current applications and future perspectives. Br. J. Cancer, 126, 4–9.
Luo, P. et al. (2019) DeepDriver: Predicting cancer driver genes based on somatic mutations using deep convolutional neural networks. Front. Genet., 10, 13.
Ma, J. et al. (2018) The therapeutic significance of mutational signatures from DNA repair deficiency in cancer. Nat. Commun., 9, 1–12.
Ma, M. et al. (2021) SMIL: Multimodal learning with severely missing modality. arXiv:2103.05677.
Martínez-Jiménez, F. et al. (2020) A compendium of mutational cancer driver genes. Nat. Rev. Cancer, 20, 555–572.
Meric-Bernstam, F. et al. (2015) A decision support framework for genomically informed investigational cancer therapy. JNCI J. Natl. Cancer Inst., 107, 107.
Molnár-Gábor, F. et al. (2017) Computing patient data in the cloud: Practical and legal considerations for genetics and genomics research in Europe and internationally. Genome Med., 9, 1–12.
Murali, N. et al. (2020) Supervised machine learning in oncology: A clinician's guide. Dig. Dis. Interv., 4, 73.
Nadauld, L. et al. (2017) Abstract 998: OPeN: The oncology precision network data sharing consortium. Cancer Res., 77, 998–998.
Nieboer, M.M. and de Ridder, J. (2020) svMIL: Predicting the pathogenic effect of TAD boundary-disrupting somatic structural variants through multiple instance learning. Bioinformatics, 36, i692–i699.
Nieboer, M.M. et al. (2021) Predicting pathogenic non-coding SVs disrupting the 3D genome in 1646 whole cancer genomes using multiple instance learning. Sci. Rep., 11, 1–13.
Nik-Zainal, S. et al. (2012) Mutational processes molding the genomes of 21 breast cancers. Cell, 149, 979–993.
Patel, S.K. et al. (2020) Artificial intelligence to decode cancer mechanism: Beyond patient stratification for precision oncology. Front. Pharmacol., 11, 1177.
Poirion, O.B. et al. (2021) DeepProg: An ensemble of deep-learning and machine-learning models for prognosis prediction using multi-omics data. Genome Med., 13, 1–15.
Porta Siegel, T. et al. (2018) Mass spectrometry imaging and integration with other imaging modalities for greater molecular understanding of biological tissues. Mol. Imaging Biol., 20, 888–901.
Raphael, B.J. et al. (2017) Integrated genomic characterization of pancreatic ductal adenocarcinoma. Cancer Cell, 32, 185–203.e13.
Rheinbay, E. et al. (2020) Analyses of non-coding somatic drivers in 2,658 cancer whole genomes. Nat., 578, 102–111.
Robinson, J.T. et al. (2011) Integrative genomics viewer. Nat. Biotechnol., 29, 24–26.

Saunders, G. et al. (2019) Leveraging European infrastructures to access 1 million human genomes by 2022. Nat. Rev. Genet., 20, 693–701.

Schrock, A.B. et al. (2019) Tumor mutational burden is predictive of response to immune checkpoint inhibitors in MSI-high metastatic colorectal cancer. Ann. Oncol., 30, 1096–1103.

Senft, D. et al. (2017) Precision oncology: The road ahead. Trends Mol. Med., 23, 874.

Sevakula, R.K. et al. (2019) Transfer learning for molecular cancer classification using deep neural networks. IEEE/ACM Trans. Comput. Biol. Bioinforma., 16, 2089–2100.

Singh, V.K. et al. (2018) Prediction of replication sites in Saccharomyces cerevisiae genome using DNA segment properties: Multi-view ensemble learning (MEL) approach. BioSystems, 163, 59–69.

Sinkala, M. et al. (2020) Machine learning and network analyses reveal disease subtypes of pancreatic cancer and their molecular characteristics. Sci. Rep., 10, 1–14.

Summaira, J. et al. (2021) Recent advances and trends in multimodal deep learning: A review, arXiv:2105.1108.

Sweeney, S.M. et al. (2017) AACR project GENIE: Powering precision medicine through an international consortium. Cancer Discov., 7, 818–831.

Tokheim, C.J. et al. (2016) Evaluating the evaluation of cancer driver genes. Proc. Natl. Acad. Sci. U. S. A., 113, 14330–14335.

Tran, K.A. et al. (2021) Deep learning in cancer diagnosis, prognosis and treatment selection. Genome Med., 13, 1–17.

Turki, T. et al. (2017) Transfer learning approaches to improve drug sensitivity prediction in multiple myeloma patients. IEEE Access, 5, 7381–7393.

Van Cutsem, E. et al. (2009) Cetuximab and chemotherapy as initial treatment for metastatic colorectal cancer. N. Engl. J. Med., 360, 1408–1417.

Vogelstein, B. et al. (2013) Cancer genome landscapes. Science, 339, 1546–1558.

Weghorn, D. and Sunyaev, S. (2017) Bayesian inference of negative and positive selection in human cancers. Nat. Genet., 49, 1785–1788.

Xiong, D. et al. (2021) A comparative study of multiple instance learning methods for cancer detection using T-cell receptor sequences. Comput. Struct. Biotechnol. J., 19, 3255–3268.

Xu, W. et al. (2003) Document clustering based on non-negative matrix factorization. SIGIR 2003: Proceedings of the 26th Annual International ACM SIGIR Conference on Research and Development in Information Retrieval, July 28 - August 1, 2003, Toronto, Canada, p. 267.

Zhang, J. et al. (2019) The international cancer genome consortium data portal. Nat. Biotechnol., 37, 367–369.

Zhang, L. et al. (2018) Deep learning-based multi-omics data integration reveals two prognostic subtypes in high-risk neuroblastoma. Front. Genet., 9, 477.

Zhou, X. et al. (2021) Exploration of coding and non-coding variants in cancer using GenomePaint. Cancer Cell, 39, 83–95.e4.

Zhu, Y. et al. (2020) Ensemble transfer learning for the prediction of anti-cancer drug response. Sci. Rep., 10, 1–11.

Chapter 15

Artificial intelligence in Precision Oncology

Ranjeet Kaur, Sabiya Fatima, Amit Doegar, and C. Rama Krishna
National Institute of Technical Teachers Training & Research (NITTTR)

Suyash Singh
All India Institute of Medical Sciences (AIIMS)

CONTENTS

DOI: 10.1201/9781003368342-15

15.1 INTRODUCTION

In the field of Biomedical Engineering, Bioinformatics and Biotechnology, treatment of cancer patients is achieving new heights with the inclusion of Target Therapies in personalized healthcare. Digital personalized treatments focus on improved patient healthcare and deliver new therapies at reasonable cost. In the BIS research study 2019, it has been revealed that Precision Medicine (PM) market will reach around $220 billion globally in the next 10 years (https://bisresearch.com/industry-report/precision-medicine-market.html). In the 21st century, though there exists chemotherapy and radiotherapy, the demand for the latest technology, i.e., next-Generation Genome Sequencing (NGS), Biomarker Testing and Precise Imaging has been increasing worldwide. Oncologists are playing a pivotal role in analysing new diagnostic tools to cure cancer patients with their in-depth knowledge and expertise. In another report (https://www.hcp.novartis.com/), 52% of pathologists and 62% of oncologists are optimistic and self-confident to make decisions by using their genetic test knowledge. Precision Oncology is one of the emerging and challenging treatments in the precision healthcare domain. It includes computational analysis [deep learning (DL), statistical analysis, etc.], clinical sciences and bioinformatics for making health-related decisions. Figure 15.1 represents different computational analysis techniques, which take biomedical data of humans as an input, process it by using AI algorithms and predict the outcomes based on which decision-making is done. These techniques are computer vision, machine learning (ML), DL, image processing, statistical analysis, and many more.

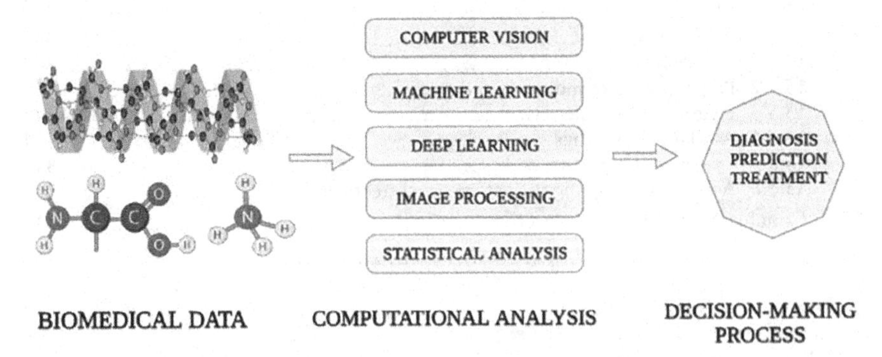

Figure 15.1 Computational analysis techniques using biomedical data.

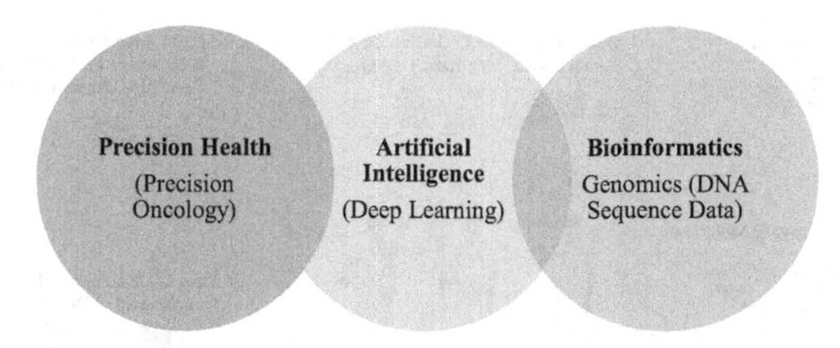

Figure 15.2 AI in Precision Oncology.

In the computational research areas, bioinformatics also plays an active and significant role in Precision Oncology when applied with prominent DL models. At the same time, genome sequencing unravels the tremendous and hidden genetic diversity among the individuals by generating the huge genomics data. This enables us to interpret and analyse the genomics data (DNA-sequence data) by applying various informatics tools such as BLAST (Basic Local Alignment Search Tool), UCSC Genome Browser, BioPerl, Clustal Omega, etc. This data is analysed so that researchers can find the variations that affect drug response, disease response and overall health. As the Genomics applications are increasing day by day, the growing trend of Genomics research in diagnosing the diseases has been observed in the last couple of years.

The collaboration of Bioinformatics, AI and Precision Oncology gives promising results in proving the best and specialized treatment to patients. This modern practice has a great impact on the prolonged survival of patients. Figure 15.2 represents the pictorial representation of AI in Precision Oncology.

15.2 PRECISION ONCOLOGY

With the molecular tumour profiling of individuals, Precision Oncology emerges as an extensive research field to deliver precision health. The basic building block of this treatment is genetic testing. Predicting cancer in a particular individual based on his genomics data is a very complex and challenging task, and this process is known as Precision Oncology [Coudray et al. 2018].

To perform this task using Artificial Intelligence (AI) models, there is a need for expert knowledge (AI experts and clinical experts), biomedical

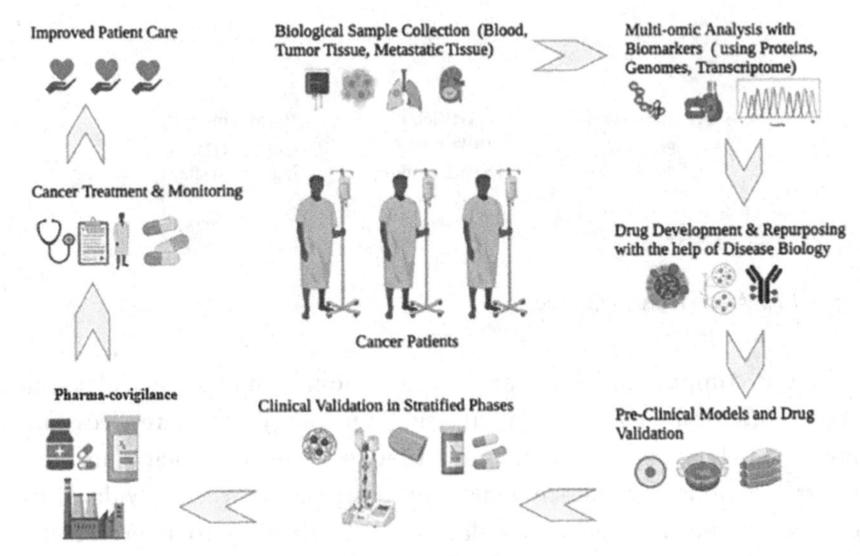

Figure 15.3 Simplified workflow of Precision Oncology.

data and sufficient infrastructure. Precision Oncology is a step-by-step procedure, which includes the following phases (Dupont et al. 2021). Figure 15.3 represents the simplified workflow of Precision Oncology. BioRender Software (Trial Version) is used for making Figures 15.1 and 15.3.

15.2.1 Sample collection

Collecting the biological samples is the foremost task to start the procedure. Blood samples, tumour tissues, metastasis tissues, etc. are a few examples of biological samples, which are utilized in precision healthcare.

15.2.2 Multi-omic analysis

In this, multiple "omes" datasets are integrated to perform the biological analysis to detect the associations and relationships between different biological entities. Multiple "Omes" dataset includes Microbiome, Genome, Transcriptome, Proteome, etc. The relevant biomarkers are then pinpointed for different diseases. This unravels the insights of the multi-omic data. There exist much software for performing multi-omic analyses such as mixOmics, omicade, bioCancer, IMAS, and many more (https://en.wikipedia.org/wiki/Multiomics/).

15.2.3 Drug development & repurposing

It involves the identification of new therapeutic use for existing approved drugs. It reduces the timeline for drug development and cuts the research & development cost. After reprofiling the drugs, it is then validated by pre-clinical models in the next step.

15.2.4 Drug validation by pre-clinical models

Before testing the drugs in humans, pre-clinical evaluation of drugs is very important. Some pre-clinical models mimic human behaviour after taking the drugs. It is performed so that safe human testing can be done.

15.2.5 Clinical validation

In this step, the documented diagnosis is reviewed to ensure whether or not the medical community has accepted the clinical criteria. There should be adequate and rigorous clinical validation in the form of documented evidence in the stratified phases.

15.2.6 Pharma-covigilance

In the lifecycle of drug or a medical device, the adverse side effects such as adverse events, drug reactions, etc. are detected and monitored over time during this step. Consumers' reactions and their sentiments about the particular drug are also recorded.

15.2.7 Treatment and monitoring

After the pharmacovigilance by the experts, patient gets the personalized treatment or therapy based on his genomes. The patients' health is monitored on daily, weekly or monthly basis.

15.3 AI MODELS

AI is one of the most powerful technologies and is utilized in many fields to get efficiency in decision-making processes. DL is the subset of AI, which includes complex architectures with hidden layers. It consists of neural networks (i.e., multiple connected neurons/nodes) which simulate the human brain to predict the outcomes. With the evolution of DL,

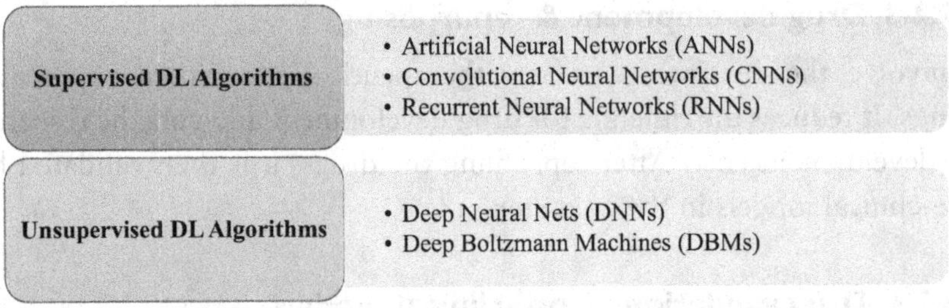

Supervised DL Algorithms

- Artificial Neural Networks (ANNs)
- Convolutional Neural Networks (CNNs)
- Recurrent Neural Networks (RNNs)

Unsupervised DL Algorithms

- Deep Neural Nets (DNNs)
- Deep Boltzmann Machines (DBMs)

Figure 15.4 Supervised and unsupervised DL algorithms.

pattern identification, prediction analysis, progression modelling, multi-class disease classification, drug discovery and repurposing, etc. have reached new heights. DL models perform the feature extraction automatically, unlike traditional or hand-crafted techniques. As the dataset size increases, DL model outperforms humans. These models are categorized into different categories, i.e., supervised DL algorithms and unsupervised DL Algorithms. Figure 15.4 depicts examples of supervised and unsupervised DL algorithms. These models incorporate neural networks into their architectures in different ways to overcome the burden of oncologists/researchers by providing the deep understanding of the cancer variants in different individuals. Acceleration in these technologies has influenced and improved the patient care by early prediction, diagnosis and treatment of cancer patients. There are many applications of DL like Forecasting & Prediction, Image Processing, Speech Recognition, Autonomous Vehicles, Computer Vision, etc.

15.3.1 Supervised DL algorithms

Supervised DL algorithms are those algorithms that use the neural networks in a supervised way by including labelled data or classes (benign/malignant, dog/cat, yes/no, etc.). In this, neural networks get trained and predict the outcomes by using the labelled dataset. Mainly, Classification and Regression problems are solved using these network architectures. ANNs, CNNs and RNNs are examples of supervised DL algorithms.

15.3.1.1 Artificial Neural Networks

Artificial Neural Networks (ANNs) (also called feed-forward neural networks) are similar to the human brain, consist of billions of connected neurons, learnable weights and biases to compute the information by applying the activation function (https://www.geeksforgeeks.org/introduction-to-artificial-neutral-networks/). It includes mainly three layers, namely, input layer → hidden layers → output layer; and an activation function. In the training phase, ANNs learn to identify and discover the patterns based on the input. When the dataset (as an input) is provided to the input layer, it extracts the features automatically. This information is processed in the hidden layers to produce the desired output. ANNs have ability to perform the computations with incomplete information and are comfortable with parallel processing. As a result, hardware dependency increases when multiple processors are required in parallel processing.

15.3.1.2 Convolutional Neural Networks (CNNs)

CNNs are also known as ConvNets. Combining two functions to generate the third function is Convolution. This process involves multiple hidden layers, which use filters or kernels to process and extract the feature map of the images. It differentiates the images by using these features. There exist five layers in CNNs i.e. Input Layer → Convolutional Layer → Relu Layer → Pooling Layer → Fully-Connected Layer. Each layer has different parameters which can be further optimized to perform different tasks on the dataset [Dupont et al. 2021]. The different architectures of CNN are AlexNet, GoogleNet, ZF Net, LeNet, VGGNet, ResNet, etc (https://cs231n.github.io/convolutional-networks/). It simplifies the computations and handles the classification of images efficiently, but it requires a large dataset for model training.

15.3.1.3 Recurrent Neural Networks (RNNs)

In RNNs, the output of the particular hidden layer is fed back as an input to predict the output (https://www.geeksforgeeks.org/introduction-to-recurrent-neural-network/). It has the internal memory, which memorizes all the calculated information of the previous and current step. It is one of the preferred algorithms for the sequential data (time series, weather, speech, financial data, etc.). This model is compatible with all input lengths but suffers from a vanishing gradient problem due to which the learning process of long data sequences takes ample time while training the model.

15.3.2 Unsupervised DL algorithms

In unsupervised DL Algorithms, the data gets trained on its own as there is no supervision or guidance. Without the human intervention, these algorithms discover hidden patterns to predict the output using the unlabeled and untrained dataset. DBNs, DBMs and Hierarchical Sparse Coding are some of the examples of Unsupervised DL Algorithms.

15.3.2.1 Deep Neural Networks (DNNs)

DNNs are the directed generative DL model, which consists of a connected series of Restricted Boltzmann Machines (RBMs) (https://www.edureka.co/blog/restricted-boltzmann-machine-tutorial/). These are also known as Deep Belief Nets (DBNs). Each of RBMs includes hidden and visible layers. They learn the complex internal representations of input data features layer-by-layer in an unsupervised manner. Then pre-training and fine-tuning of the model are done to get the better outcome. They solve speech recognition and object recognition problems accurately (https://data-flair.training/blogs/deep-neural-networks-with-python/), but the learning process is very expensive.

15.3.2.2 Deep Boltzmann Machines

Deep Boltzmann Machines (DBMs) are the undirected deep-generative models. The working of DBMs is similar to DNNs, but DBMs are more robust than DNNs (http://www.cs.toronto.edu/~fritz/absps/dbm.pdf). These deep models are the future of AI on which the data scientists are focusing more to deal with very high-dimensional data.

15.4 LITERATURE REVIEW

DL models are providing great support and benefits to the researchers to deal with Precision Oncology in both supervised and unsupervised manner. As they deal with multi-dimensional and multi-modality data, they are able to handle the multi-omic dataset efficiently. After screening PubMed from 2018 to 2021, original peer-reviewed articles are presented and compared in Table 15.1. Keywords used while searching the papers on digital platforms are 'Deep Learning in Genomics' or 'Precision Oncology' or 'AI in Precision Medicine' or 'Deep Learning in Oncology' or 'Cancer Genomics'. Metrics like Cancer type, Number of patients,

Table 15.1 Summary of the state-of-the art models

References	*Journal name*	*Year*	*Cancer type*	*No. of patients*	*Methodology*	*Accuracy (%)*	*AUROC*	*Other metrics*
Bychkov, D et al. (2018)	Scientific Reports	2018 2018	Colorectal Cancer	420	Survival prediction	-	0.96	Hazard Hazard
Coutureet al. (2018)	NPJ Breast Cancer	2018	Breast Cancer	859	Mutation detection	84	- -	Specificity = 76%, sensitivity = 88%
Coudray et al. (2018)	Nature Medicine	2018	Lung Cancer	-	Mutation detection	-	0.68	-
Harder, N et al. (2019)	Scientific Reports	2019	Melanoma (Skin Cancer)	31	Therapy-response prediction	70.9	-	-
Courtiolet al. (2019)	Nature Medicine	2019	Mesothelioma (Lung Cancer)	3,037	Survival prediction	-	-	C-score = 0.66

(Continued)

Table 15.1 *(Continued)* Summary of the state-of-the art models

References	*Journal name*	*Year*	*Cancer type*	*No. of patients*	*Methodology*	*Accuracy*	*AUROC*	*Other metrics*
Sun et al. (2019)	Cancers	2019	Melanoma (Skin Cancer)	47	Mutation detection	92.8	-	Specificity = 92.1%, sensitivity = 91.1%, F-score = 0.93
Turkki et al. (2019) (2019)	Breast Cancer Research	2019	Breast Cancer	1,299	Survival prediction	-	0.58	Hazard ratio = 1.74
Yip et al. (2019)	Journal of Pathology Informatics	2019	Lung Cancer	130	Mutation detection	-	0.8	-
Schmauch et al. (2020)	Nature Communication	2020	Pan-Cancer (related to genomics)	8,725	Mutation detection	-	0.81	-
Saillard et al. (2020)	Hepatology	2020	Carcinoma	522	Survival prediction	-	-	C-score = 0.7, hazard ratio = 4.3
Wulczyn et al. (2020) (2020)	PLoS One	2020	Multiple cancer types	4,880	Survival prediction	-	0.64	C-score = 65.1, hazard ratio = 1.48
Skrede et al. (2020)	Lancet	2020	Colorectal Cancer	3,595	Survival prediction	76	-	Specificity = 78%, sensitivity = 52%, hazard ratio = 3.83

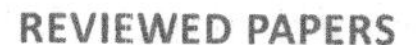

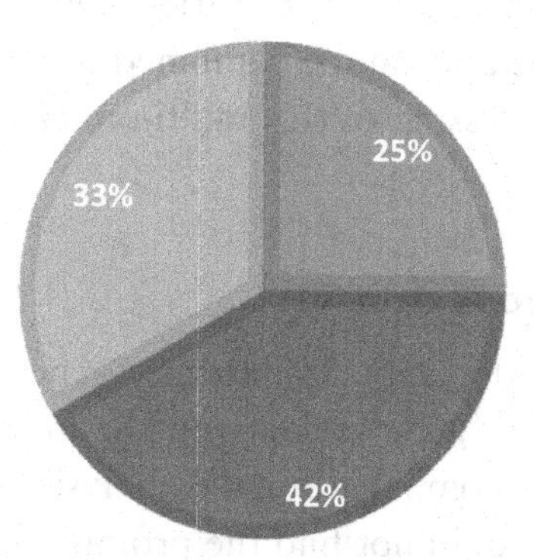

Figure 15.5 Literature review from 2018 to 2020.

methodology, accuracy, Area under Receiver-Operating curve (AUROC), sensitivty and hazard ratio are used for performance evaluation of the DL models.

Figure 15.5 represents the percentage of papers that are included in the literature review from the year 2018 to 2020.

15.5 RESEARCH CHALLENGES

Although Precision Oncology provides a way to get the targeted therapies and personalized treatment using AI, there are some challenges faced by researchers in the real-time and clinical diagnosis. As per the reviewed literature, the limitations of AI models in Precision Oncology are discussed below:

15.5.1 Black-box nature of AI

In clinical decision-making, where patients are vulnerable to health-related risks, it is not enough to depend on AI models completely. Sometimes, AI doesn't predict the exact outcome in the case of clinical diagnostics (Ghorbani et al. 2019). The predictions generated by the AI models should be justifiable and explainable to start the treatment (Graham et al. 2020).

15.5.2 Preprocessing of multi-omics dataset

Most of the AI models utilize multi-scale and multi-omics data to predict the outcomes. There exist data repositories of multi-omic dataset, which are publicly accessible and can be combined to provide the input to the AI model. But preprocessing of this multi-omics data is required to get the effective results.

15.5.3 Heterogeneous dataset

Genomics data includes gene transcripts, genes expressions profiles, alterations in genomes, gene variants on the individual level, etc. This heterogeneous data is combined for the analysis and prediction. Unfortunately, researchers could not find the promising results in most of the cases (Ceri and Pinoli 2019).

15.5.4 Availability of drugs

Drug availability for the patients having personalized therapies are also very limited. Sometimes, there may be cases like no personalized drug is available in stock that is relevant to particular DNA or other alternate drugs may not be given to patient due to lack of testing on DNA.

15.5.5 Expensive treatment

As biomarkers are utilized for these targeted therapies, it makes this treatment very expensive for the patients. Government funding, charitable trusts, donors, scientific communities, etc. are required to help needy patients.

15.5.6 Awareness & opting the personalized treatment

Although technology has geared up, poor patients are still lacking the knowledge of targeted therapies and personalized treatment. Sometimes, they may be reluctant due to lack of knowledge, financial support, etc. to have PM or treatment. Therefore, there should be awareness programmes for motivating people to opt for personalized treatments.

15.6 CONCLUSION & FUTURE PERSPECTIVES

In this chapter, an overview of Precision Oncology is discussed and various DL models, which are utilized in the genomics area, are outlined.

It is evident from the state-of-the-art approaches that DL models can work effectively with multi-modal genomics data to predict the cancer. DL algorithms are more effective than genomics algorithms as these traditional models are prone to more errors and take ample time to learn while training the model. The predictive power of DL models is incomparable in genomics field, but developing an explainable or justifiable DL model is still challenging. Integrating and handling heterogeneous big dataset is also one of the concerns to be dealt with. This data should be handled with the utmost care by DL models. One of the major challenges is to extract and clinical validation of the subtypes of genes with DL. Clinical experts and data scientists should perform collaborative assignments and experiments to overcome the research challenges. Patient-based comprehensive tumour evaluation is most required for promising treatments. Social, economic and physical factors affecting the tumour patients should be explored more.

REFERENCES

Bychkov, D., Linder, N., Turkki, R., Nordling, S., Kovanen, P., Verrill, C., Walliander, M., Lundin, M., Haglund, C. and Lundin, J., 2018. "Deep learning based tissue analysis predicts outcome in colorectal cancer". *Scientific Reports*, 8 (1): 1–11.

Ceri, S., and Pinoli, P. 2019. "Data science for genomic data management: Challenges, resources, experiences". *SN Computer Science* 1 (1). doi:10.1007/s42979-019-0005-0.

Coudray, N., Ocampo, P., Sakellaropoulos, T., Narula, N., Snuderl, M., Fenyö, D., Moreira, A., Razavian, N. and Tsirigos, A., 2018. "Classification and mutation prediction from non–small cell lung cancer histopathology images using deep learning." *Nature Medicine*, 24 (10): 1559–1567.

Courtiol, P., Maussion, C., Moarii, M., Pronier, E., Pilcer, S., Sefta, M., Manceron, P., Toldo, S., Zaslavskiy, M., Le Stang, N., Girard, N., Elemento, O., Nicholson, A., Blay, J., Galateau-Sallé, F., Wainrib, G. and Clozel, T., 2019. "Deep learning-based classification of mesothelioma improves prediction of patient outcome." *Nature Medicine*, 25 (10): 1519–1525.

Couture, H., Williams, L., Geradts, J., Nyante, S., Butler, E., Marron, J., Perou, C., Troester, M. and Niethammer, M., 2018. "Image analysis with deep learning to predict breast cancer grade, ER status, histologic subtype, and intrinsic subtype." *NPJ Breast Cancer*, 4 (1): 1–8.

Dupont, C., Riegel, K., Pompaiah, M., Juhl, H. and Rajalingam, K., 2021. "Druggable genome and precision medicine in cancer: Current challenges." *The FEBS Journal*, 288 (21): 6142–6158.

Ghorbani, A., Abid, A. and Zou, J., 2019. "Interpretation of neural networks is fragile." *Proceedings of the AAAI Conference on Artificial Intelligence*, 33: 3681–3688.

Graham, G., Csicsery, N., Stasiowski, E., Thouvenin, G., Mather, W., Ferry, M., Cookson, S. and Hasty, J., 2020. "Genome-scale transcriptional dynamics and environmental biosensing." *Proceedings of the National Academy of Sciences*, 117 (6): 3301–3306.

Harder, N., Schönmeyer, R., Nekolla, K., Meier, A., Brieu, N., Vanegas, C., Madonna, G., Capone, M., Botti, G., Ascierto, P. and Schmidt, G., 2019. "Automatic discovery of image-based signatures for ipilimumab response prediction in malignant melanoma." *Scientific Reports*, 9 (1): 7449.

Saillard, C., Schmauch, B., Laifa, O., Moarii, M., Toldo, S., Zaslavskiy, M., Pronier, E., Laurent, A., Amaddeo, G., Regnault, H., Sommacale, D., Ziol, M., Pawlotsky, J., Mulé, S., Luciani, A., Wainrib, G., Clozel, T., Courtiol, P. and Calderaro, J., 2020. "Predicting survival after hepatocellular carcinoma resection using deep-learning on histological slides." *Journal of Hepatology*, 73: S381.

Schmauch, B., Romagnoni, A., Pronier, E., Saillard, C., Maillé, P., Calderaro, J., Kamoun, A., Sefta, M., Toldo, S., Zaslavskiy, M., Clozel, T., Moarii, M., Courtiol, P. and Wainrib, G., 2020. "A deep learning model to predict RNA-Seq expression of tumours from whole slide images." *Nature Communications*, 11 (1): 3877.

Skrede, O., De Raedt, S., Kleppe, A., Hveem, T., Liestøl, K., Maddison, J., Askautrud, H., Pradhan, M., Nesheim, J., Albregtsen, F., Farstad, I., Domingo, E., Church, D., Nesbakken, A., Shepherd, N., Tomlinson, I., Kerr, R., Novelli, M., Kerr, D. and Danielsen, H., 2020. "Deep learning for prediction of colorectal cancer outcome: A discovery and validation study." *The Lancet*, 395 (10221): 350–360.

Sun, M., Zhou, W., Qi, X., Zhang, G., Girnita, L., Seregard, S., Grossniklaus, H., Yao, Z., Zhou, X. and Stålhammar, G., 2019. "Prediction of BAP1 Expression in Uveal melanoma using densely-connected deep classification networks." *Cancers*, 11 (10): E1579.

Turkki, R., Byckhov, D., Lundin, M., Isola, J., Nordling, S., Kovanen, P., Verrill, C., von Smitten, K., Joensuu, H., Lundin, J. and Linder, N., 2019. "Breast cancer outcome prediction with tumour tissue images and machine learning." *Breast Cancer Research and Treatment*, 177 (1): 41–52.

Wulczyn, E., Steiner, D., Xu, Z., Sadhwani, A., Wang, H., Flament-Auvigne, I., Mermel, C., Chen, P., Liu, Y. and Stumpe, M., 2020. "Deep learning-based survival prediction for multiple cancer types using histopathology images." *PLoS One*, 15 (6): e0233678.

Yip, S., Sha, L., Osinski, B., Ho, I., Tan, T., Willis, C., Weiss, H., Beaubier, N., Mahon, B. and Taxter, T., 2019. "Multi-field-of-view deep learning model predicts nonsmall cell lung cancer programmed death-ligand 1 status from whole-slide hematoxylin and eosin images." *Journal of Pathology Informatics*, 10 (1): 24.

Chapter 16

Computer-aided breast cancer diagnosis using machine learning and deep learning methods

A comprehensive survey

Ritika Singh, Vipin Kumar, Prashant Prabhakar, and Ibrahim Momin
Mahatma Gandhi Central University

CONTENTS

16.1 INTRODUCTION

Early detection is critical in treating Breast Cancer (BrC), as it can prevent the disease from spreading. Machine learning (ML) is a commonly used research technique involving learning algorithms designed to perform specific tasks. Various algorithms are used in this field, such as decision

DOI: 10.1201/9781003368342-16

trees, K-Nearest neighbour (KNN), support vector machine (SVM), and naive bays. Due to the limitations of ML, DL is being used in the field of BrC detection. It is mainly used in data science to develop algorithms such as convolutional neural network (CNN), recurrent neural network (RNN), and deep belief network (DBN) [1].

BrC is usually curable in about 70% of cases. However, it can be challenging to treat with currently available therapies [2]. The molecular characteristics of BrC are complex. Some of these include the activation of various receptors, viz., progesterone and estrogen receptors [3]. Different treatment strategies are utilised for different types of BrC. There are multiple options available, such as systemic therapy and radiation therapy. Various systemic therapy options are also available for patients with hormone receptor-positive BrC. These include chemotherapy, anti-HER2 therapy, and bone stabilising agents. According to the WHO, BrC is prevalent cancer affecting women. It is expected to account for about 15% of all cancer deaths worldwide in 2020 [4]. Figure 16.1 displays the number of deaths and new kinds of cases from different types of cancer that affect females in 2020.

Various early research studies have been conducted to minimise the risk of developing BrC. This has led to a steady decline in the mortality rate. According to the Center of Cancer Research UK[6], the five-year survival

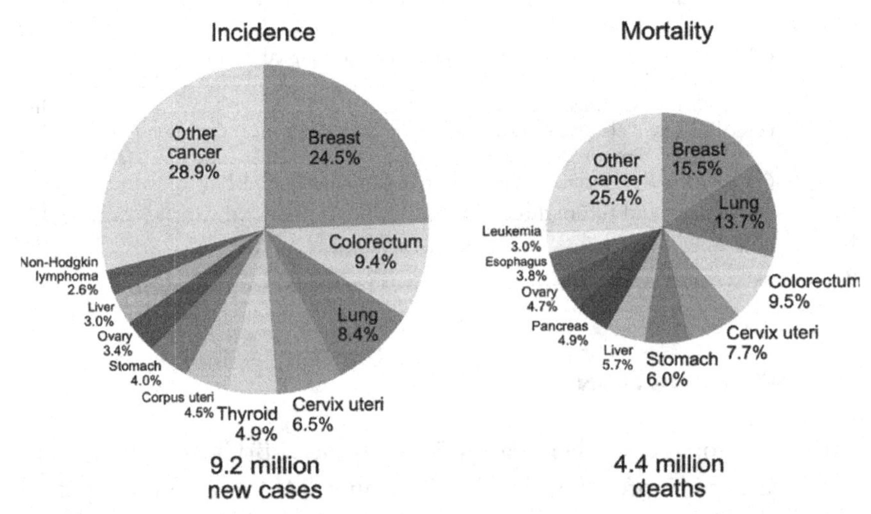

Figure 16.1 The sectoral % age of deaths and cases from the ten highly prevalent cancers among females in the year 2020 [5].

rate for BrC is around 100%, possibly if detected early. However, it can be as low as 15% if seen later. Techniques such as ML are being utilised for diagnosing and prognosing BrC. They can help identify people with the disease and predict their chances of survival.

Epigenetics has revolutionised the understanding of BrC, as it allows us to recognise and understand various factors that put up the development of this disease [7]. The mechanisms by which epigenetic regulation is carried out involve interactions between different genes. These interactions regulate the structure and function of the genes, which activates or silences gene expression. A change in the face of key genes in breast cells can lead to cancer development and the maintenance of drug resistance. With comprehensive information about their disease, patients with BrC can make informed decisions regarding their treatment. Complete details on BrC are essential for patients and healthcare providers. It can help them make informed decisions regarding their treatment and improve their quality of life. Electronic health records (EHRs) have a large amount of clinical information that has been utilised to enhance the quality of care for patients. Aside from providing comprehensive information about patients, EHRs can also be further used to improve the quality of care by monitoring various aspects of a patient's health [8]. This study referred to around 80 research papers that analysed the multiple aspects of BrC diagnosis and treatment. Some articles focused on deep learning alone, while others used ML and DL. The source was scientific databases such as ScienceDirect, Nature, IEEE, Science citation indexing, Google Scholar, and Springer to download the research paper. The number of studies published in BrC studies peaked between 2012 and 2022.

The various challenges the models face in detecting the masses are some factors that affect their performance. The introduction of DL has revolutionised the interpretation of imaging studies. However, this technology is also being used to transform the field of breast imaging. One example of this is DBT [9]. The emergence and evolution of DBT and the use of AI in the imaging of breasts have highlighted the need for systems to adapt to new imaging methods [10]. DL has many advantages over traditional medical imaging methods, but some significant issues still need to be addressed. One is the lack of annotations for regions of interest in huge images. Multi-column CNNs that can perform multiple scans simultaneously can be tried, and inter-nuclear arrangements can also be modelled using graph-based techniques. A method that accounts for variation in staining variation can be used. It involves extracting nuclei-based patches and estimating the patient class of each patch. Using nuclear-based patches aims to identify inter-nuclear arrangements and nuclear structure in an image. In addition, approaches based on multiple instances of earning operating with weakly supervised data can be tested [11].

The first step was to collect the preliminary information about the paper, such as the author's name, the list of the publishers, and the year of publication. Then, it includes a few more details about the algorithm used and the features of the paper. Some of these include the accuracy of the results, the dataset, the elements, and performance evaluation parameters. Broadly, the selection of research articles has been made based on the following research questions:

- What steps are being taken to establish a BrC CAD system?
- Various screening modalities methods and publicly available mammographic datasets used for BrC.
- What evaluation criteria are used to determine the viability of building a BrC CAD system?
- How to use imaging modalities and deep learning models to investigate the numerous aspects that influence BrC classification?
- How to identify the types of datasets used to build these models?
- What are the drawbacks, issues, and research needs for detecting a categorising BrC?

The novel about survey papers is in the following section:

- Most of the studies on the identification of BrC primarily relied on the use of old-fashioned ML techniques and generic classifiers such as ANNs and SNNs. Existing review studies on the identification of BrC only relied on grayscale images.
- They also discussed deep learning techniques. This research examines current standard image classification methods in CAD. It focuses on various aspects of this field, such as image pre-processing, image datasets, image performance measurements, and DNNs. The review is conducted through a systematic review process to identify the most relevant studies and their quality.
- It also offers a critical assessment of DL algorithms' performance on various datasets. Finally, this article thoroughly examines the

Table 16.1 List of abbreviations used

Abbreviations	*Full form*	*Abbreviations*	*Full form*
BrC	Breast Cancer	CM	Confusion Matrix
AI	Artificial intelligence	Acc	Accuracy
ML	Machine learning	Pr	Precision
DL	Deep learning	Re	Recall
DBN	Deep Belief Network	Se	Sensitivity
ANN	Artificial neural network	Sp	Specificity
CNN	Convolutional neural network	ROI	Region of interest
DCNN	Deep Convolutional Neural Network	AUC	Area Under Curve
FFNN	Feed Forward Neural Network	PPV	Positive Predictive Values
PCNN	Pulse Coupled Neural Network	NPV	Negative Predictive Values
SVM	Support vector machine	FPR	False-Positive Rate
KNN	K-nearest neighbour	FNR	False-Negative Rate
LR	Logistic regression	TPR	True-Positive Rate
DT	Decision tree	TNR	True-Negative Rate
HP	Histopathology	MCC	Medical Counselling Committee
MRI	Magnetic resonance imaging	WBCD	Wisconsin Breast Cancer Dataset
DCE-MRI	Dynamic Contrast-Enhanced-MRI	WDBC	Breast Cancer Wisconsin (Diagnostic) Data Set
CE-MRI	Contrast-Enhanced Magnetic Resonance Imaging	DDSM	Digital Database for Screening Mammography
US	Ultrasound	MIAS	Mammography Image Analysis Society
BUS	Breast ultrasound	WPBC	Wisconsin Prognostic Breast Cancer Data
SFM	Screen film mammography	IRMA	Image Retrieval in Medical Application
FFDM	Full-field digital mammography	UCI	University of California Irvine
DM	Digital Mammography	SEER	Surveillance Epidemiology and End Result
CT	Computerised Tomography	WEKA	Waikato Environment for Knowledge Analysis
PET	Positron Emission Tomography	CLAHE	Contrast Limited Adaptive Histogram Equalisation
CADx	Computer-aided diagnosis	DBT	Digital Breast Tomosynthesis
CADe	Computer-aided detection	DET	Data Exploratory Techniques
GPU	Graphical processing unit	RBF	Radial basis function

(Continued)

Table 16.1 (Continued) List of abbreviations used

Abbreviations	*Full form*	*Abbreviations*	*Full form*
HER2	Human Epidermal growth factor Receptor 2	GONN	Genetically optimised neural network
EHR	Electronic Health Record	DLS	Deep Learning Software
LESSO	Least Absolute Shrinkage and a Selection Operator	EIT	Electrical Impedance-based mapping
PCA	Principal Component Analysis	DWI	Diffusion-Weighted Imaging
LDA	Linear Discriminant Analysis	DCE	Dynamic Contrast Enhanced
CSAE	Convolutional (sparse) Autoencoders	RDN	Recovery Database Network
FCN	Fully Convolutional Networks	IOU	Intersection Over Union
WSIO	Watershed Index Online	NIR	Near Infrared
RFE	Recursive Feature Elimination		

many research directions and issues confronting the area of image classification for BrC detection and diagnosis (Table 16.1).

The organisation of the paper: Following this introduction, the study begins with "Breast Cancer", which introduces various stages of the disease and its imaging modalities. Then, the focus goes to the description of the datasets in Section 16.3. Section 16.4 summarises the literature survey on BrC diagnosis, and Section 16.5 focuses on CADx. This study uses ML algorithms and deep learning algorithms to analyse images. Section 16.6 explains various methodologies used by researchers for BrC detection. Later, this presents the survey's findings and discusses the multiple research gaps and future directions that will be pursued in CADs. In Section 16.7, this chapter concludes that information on various aspects of BrC diagnosis is the primary goal of this survey.

16.2 BREAST CANCER (BrC)

The ducts and lobules of the breast are the primary sites where BrC begins. This type of cancer can potentially expand to other tissues and body organs. The lymphatic system does the movement of cancer cells from one site to another. Some signs of BrC include pain in the breast, breast size, and a discharge from the breast. Individuals with certain risk factors such as being overweight or having a family history of BrC are more prone to developing this type of cancer. In a study conducted by Ref. [9], they analysed various factors in the development of BrC. They then used LR and an ANN to monitor these effects. Although age and overall health were considered important factors in assessing a patient's survival, these factors might not contribute as much to predicting a patient's future survival. Instead, they should be considered part of a model that can indicate a patient's survival. Figure 16.2 shows the placements of the duct, areola, nipple, lobules, lobe, and fat.

16.2.1 Categorisation

The differences between malignant and benign tumours are the major goal of BrC diagnosis. To diagnose these two forms of cancers, a trustworthy method is required. BrC is distributed majorly into two types, particularly non-invasive and invasive. Tumours of Invasive type usually get generated in the milk ducts and could migrate to other regions of the organ rest. Non-invasive tumours cannot spread to other areas of the body [10].

1. *Lobular carcinoma in situ:* This type of BrC does not spread to other body parts. Instead, it is created in the glands(milk) of the organ breast.
2. *Invasive lobular carcinoma:* Starting from lobules and it spreads towards neneighbouring issues.
3. *Ductal carcinoma in situ:* it is a non-invasive type of BrC that doesn't spread to other body parts. It can only be found in the breast ducts.
4. *Invasive ductal carcinoma:* it is the most prevalent type of BrC. It usually starts in milk ducts and could mainly spread to various other breast parts.

The Phyllodes tumour, as well as angiosarcoma, are two less typical kinds of BrC. Angiosarcoma is a particular kind of cancer that could grow in the lymph of breast vessels or blood vessels. Inflammatory breast cancer is the most uncommon kind of BrC, accounting for 1%–5% of all patients. It can cause the breast to swell and feel hot. Triple-negative BrC is also a triple-negative tumour; this type of cancer usually grows in the breast without specific proteins [2].

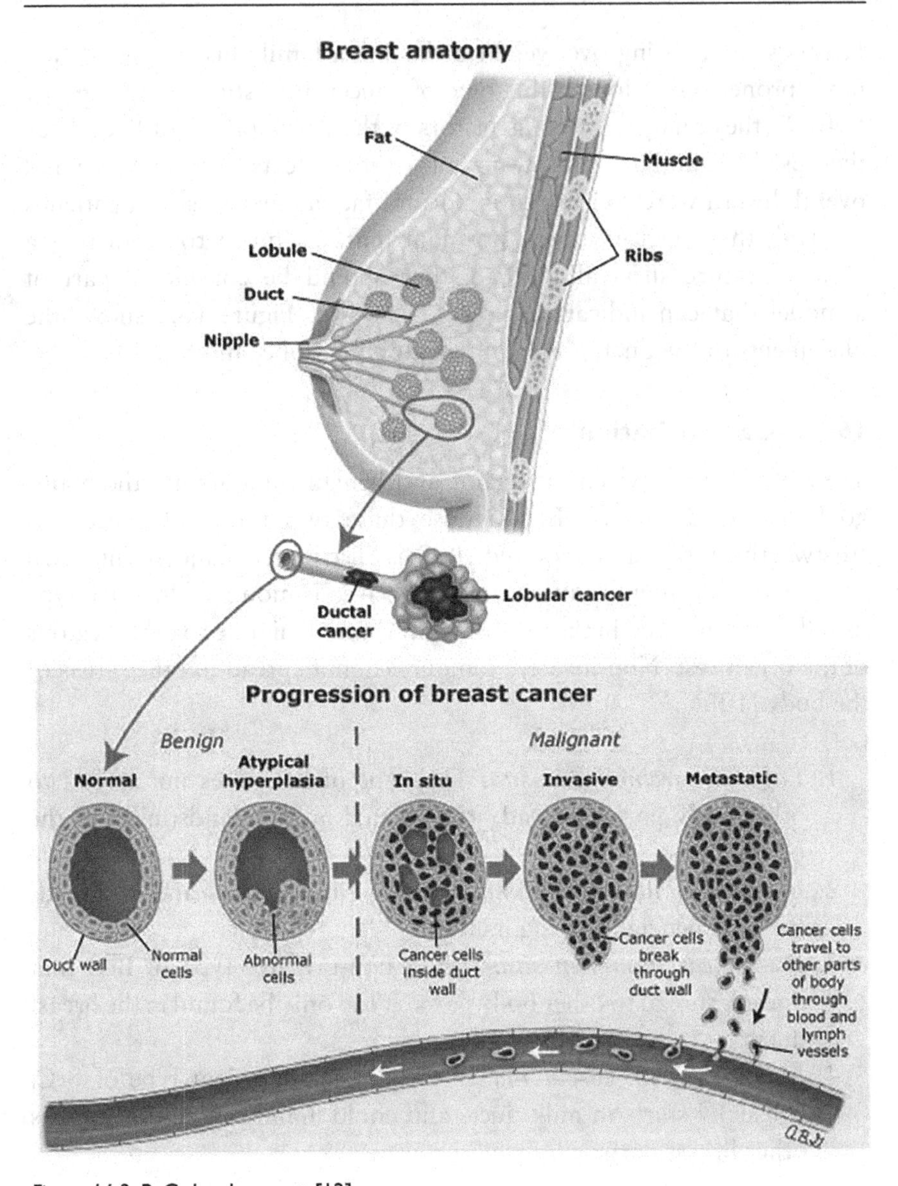

Figure 16.2 BrC development [12].

16.2.2 Evolution of breast cancer stages

BrC is classified into four phases based on the size of the tumour and how much it has expanded in the adjacent tissues. Table 16.2 depicts the classification of BrC into four major stages [11].

Table 16.2 Progression stages of breast cancer

Stages	*Description*
Stage 0	In surrounding tissues, defective cells are present, but they are not growing
Stage 1: In situ	BrC cells can only be found in the lobules and ducts of the body
Stage 2: Localised	There are few lymph nodes engaged, and the tumour is between 20 and 50 mm in size
Stage 3: Regional	The tumour is larger than 50 mm, and the malignancy is growing in the skin or chest wall, with lymph node involvement
Stage 4: Distant	tumours can grow to any size and spread to anybody

16.2.3 Breast cancer imaging modalities

BrC screening begins with imaging modalities such as MRI and CT. It is usually easy to treat when an abnormality is detected, but if it shows evidence of cancer later, it can lead to treatment delays. Some of the screening methods discussed in this article are also used in Ethiopia. BrC screening employs a variety of imaging modalities [13]. Figure 16.3a demonstrates frequently used medical multi-image modalities for BrC diagnosis. Evaluation of their performance is carried out by multiple factors such as Se, Re rates, and Acc.

- *Screen film mammography (SFM):*The standard imaging method for detecting suspicious lesions in women is SFM3 [14] and it has been a suitable medium for breast screening in the past few decades.
- *Digital mammography (DM):* DM is a valuable imaging technique for detecting BrC in its early stages [15]. It is commonly used to diagnose abnormalities of the female breast.

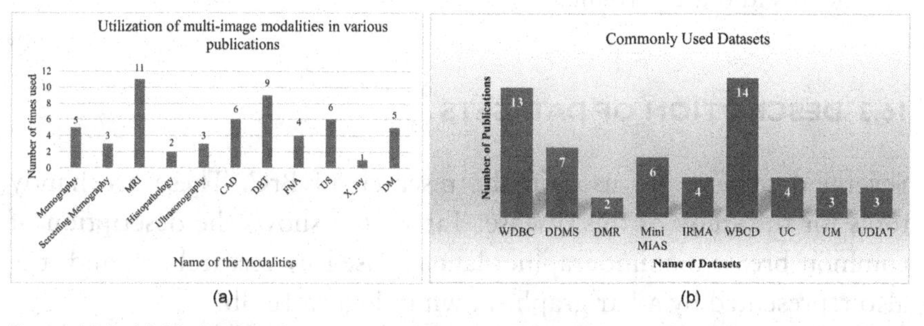

Figure 16.3 (a) Medical multi-image modalities widely utilised in the diagnosis of BrC. (b) Commonly used dataset for BrC detection.

- *Ultrasound (US):* For the identification of lesions of the breast as well as for virtual differentiation, it has been functionally used on an enormous scale, despite its operator-dependent nature [14].
- *MRI:* Magnetic Resonance Imaging is imaging that uses radio frequency to visualise the presence of nuclei in the body. It is commonly used to evaluate BrC and the finite touring patients with high risk.
- *DBT:* DBT is a kind of imaging method that uses deeply low-dose X-rays to create 3D images of the breast. It is a recent imaging technique that uses the same principle as a mammogram but with a tube that moves in a circular direction [16].
- *Breast thermography:* The metabolic rate of pre-cancerous and cancerous tissues increases due to new blood vessels. It supplies nutrients to the cancer cells.
- *Positron emission tomography:* Nuclear medicine imaging, known as positron emission tomography, is commonly utilised to detect and treat cancer. It uses a pair of rays to detect the presence of a tumour.
- *Scintimammography:* The use of a radioisotope to visualise BrC is known as scintimammography. This imaging technique can help detect BrC in dense tissue.
- *Optical imaging:* NIR light is used to find breast lesions using optical imaging. Optical imaging in various types utilises this light, such as diffuse optical imaging and optical mammography [14].
- *Electrical impedance-based imaging:* EIT is a process that visualises the electrical flow through a breast tissue using a series of circular electrodes placed around its surface.
- *Computer tomography (CT):* X-ray CT uses various techniques to capture 2D and 3D images of examined body parts. Several algorithms are utilised to produce 3D pictures that reveal anatomical details about the tissue.

16.3 DESCRIPTION OF DATASETS

Several databases are used in the research of BrC. These are handy tools for the study of this disease. Table 16.3 shows the description of common breast mammographic datasets used by researchers, and it is also represented by a bar graph shown in Figure 16.3b.

Table 16.3 The most prevalent mammographic datasets for cases (B: benign, M: malignant, N: normal)

Dataset name	*Cases number*	*Images available*	*Classes available*	*Format of image*	*Available publicly*
MIAS [17, 18]	-	322	B, N & M	PGM	Yes
BCDR [18]	1734	3,612 DM -3,703 FM	M, B & N	TIFF	Yes
DDSM [18]	2620	10,480	B, N & M	JPEG	Yes
INbreast [19]	115	410	N, B & M	DICOM	No
CBIS-DDSM [20]	6,775	10,239	M, B & N	DICOM	Yes
WDBC [21]	32	569	M& B	CSV	Yes
DMR [22]	141	3,534	B & M	JPEG & BMP	Yes
WBCP [23]	-	198	Recur, Non-recur	-	Yes
UC [24]	-	306	N, B & M	CSV	No
UDIAT [25]	6,775	630	B & M	JPEG	Yes
IRMA [26]	-	1,515	N, B & M	JPEG	No
UM [27]	-	2,606	N, B & M	JPEG	No

16.4 LITERATURE REVIEW

This study looked at 80 peer-reviewed papers, 21 of which utilised ML classification algorithms to identify BrC, while the rest applied DL approaches. This section contains information about previous research that has been done in this area. BrC is diagnosed using two methods. Machine learning is the first, while DL is the second. ML is used in a variety of research projects. However, ML techniques have some flaws that deep learning solves. This section describes ML and DL techniques. where abbreviations used throughout the papers are shown in Table 16.1. Shen et al. [28] developed a training algorithm to identify breast cancer lesions based on images taken during the initial training stage. Four different models improved the accuracy of their training algorithm (AUC to 0.91. AUC of 0.88). They also demonstrated that it could transfer the classification of images from the film to digital formats.

Furthermore, data about BrC tumours were analysed to predict their characteristics. MF, Ak [29] performed a comprehensive analysis of the data collected from the BrC tumour database to predict the features of the tumours. They then used machine learning techniques such as random forest, logistic regression, and DT to visualise the data. The goal of this study was to identify the most accurate and valuable tools for the detection of breast cancer. According to the findings, the proposed logistic regression method outperformed the standard method regarding classification accuracy, i.e. (98.1%). A team of researchers Hu et al.

[30] have used a combination of ML and statistical models to identify different kinds of BrC tumours. The researchers were able to assess the accuracy of their models using cross-validation, particularly of varying sizes ten-fold. They also evaluated their overall effectiveness in terms of various measuring methods. The researchers performed the most effective extraction strategy by extracting multiple features, such as texture, morphology, and EFDs. Moreover, Sharma et al. [31] uses a dataset from Wisconsin's BrC diagnosis to train various ML methods. The results reveal that the procedures are capable of high precision and accuracy. Wu et al. [32] have proposed a thorough review of various techniques used for the initial identification of BrC. It also explores the use of DL models and computer vision techniques. Infrared imaging was also a potential technique to improve detection accuracy. This method involves combining an existing agent with a new one. A model could be developed (using a thermal sensitivity camera of 0.5) for the breast to aid in diagnosis.

Furthermore, Mambou et al. [33] offered an approach based on ML for distinguishing between non-triple-negative and triple-negative patients BrC. To identify the models' construction traits, we looked at data from The Cancer Genome Atlas. The SVM model was more accurate than the other models in classifying BrC patients into three kinds. There were also fewer categorisation errors. The objective of Naranjo et al. [34] was to assess the performance of ML in the analysis and detection of BrC using radionics and diffusion-weighted imaging. The models were evaluated using an SVM. The models that were selected exhibited the best overall performance. They were able to produce an average AUC of 0.83. The study outcomes indicated that combining ML and radionics could help identify more BrC patients for a possible biopsy.

Masud et al. [35] proposed pre-trained neural network models to improve the screening rate for BrC in ultrasound pictures. They then studied the effects of various techniques on the models' performance. After fine-tuning them, they were able to show a 100% accuracy in identifying healthy individuals and breast cancer patients. They then created a customised model that uses a convolutional layer system. Similarly, Kavitha et al. [36] introduced a new type of segmentation model that combines the advantages of a multi-level thresholding approach and a capsule network approach. It can also detect the presence of BrC in the environment by implementing a backpropagation model. The study results posed model performed better than the previous ones. According to Chouhan et al. [37], a BrC detection system can automatically classify a mammogram as normal or abnormal. It can generate four different feature types using a deep convolutional network. The study's results suggest that this method effectively identifies cancer cells early. The system's four features can be trained on an IRMA dataset. Tajane et al. [38] will implement various methods to find the best approach. One of these is the ResNet-34 model. One of the most challenging aspects of such systems is the high dimensionality of data. It is quite hard to classify genes. Rasool et al. [39] proposed four models that can be used to classify BrC patients into two categories: benign and malignant. DL methods were then used to identify various features that can be used to classify patients. The study's results revealed that the proposed models could improve their capabilities by almost 100%. To better BrC diagnosis, Chowdhury et al. [40] recommend combining CNN and transfer learning (TL). The research uses the ResNet101 framework to create a TL model. It performed well with the ImageNet dataset and had an accuracy of 99.58%.

Mohamed et al. [41] offered a fully automatic approach to detect BrC employing thermography imaging in this work. This method, which is mainly recommended for the U-Net network, can automatically separate breast tissue from other body parts. To improve its efficiency, the authors trained a two-class DL model. It achieved an accuracy of 99.33%, specificity of 99% and sensitivity of 100%. The goal of Pillai et al. [42] is to evaluate and train the VGG16 model on images numbered 322 from the dataset of MIAS to detect BrC. It attains better results than GoogLeNet, EfficientNet, and AlexNet models. It will help enhance the screening process's efficiency and enable radiologists to provide better care. In this work, Jabeen et al. [43] develop a framework that combines the best features of various ultrasound images to classify BrC. The DarkNet-53 model is then trained using TL. The framework was tested on an image dataset having augmented breast ultrasound. It performed well and classified BrC with 99.1% accuracy. In Ref. [44] presents a framework for building a decision support system that uses a combination of a radial basis function and a Bayesian network. Experiments were carried out on the Wisconsin BrC Data set. The proposed model was tested on various metrics by M. A. Jabbar [44] to measure its performance. The results show a remarkable 97% accuracy in classifying BrC data. Cancer specialists could utilise the proposed system to improve the accuracy of their decisions regarding treating patients with BrC.

The authors of Ref. [45] introduced ML techniques mainly to increase the accuracy of the diagnosis of BrC. Using various learning algorithms, such as multi-layer perceptron, Gupta & Gupta [45] were able to show that it performed better than other techniques [46]. The authors utilised three different CNNs to recognise the availability of axillary lymph nodes in US images. The models achieved a sensitivity of 85% and specificity of 73% compared to radiologists. The Inception V3 model was the best-performing CNN. The models could identify axillary lymph nodes in more than 30 images. The study outcomes [46] indicated that the particular models could perform a better job than radiologists at detecting axillary lymph nodes in BrC patients. In Ref. [47], Bhattacherjee et al. are to investigate the features of the backpropagation neural network that can be trained on the WBCD, which has 683 patients. Out of the nine features used, the network could classify BrC with a sensitivity of 99.27%. In Ref. [48], Sha et al. have developed an overall method to identify the cancer region in an image of the mammogram. The proposed method was tested upon two DM databases. The proposed system's efficiency was compared to ten approaches which are of state-of-the-art nature. Results indicated that the proposed method had a sensitivity of 96%, specificity of 85%, and a PPV of 97%. It performed better than other methods.

DL could be used to improve the accuracy of digital mammograms. In Ref. [49], Eskreis-Winkler et al. developed a deep learning algorithm that can identify the tumour-infiltrating axial slices in breast MRI images using predefined parameters. During the first post-contrast phase, the slices were divided into two sub-images. One sub-image was labelled with cancer, and the other was without cancer. The accuracy of the DL algorithm for detecting the presence of tumour-associated axial slices was 92.8%. Bhardwaj et al. [50] proposed a new generation of genetically optimised neural network (GONN) algorithms that can solve classification problems. The new algorithm features a variety of mutation and crossover operators designed to reduce these operators' destructive effects. The results show that GONN can classify BrC tumours with a classification accuracy of almost 100% by using ten-fold cross-validation. In Ref. [4] authors Wang et al., were able to achieve a score of 0.7051 and an AUC of 0.925 for the localisation task of the tumour.

The system then predicted the diagnoses of the human pathologist, which resulted in a significant reduction in the pathologist's error rate. This study demonstrates the potential of DL to improve the accuracy of a BrC diagnosis.

Using a DNN and a backpropagation supervised path, a CAD for diagnosis of BrC is presented by Abdel-Zaher & Eldeib [51]. The proposed system was tried on the WBC dataset. The results indicate the proposed method detects BrC with an accuracy closer to 99.6%. Ragab et al. [52] developed a CAD system to perform segmentation based on the target area of interest. It can be done through two techniques: the first involves manually selecting the target area. In contrast, the second one uses a threshold and region-based strategy for performing the segmentation. The results show that it can accurately classify BrC data with an accuracy of 87.2%. The proposed system [53] has been implemented by Kassani et al., and is trained on various VGGNet models, and their overall prediction accuracy evaluates the performance of different architectures. For instance, the InceptionV3 and Xception architectures have an overall prediction accuracy of 84.50% and 88.50%, respectively. In Ref. [54], Bayrak et al. presented a comparison of the performance of two ML methods(SVM & ANN) for classifying Wisconsin's BrC dataset With the WEKA machine learning tool. The results show that SVM delivers the best accuracy and recall.

Dhahri et al. [55] have developed a system that could distinguish between breast tissues that are normal and cancerous. It was built using ML and genetic programming techniques. In Bhardwaj et al. [56], developed a featured ensemble learning framework which revealed that the proposed method could produce better outcomes than the current classification system, with an absolute accuracy of 98.60%. The study [57] classifies BrC in photos; the researchers Islam et al., suggested a new DL framework that integrates the ideas of TL and CNN. The proposed framework consists of three CNN architectures: VGGNet, ResNet, and GoogLeNet. They say these networks can extract the essential parameters from images and connect them to a fully connected layer for classification. The results of these experiments were compared with those of other DL frameworks. In R. K. Samala, Chan, Hadjiiski, Cha et al. [58] have used DCNN and CNN as a classifier; the dataset used is UM of size 64. The best model was able to attain an AUC of 0.93 and 0.89 on the different classifiers using the modality DBT; the CAD system's processing phases include repeated thresholding and region growth to identify microcalcification candidates false-positive reduction (FP) and clustering.

Moreover, in R. K. Samala, Chan, Hadjiiski, Cha et al. [59] have used DCNN as a classifier with a dataset size of 324; the best model was able to attain 0.80 AUC. The results indicate that the system proposed can find BrC having a sensitivity of 80%. The dataset and modality used are UM and DBT. BrC screening has traditionally relied on mammography, a two-dimensional (2D) imaging method. Mammography images can train a DCNN for bulk detection in DBT. In another paper [60], Kim et al. have used the classifier SVM, having a feature size of 160, and thus the best model was able to attain an AUC of 0.847, and the dataset and modality they have used are SMC and DBT. In this study, the author proposes a representation of bilateral features based on DBT that is latent. The results of the experiments suggest that the representation of the latent bilateral feature could increase classification performance at DBT based on AUC and ROC.

In Ref. [61], Fotin et al. have applied the classifier as DCNN with dataset size 344 using which the best model has attained the accuracy as 86.40% and sensitivity achieved is 89%, DBT is the modality used. At four detection markers per volume, detection sensitivity was assessed on an area of interest (ROI) basis. Further, In Ref. [62], Zhu et al. have used a classifier as DCNN; the dataset size is 40. The results indicate that the system proposed detects BrC has a Sensitivity of 0.41. The dataset they used is DDSM, and Modality is used in DBT. R. Samala et al. [63] have used a classifier as DCNN with dataset size as 324, through which the model successfully achieved an AUC of 0.76, the dataset used is UM and modality used in DBT. The DM photos were captured in raw format at 14 bits per pixel rate and measured to 12 bits/pixel using a simple inverse logarithmic adjustment. At Reiser et al. [64] have used a classifier as LDA, and the dataset size was 36; the model was capable of achieving a sensitivity of 90%, and the Modality they have used was DBT. CAD can be implemented using projected data or volumes of pictures rebuilt from projections. LDA is utilised to integrate features.

In this study [65], van Schie et al. have used a classifier neural network with a dataset size of 752, and the suggested system can detect BrC with a sensitivity of 80% modality used in DBT. The authors have created a method for detecting masses using CAD, reconstructed in DBT volumes. It was discovered that using slabs enhances detection performance. Furthermore, [66], Chan et al. have used classifier as LDA with dataset size as 100 and thus sensitivity achieved by the model is 80%, Modality used in DBT. Due to the enormous dynamic range and high detective photon energy of digital detectors, each PV picture could be attained with a proportion of the exposure of X-ray required for regular mammography. The 3D technique was shown to have a much greater detection perfection than the 2D approach, with a $p = 0.02$ difference. Further, Mendel et al. [67] have used an SVM classifier, and the dataset size used is 76; thereby, the best model is capable of achieving an AUC of 0.832. And Modality is used as DBT. Many studies have proven Tomosynthesis to lower screening retention rates while raising cancer detection accuracy. Moreover, Antropova et al. [68] have used classifiers such as SVM (handcrafted), SVM (CNN), And SVM (fused) with a dataset size of 245; the model was capable of achieving an AUC of 0.79,0.81, 0.86, respectively, using all the three different classifiers, where the dataset used here is UC. The modality used in DBT. In the problem of breast lesion identification, deep features applied on classifiers and current regular CADx characteristics may be combined to dramatically increase prediction performance across three different imaging modalities.

In Ref. [69], Debelee et al., have used classifiers such as KNN (DDSM) and KNN (MIAS) with a dataset size of 320; the proposed system can detect BrC with an accuracy of 98.90% and 98.75%, respectively. The dataset used here as DDSM, MIAS, and Modality used is DM. The experiment aimed to see how well KNN with a K value of 3 performed on the MIAS and DDSM databases. The experimental results suggest that KNN performs better in terms of classification accuracy. The CNN + augmentation, CNN + augmentation + manual features, and CNN- augmentation has been proposed by Kooi et al. [70]. The author has used 45,000 sized datasets. Thereby best model attains AUC of 0.929, 0.94, and 0.875, respectively. RDN was utilised as the dataset, while DM was used as the modality. Both models were trained on a vast dataset of having images 45,000. According to the data, the CNN outperforms the old fashioned CAD system at low sensitivity while performing comparably at high sensitivity. Further in Ref. [71], Lawson et al. have used classifier (features) as CNN and SVM, having dataset size as 4,863, using which best model was able to achieve AUC as 0.91 and 0.81 respectively. The proposed system developed by Lawson et al. [71] can detect BrC with 83% and 73% accuracy, respectively, and specificity of 82% and 68%, respectively, and sensitivity of 84% and 77%, respectively. In the final step, the author has a CNN of minimal size, which can learn to categorise photos of benign and malignant tumours quickly. In Ref. [72], BeCkeR et al., have used the classifier DL, Experts, and Experts(inexperienced); the size of the dataset used is 632. The model attained AUC of 0.84, 0.88, and 0.79; the dataset used is ZUH, and the US modality was used. The goal of BeCkeR et al. [72] was to build a generic DL software to diagnose BrC on images of US. Its performance is comprised of human readers with varying levels of experience in breast imaging.

Fei et al. [13] have used a classifier as DCNN; the number of images in the dataset is 5,151. Thus the proposed system was able to attain an AUC of 0.90. The proposed method can detect BrC with an accuracy of 90%, specificity achieved is 96%, and sensitivity achieved is 86%. The modality used is the US. The categorisation of malignant lesions showed encouraging results, even though target ROIs were chosen by radiologists, suggesting that radiologists should have to find the location of ROIs. If radiologists employ this strategy in a clinical setting, it can quickly categorise malignant lesions and aid radiologists' diagnosis in distinguishing malignant lesions.

In Ref. [73], Yap et al. have used a classifier as CNN(LeNet), dataset used is size 469(A+B, the dataset used is UDIAT, and the modality used is the US. This study investigated three alternative methods: a U-Net, Patch-based LeNet, and a TL approach using a pre-trained FCN-AlexNet. This research studied the application of three DL algorithms (Patch-based LeNet, U-Net, TL FCN-AlexNet) for breast ultrasound (BUS) lesion identification and a full assessment of the most representative lesion detection strategies. Moreover, Shin et al. [74] have used a classifier as CNN, having a dataset size of 5,424, and the dataset used is UDIAT. And modality used is the US. BUS pictures present mass localisation and categorisation framework. It offers a semi-supervised and poorly supervised method with proper training loss selection. Furthermore Li et al. [75] have used classifiers such as 2D CNN and 3D CNN, the dataset used is of size 143. The model was capable of attaining an AUC of 0.752 and 0.841, respectively. The system proposed can detect BrC with 71.1% and 80.40% accuracy, specificity of 67.41% and 77.30%, respectively, and sensitivity of 76.1% and 81.40%. Dataset used are ZCH and modality used as MRI. The MRI scans were pre-processed to remove noise and segment the breast tumour area. The findings demonstrate that by including additional information from the tumour ROI, CNN may achieve excellent accuracy.

Jadoon et al. [76] have used a classifier as an SVM. Using the proposed system can detect BrC with an accuracy of 83.74%. The dataset used is IRMA, and Modality used is DM. In Ref. [77], Kallenberg et al. have used a classifier as Convolutional (sparse) autoencoders (CSAE), the model can achieve an AUC of 0.61, and the modality is used as DM. A method for learning a feature hierarchy from unlabelled data is shown.

The SVM classifiers used in Ref. [78] and dataset size is 101. Thus the proposed system developed by Palma et al. [78] can detect BrC with a sensitivity of 90% and the modality used in DBT. This is a revolutionary 3D imaging technology which overcomes some of the drawbacks of standard DM. As the technology advances, more data must be analysed, necessitating a computer-assisted detection system to assist the radiologist. Yousefi et al. [79] have used classifiers such as MI-RF, DCaRBM MI-RF, and DCNN MI-RF with a dataset size of 87. The model can achieve AUC of 0.87, 0.70, and 0.75, respectively, and the proposed system can detect BrC with an accuracy of 86.81%,78.50%, and 69.20%, and specificity achieved as 87.5%, 66.6%, 75% respectively. The system proposed can detect BrC with a sensitivity of 86.6%,81.8%, and 66.6%. Dataset used is MGH, and the modality is used in DBT. The suggested CAD framework benefits from learning complicated patterns from the 2D slices of DBT data and analysing DBT pictures using all of the information gained from the slices.

16.5 COMPUTER-AIDED DIAGNOSIS

MIP(Medical image processing) has been computed using the manual approach. However, it still faces various issues, such as the unavailability of multiple pathologists in one place and the complexity of the task. Also, the professional pathologist's knowledge is quite essential for BrC diagnosis. Computer-aided design (CAD) has evolved as a method that can help diagnose BrC in its early stages [80]. This concept is a second notion that addresses the need for complex computational algorithms to process medical images. Although it is generally good at detecting early stages of BrC, it can also increase the chances of false-positive results. Before implementing this technology in clinical practice, it is essential to consider its various limitations and capabilities. Usually, two types of CAD systems are available that can be utilised for BrC diagnosis [81]: computer-aided detection (CADe) and computer-aided diagnosis (CADx). These systems can perform various tasks, such as detecting and classifying medical images. This technology can also be utilised as a next step for identifying the model, providing enough information and helping make decisions.

16.5.1 Common framework for breast cancer diagnosis using ML

This section discusses several steps for implementing a CAD system utilising an ML pipeline. The classification is used in the evaluation of a lesion. It is performed to determine if it is a cancerous or a normal region. Further evaluation is performed to identify cancer pathology if it is categorised as a cancerous zone. Several types of classifiers are commonly used for BrC classification [82, 83]. These include the KNN, SVM, ANN, binary-DT, and simple logistic classifiers. Figure 16.4a illustrates a chart of different ML techniques discussed in this review for BrC classification. The performance of these systems can be improved by removing the redundant features and keeping the most discriminative ones.

Various studies [59, 64, 65, 79, 84] have been conducted on various aspects of breast mass and microcalcification detection. The most challenging aspect of this field is finding masses like those of normal breast tissue. One of the most challenging aspects of the process is finding masses like those of normal breast tissue. Due to the varying size of the masses, it is impossible to determine the appropriate scale for the range

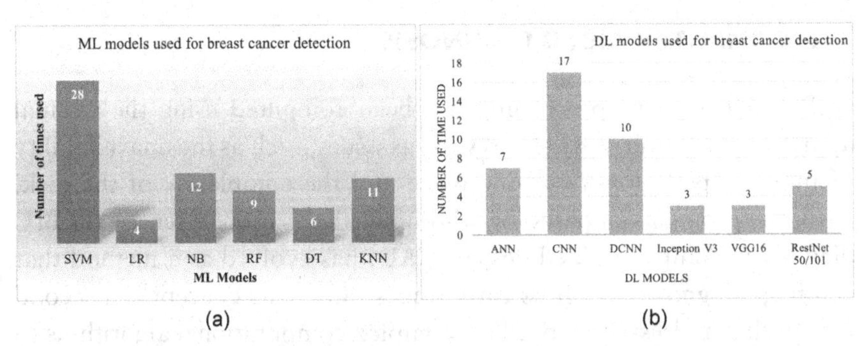

Figure 16.4 (a) Different ML techniques used in BrC classification. (b) Different DL techniques used in BrC classification.

of sizes. Therefore, the researchers must define the range of sizes instead of doing mass analysis. Since the boundaries of the masses are not always detected. A more confined approach is also needed to detect the varying densities and lengths of the masses. Aside from mass detection, other studies related to the detection of asymmetry and architecture distortion are also being conducted. New developments in BrC detection should also focus on improving existing algorithms' performance. Currently, commercial systems are capable of detecting masses and calcifications. One of the steps in developing a CAD system is the extraction of features. This process involves identifying various features utilised in a system. The goal is to find the optimal feature subset for a given problem for a given task. Although some features are useful for a given task, some are irrelevant or even redundant. Therefore, most cases use automatic extraction to develop mammography CAD systems.

16.5.2 Common DL framework for CAD of breast cancer

DL has made observable improvements in its overall performance compared with other artificial intelligence and ML techniques. It has gained widespread applications in enormous fields, such as the classification of images and NLP. Various categories of DL networks are described in their architecture. These include unsupervised networks, discriminative networks, and hybrid networks. The most prevalent type of DL network commonly used is CNN. This technique consists of most of the convolutional layers which are stacked. This collection of layers is aligned in the order on top of one another to form a deep network capable of handling 2D and 3D images. The network's field of view is increased by various factors, such as a maximum pooling layer.

The general modern design of the DL-CAD system consists of four sections. The first one is the input data analysis, while the second one focuses on post-processing. The articles about the CNNs used in the DL architecture were analysed in the third part. The top assessment metrics were also evaluated for accuracy. Finally, an explanation of these algorithms is provided. Figure 16.4b illustrates a chart of different DL techniques discussed in this review for BrC classification.

General Figure 16.5 shows how a modern CAD system can be used with images from public and private sources. Usually, the system has multiple stages, including feature extraction and classification segmentation. DL-CAD systems are built on CNN models and architectures for

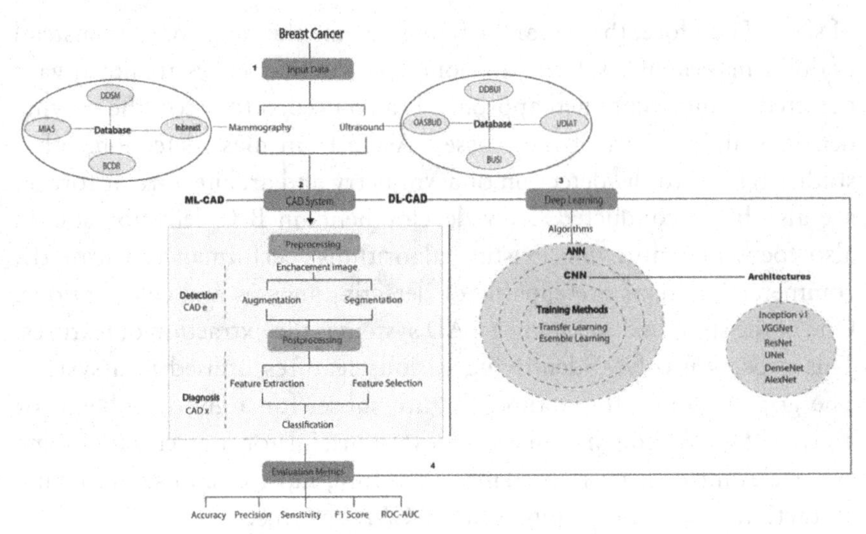

Figure 16.5 A generalized flowchart of the DL process [85].

automatic feature extraction and classification. Some of these include the BCDR, BUSI, and the DDBUI. These organisations provide the most comprehensive set of digital BUS images.

These are some essential steps that are inherently involved in implementing a CADx system using the DL pipeline.

1. *Step -1: (Databases)* The first step for diagnosis has relevant data for the effective model to be trained. The dataset should be mainly classified into two DM and US.
2. *Step -2 (Pre-processing of dataset):* A particular processing technique, as well as the performance of the computer program, will be hugely affected by the characteristics of this specific database. Due to noise and other factors that could alter the interpretation of medical images, a database can develop a scheme that produces erroneous results. Many approaches to preprocess the dataset include image enhancement, image augmentation, image segmentation, etc.
3. *Step -3: Post-processing:* After segmentation, the next step is retrieving the data's relevant information. This process can be performed through the selection and segmentation of features.
4. *Step-4: Classification:* In this process, the features of breast US images are divided mainly into four general types. They are then

input into a classification program to classify them into different classes. Multiple applications commonly use various classifiers, such as decision trees, ANN, and linear. Recently, deep CNNs have shown impressive performance in detecting and recognising objects on large datasets. It could improve the accuracy of both the US and DM breast lesion detection methods. Some researchers are interested in classifying mass and lesion images based on CNN models. They also study microcalcification and lesion calculations.

16.6 METHODOLOGIES

This section discusses the different methodologies used in detecting breast cancer using DL concepts such as a CNN, TL, etc., to be applied by different kinds of modalities having different types of datasets. Further, the results have also been discussed, corresponding to the methodology.

16.6.1 Combined DL model based on TL and Pulse-coupled Neural Networks (PCNN) for breast cancer [86]

16.6.1.1 Modified PCNN

Multiple variations of the PCNN training algorithm are available. Variations of such kind seek to copy the physiological pulse-coupled neuron. Every variation represents different simplifications made to the computational part, but it still retains the essential features of the theory.

In this model, each neuron is governed by the following sequence of equations:

$$L(i) = L(i-1)e^{-\alpha L} + Vl.(W * Y_{sur}(i-1)) \tag{16.1}$$

$$F(i) = P + F(i-1) + e^{-\alpha F} + VF.(W * Y_{sur}(i-1)) \tag{16.2}$$

$$Y(i) = F(i).[1 + \beta.L(i)] \tag{16.3}$$

$$\theta(i) = \theta(i-1)e^{-\alpha q} + V\theta.YO(i-1) \tag{16.4}$$

$$YO(i) = \begin{cases} 1, & Y(i) > \theta(i) \\ 0, & otherwise \end{cases} \tag{16.5}$$

where $F(i)$ stands for feeding,$L(i)$ stands for input linking, P is image's pixel intensity, $U(i)$ stands for neuron activation potential, and $\theta(i)$ stands for neuron threshold. it consists of multiple hyperparameters, including αL, αF, and αq, as well as the decay coefficients apart from (β), which mainly defines the linking coefficient. VL and VF are the threshold potential and linking hyperparameters. The output of the neuron, Y, presents the firing information in and around the surrounding neurons, while YO mostly indicates the neuron firing information. W represents the weight matrix. The "Modified PCNN" neuron architecture is illustrated in Figure 16.6.

The firing status of each neuron(The output of each iteration) is used to form a signature almost like a time series. The formula for standard feature generation G(n) for the iteration (i) is calculated as

$$G(n) = \sum_{i=0}^{n} Y(i) \tag{16.6}$$

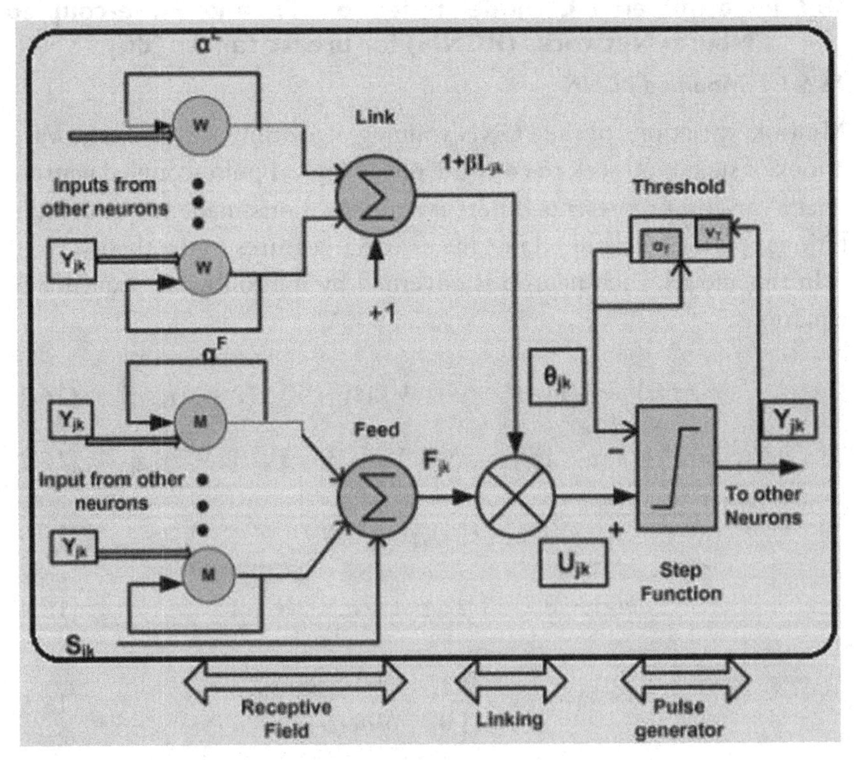

Figure 16.6 Modified PCNN neuron model [86].

The actual to be achieved by the system is to create a model based on classification, which will segregate the image input into three main categories, viz. abnormal benign, abnormal malignancy and regular. Several TL models are used for the dense layers to identify the input image to offer increased features. The fundamental problem, and the real purpose for utilising PCNNs, is to neutralise the influence of qualitative acquisition on the obtained model. PCNNs generate image signatures without the requirement for segmentation or pre-processing. Besides CNN features, The image signature is fed into feed-forward neural layers (Figure 16.7).

For classification, the vector, fused features, is incorporated into a deep feed-forward network. Most prior studies employed a segmentation stage to identify the Region of Interest (ROI). The main motivation is to lower the CNN's computing effort and remove the influence of small training datasets. In the meantime, the suggested approach receives the whole image without pre-processing or segmentation. The PCNN's capacity to produce signatures of the image, which are generally invariant to the scaling, rotation, acquisition quality, and translation, turned out to be a key concept.

The possibility of multi-level feature illustration in any hidden layer distinguishes DL and PCNN from other machine learning algorithms. Furthermore, DL and PCNN can effectively mitigate the impacts of the resolution, which are low images and predicted noise.

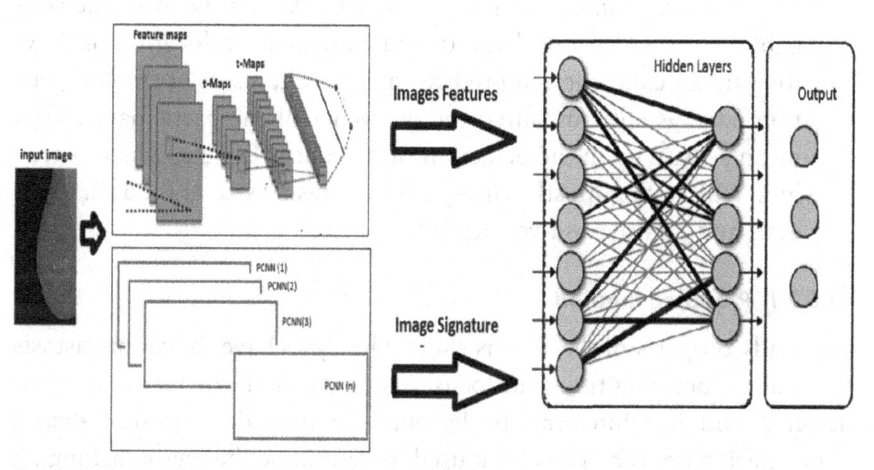

Figure 16.7 Modules of the proposed system [86].

In this research, the author has proposed different types of DL pre-trained models, which were mainly exploited in a blend of PCNNs to categorise the candidate images of breast cancer. The model has been tested and trained on many different types of datasets, achieving an AUC of 0.99 and an accuracy of 98.77%. The main helpful aspect of the model proposed is that it could be generalised to any application of computer vision. The merged CNN and PCNN can be used as matching feature extractors for videos and images.

16.6.2 Slide-based classification and lesion-based breast cancer detection [4]

Camelyon16 is a dataset that contains whole slide images (WSIs) of nearly 400 in size, comprising training 270 in size and testing 130 in size. On The following two metrics, the evaluation is based on the submissions to the competition:

- *Slide-based evaluation:* To distinguish among slides with regular slides and metastasis using the parameter, Teams are adjudicated on their ability. For each test slide, a definite probability has been submitted by the participants of the competition, which indicated the prediction of the likelihood of cancer contained. To assess the participant's performance, competition organisers use the area under the receiver operator score.
- *Lesion-based evaluation:* For this metric, Within the WSI, the contributors provides a probability and an equivalent location of (x; y) for various cancer lesion prediction. The organisers of the competition have usually measured the outcomes of the participant as the mean sensitivity in the detection of all cancer lesions, which is true in a WSI having mostly false-positive rates of size 6: 0.25, 0.50, 4, 1, 2, and 8 false positives per WSI.

16.6.2.1 Proposed method

The study on parts of the slide is usually likely to have cancer metastasis to reduce processing time and focus. Inside the WSI, the tissues are first detected, and the white space background is removed. A threshold-based segmentation approach has been used to determine the region belonging to its background automatically. According to the detection findings, the average proportion of backdrop region per WSI is around 82%.

- *Cancer metastasis detection framework:* As shown in Figure 16.8, the detection of cancer metastasis methodology includes a classification based on the patch step and a stage based on the post-processing stage of the heatmap-based. The supervised classification model is trained to differentiate among the patches of two different classes after selecting positive and negative training samples. We integrate the prediction findings into an image based on the heatmap. At the post-processing stage, which is based on the heat map, the researcher uses the tumour probability heatmap to calculate the evaluation scores, which are lesion and slide based on each WSI.
- *Patch-based classification stage:* At the time of training, this particular stage mainly uses 256 × 256-pixel patches both from negative and positive areas of the WSI and trains the classification model to differentiate both negative and positive patches.

The performance of the four well-known architectures of deep learning networks has been evaluated for the classification task of VGG16 AlexNet, GoogLeNet and a deep network with face orientation, as shown. The best performance classification is based on a patch that has been achieved by the two deeper networks, viz. VGG16 and Google Net. Deep network structures like GoogLeNet, have been adopted for this particular framework. The sole reason for using this particular structure is that it is usually more stable and faster than VGG16. A total of more than 6 million parameters

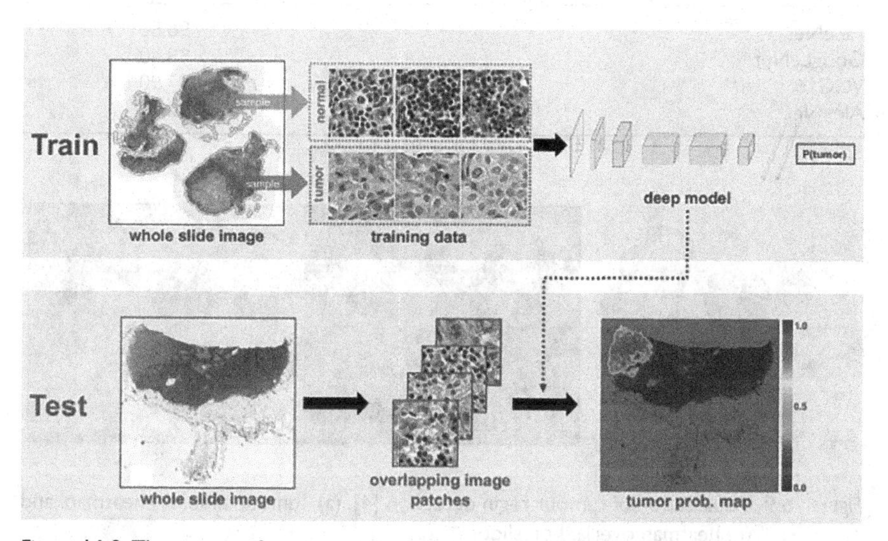

Figure 16.8 The strategy for recognising cancer tumours [4].

and 27 layers constituted the network structure of GoogLeNet (Table 16.4).

A range of magnification levels, including 20,10 and 40 has been evaluated in these experiments. And the super best results with 40- magnification have been obtained. For the competition of Camelyon the magnification of only 40- value has been reported in the experimental results.

Whole Slide image has been given (Figure 16.9a) and a classification model based on patches of deep learning. Highlighting the tumour area, The Corresponding tumour region heatmap has been generated (Figure 16.9b),

- *Post-processing of tumour heatmaps to compute Slide-based and lesson-based probabilities*:

  We generate a tumour probability heatmap for each WSI when the patch-based classification stage has been completed. Each pixel on these heatmaps has a value range between 1 and 0, which indicates the probability that the pixel contains a tumour. A value range between 1 and 0 on the heatmaps represents a pixel, wherein the probability value indicates that each pixel consists of the tumour.

Table 16.4 Evaluation of various deep models [4]

DL models	*Patch classification accuracy (%)*
FaceNet	96.80
GoogLeNet	98.40
VGG16	97.90
AlexNet	92.10

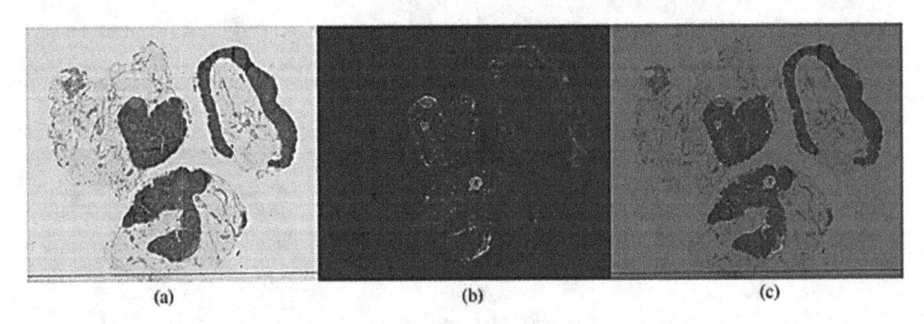

Figure 16.9 Visualisation of tumour regin detection [4]. (a) Tumour slide, (b) heatmap, and (c) heatmap overlaid on slide.

- *Slide-based classification:* For the task of slide-based classification, the post-processing for every WSI takes a heatmap as input and, in turn, gives outputs a particular single probability of tumour for the whole WSI. An AUC of 0.925 has been achieved for the slide-based classification of the entire test cases.,thus it has made the system performance the best in the challenge of Camelyon Grand for the slide-based classification task.
- *Lesion-based detection:* In the post-processing of lesion-based detections, all cancer lesions residing inside each WSI have been identified with very few false positives. For the dataset Camelyon 16, The metric score is calculated as the mean sensitivity for the six predefined false-positive rates 0.75, 0.50, 1, 2, 4 and 8 FPs per the entire slide image. The proposed system has achieved a metric score of 0.7051.

For the task of classification. The human pathologist attained an AUC of 0.9664, showing an error rate of 3.4%. The predictions resulted by a human pathologist as well as by the use of DL systems got combined, which resulted in the enhancement of 0.9948, thus indicating the error rate of 0.52

16.6.3 Genetically Optimised Neural Network (GONN) model

In paper [50], Bhardwaj et al. created a GONN architecture to grow the ANN structure using GP (Genetic Programming), which is also treated like an ANN structure. The following sections cover the steps involved in the GONN architectures.

- *Initialisation:* The initialisation of GP involves transforming computer functions into tree structures that are stored in memory. Every node in the tree has an operator function, making it easy to evolve and evaluate various mathematical expressions, then limit the tree formation in GP to preserve the neural network's architecture. Allow a feasible function set F and terminal set T for a GP tree to be as follows:

$$F = \{P, W, +, -, \times, \%\} \tag{16.7}$$

T ={ dataset of feature variables, R''}wherein P stands for activation function which is a standard sigmoid function in our case whose range is $[0, 1]$. W stands for the weighting function for a signal and % are normal arithmetic functions $D_0, D_1, ..., D_n$ is the dataset's feature variables (input data signal).

The R framework considers the input variables' values in the range of 1 to 10 and randomly generates floating-point constants. The activation function then outputs a discrete signal. The basic sigmoid function, with a range of [0], is utilised as an activation function in this

$$Y = \frac{1}{1 + e^{-x}} \tag{16.8}$$

where x is between -1 and 1, the function P returns a one if the sum of its two weighted input lines is more significant than 0.5, and it also outputs a 0 if the sum is less. The four arithmetic procedures used to generate and alter the numerical constants of an ANN are performed in GP. Authors must follow certain principles to evolve the ANN using GP.

- *Fitness function:* The fitness function is the most crucial topic in GP and is responsible for determining a program's capacity to per tasks efficiently. The mean-square error of the output of the GONN algorithm is then used to determine the model's fitness.

$$\text{fitness}_{\text{GONN}} = \frac{1}{1 + \frac{1}{x}\sum_{x}^{y}(DES_y - ACT_y)^2} \tag{16.9}$$

Here, x denotes the total size of the training dataset, DES_y denotes the desired output when using the train dataset number y as input, and subscripted ACT_y denotes the GON output from using the training dataset number y as an input.

- *Modified crossover operator:* The GP life cycle is usually performed in two phases: the first involves selecting the top fitness individuals, and the second involves transferring those individuals to the next generation. Consider all the still alive individuals after the reproduction process for the crossover operation. The operator for the crossover operation must follow the tree structure criteria specified by the tree structure. In this process, the functional nodes of the tree are given a 90% chance of being exchanged with the other subtrees. The fitness value of the newly created offspring is then compared with that of its parent. If its value is higher than the parent's, it can enter the next generation. The percentage of new individuals chosen to be passed down to the next generation is known as the percent. The parent trees that did not produce high-quality offspring are then selected for mutation. The goal of this operation is to avoid the harmful tendency of cross-pollination. Only kids better than their parents are admitted into the next generation.

- *Modified mutation operator:* The modified mutation operator can also introduce diversity into a tree by selecting trees that have not been able to produce high-quality offspring.
- *Termination criteria:* The GONN approach is designed to terminate the learning/evolutionary process if it meets certain conditions. If the number of fitness evaluations exceeds its maximum count, the fittest individual will determine the optimal GONN architecture. After the GONN tree has been mapped to its FNN equivalent, the data collected by the system is then tested.

16.7 RESEARCH GAPS AND FUTURE DIRECTIONS

The following issues must be addressed when employing DL for BrC detection:

- *Lack of large-scale, credible datasets from professional clinicians for BrC diagnosis:*

  Due to the lack of accurate large-scale databases to diagnose BrC, most of the authors of DL models rely on publicly available datasets. These are the ones that have been published and are open to the public. Unfortunately, the algorithms constructed using public datasets are not as accurate as those trained on medical images. This issue could be solved by providing extensive, annotated datasets from medical experts.
- *There are fewer models available that have been pre-trained on medical images [2]:*

  Most research has been published in the field of BrC diagnosis using pre-trained models that have been trained on various types of non-medical imagery. The next step involves re-training the model on medical images. This procedure takes time and involves a vast number of resources. Since only so many images can be trained on a given dataset, pre-trained networks are prone to experience issues if the data is too narrow. Therefore, there is a need for specialised models trained on medical images [80].

- *Breast carcinoma categorisation using many imaging modalities and multiple modalities [2]:*

  Most BrC researchers use conventional imaging techniques such as mammography and histopathology to diagnose BrC. Although digital breast imaging (DBT) has shown great promise in detecting tumours, it is still very costly. With various imaging techniques, a patient could be diagnosed with cancer even if previously treated. It is a promising idea, but more research is needed to improve these techniques' reliability and classification capabilities.
- *Mammography craniocaudal (CC) and mediolateral oblique (MLO) views:*

  The authors of [87] and [88] compared the performance of the MLO and CC views on different types of BrC. They found that the CC view performed better than the MLO view when used with dense breasts. However, the results across the whole breast area were reversed. Because breast tissue is so complicated, more study is needed to compare the efficacy of surgical and non-surgical methods for thick breasts.
- **BrC classification through Unsupervised methodology** [2]**:**

  The enormous amount of research which analysed the performance of unsupervised BrC classification systems relied on large, annotated datasets. Due to the complex nature of breast tissue, more research is required to develop models that can capture unlabelled images. These images are a valuable resource when it comes to studying BrC.
- **BrC survival prognosis based on stage:**

  The authors of [89] presented a data-driven knowledge model for predicting the 5-year survival of BrC patients on the SEER database. They compared the models with various ML algorithms. They noted that it is essential to collaborate with the other models to improve their results. More research is needed to develop a more accurate prediction of BrC survival rates.
- **Combining non-imaging data with imaging data:**

  Only a few CAD models can integrate non-imaging features with imaging data. The authors of [90] examined how many models combining non-imaging factors such as analytical information, cancer history, genetic information, and image data will be needed in the future. This could allow them to give advanced detection, usually for women at high risk of getting affected by BrC.

- **Future of CAD in medicine:**
  In Refs. [91, 92] discussed the future of CAD in medicine. They talked about various aspects of the technology, such as data acquisition, quality estimation, and trading with big data.
- *DL using fewer datasets in medical applications:* In addition, they talked about the need for new deep models to be trained on smaller medical image datasets due to the lack of available resources. Currently, no deep models are being used on these smaller datasets.

16.8 CONCLUSION

BrC is the most deadly kind of malignancy cancer in women. It requires immediate identification and treatment to reduce its death rate. Clinical image processing has become a critical tool for early diagnosis and prognosis. This survey aims to present the new state-of-the-art research on BrC that is being conducted using ML and DL techniques. Early identification is essential for BrC patients to prevent the disease from spreading. BrC detection by mammography is the standard method. Unfortunately, imaging techniques such as ultrasound are often criticised for low effectiveness in BrC detection in women with dense breasts. Researchers need to combine a variety of imaging modalities such as CT, MRI, and digital breast imaging to improve their effectiveness. Machine learning has been identified as the primary classifier for BrC diagnosis. DL techniques have shown their ability to perform better on various evaluation parameters such as specificity, sensitivity, and F-measure. Due to the complexity of training, deep learning models have proven more effective than conventional machine learning models when the data is significant. The increasing number of DL techniques and healthcare studies have highlighted the need for more practical and scientific research.

REFERENCES

1. K. S. Priyanka, "A review paper on breast cancer detection using deep learning," *in IOP Conference Series: Materials Science and Engineering*, Rajpura, India, vol. 1022, p. 012071, IOP Publishing, 2021.

2. G. Chugh, S. Kumar, and N. Singh, "Survey on machine learning and deep learning applications in breast cancer diagnosis," *Cognitive Computation*, vol. 13, no. 6, pp. 1451–1470, 2021.
3. S. Cleator, W. Heller, and R. C. Coombes, "Triple-negative breast cancer: therapeutic options," *The Lancet Oncology*, vol. 8, no. 3, pp. 235–244, 2007.
4. D. Wang, A. Khosla, R. Gargeya, H. Irshad, and A. H. Beck, "Deep learning for identifying metastatic breast cancer," arXiv preprint arXiv:1606.05718, 2016.
5. N. M. Hassan, S. Hamad, and K. Mahar, "Mammogram breast cancer cad systems for mass detection and classification: A review," *Multimedia Tools and Applications*, vol. 81, pp. 20043–20075, 2022.
6. L. Fallowfield, V. Jenkins, V. Farewell, J. Saul, A. Duffy, and R. Eves, "Efficacy of a cancer research UK communication skills training model for oncologists: A randomised controlled trial," *The Lancet*, vol. 359, no. 9307, pp. 650–656, 2002.
7. Y. Huang, S. Nayak, R. Jankowitz, N. E. Davidson, and S. Oesterreich, "Epigenetics in breast cancer: What's new?," *Breast Cancer Research*, vol. 13, no. 6, pp. 1–11, 2011.
8. A. W. Forsyth, R. Barzilay, K. S. Hughes, D. Lui, K. A. Lorenz, A. Enzinger, J. A. Tulsky, and C. Lindvall, "Machine learning methods to extract documentation of breast cancer symptoms from electronic health records," *Journal of Pain and Symptom Management*, vol. 55, no. 6, pp. 1492–1499, 2018.
9. S. Simsek, U. Kursuncu, E. Kibis, M. AnisAbdellatif, and A. Dag, "A hybrid data mining approach for identifying the temporal effects of variables associated with breast cancer survival," *Expert Systems with Applications*, vol. 139, p. 112863, 2020.
10. I. Mihaylov, M. Nisheva, and D. Vassilev, "Machine learning techniques for survival time prediction in breast cancer," in *International Conference on Artificial Intelligence: Methodology, Systems, and Applications*, pp. 186–194, Springer, 2018.
11. R. J. Kate and R. Nadig, "Stage-specific predictive models for breast cancer survivability," *International Journal of Medical Informatics*, vol. 97, pp. 304–311, 2017.
12. UpToDate, "Breast cancer development - uptodate." https://www.uptodate.com/contents/image/print?imageKey=PI%2F53453, May 2022.
13. X. Fei, S. Zhou, X. Han, J. Wang, S. Ying, C. Chang, W. Zhou, and J. Shi, "Doubly supervised parameter transfer classifier for diagnosis of breast cancer with imbalanced ultrasound imaging modalities," *Pattern Recognition*, vol. 120, p. 108139, 2021.
14. G. Meenalochini and S. Ramkumar, "Survey of machine learning algorithms for breast cancer detection using mammogram images," *Materials Today: Proceedings*, vol. 37, pp. 2738–2743, 2021.
15. Z. Sedighi-Maman and A. Mondello, "A two-stage modeling approach for breast cancer survivability prediction," *International Journal of Medical Informatics*, vol. 149, p. 104438, 2021.
16. S. J. S. Gardezi, A. Elazab, B. Lei, and T. Wang, "Breast cancer detection and diagnosis using mammographic data: Systematic review," *Journal of Medical Internet Research*, vol. 21, no. 7, p. e14464, 2019.

17. R. S. Lee, J. A. Dunnmon, A. He, S. Tang, C. Re, and D. L. Rubin, "Comparison of segmentation-free and segmentation-dependent computer-aided diagnosis of breast masses on a public mammography dataset," *Journal of Biomedical Informatics*, vol. 113, p. 103656, 2021.
18. "Cancer Imaging Data," *medicmind*. [Online]. Available: https://www.medicmind.tech/cancer-imaging-data.
19. R. Subramanian, "INbreast dataset," *Kaggle*, 27-Mar-2021. [Online]. Available: https://www.kaggle.com/datasets/ramanathansp20/inbreast-dataset.
20. Awsaf, "CBIS-DDSM: Breast Cancer Image Dataset," *Kaggle*, 24-Jan-2021. [Online]. Available: https://www.kaggle.com/datasets/awsaf49/cbis-ddsm-breast-cancer-image-dataset.
21. Dr. William H. Wolberg, W. Nick Street, and O. L. Mangasarian, "Breast Cancer Wisconsin (Diagnostic) Data Set," *UCI Machine Learning Repository: Breast Cancer wisconsin (diagnostic) data set*, 11-Jan-1995. [Online]. Available: https://archive.ics.uci.edu/ml/datasets/breast+cancer+wisconsin+(diagnostic).
22. D. A. S, "Thermal images for breast cancer diagnosis DMR-IR," *Kaggle*, 13-Apr-2020. [Online]. Available: https://www.kaggle.com/datasets/asdeepak/thermal-images-for-breast-cancer-diagnosis-dmrir.
23. Dr. William H. Wolberg, W. Nick Street, and O. L. Mangasarian, "Breast Cancer Wisconsin (Prognostic) Data Set," *UCI Machine Learning Repository: Breast Cancer wisconsin (prognostic) data set*, 01-Dec-1995. [Online]. Available: https://archive.ics.uci.edu/ml/datasets/breast+cancer+wisconsin+(Prognostic).
24. GilSousa, "Haberman's survival data set," *Kaggle*, 30-Nov-2016. [Online]. Available: https://www.kaggle.com/datasets/gilsousa/habermans-survival-data-set.
25. Yap MH, Pons G, Marti J, et al. Automated breast ultrasound lesions detection using convolutional neural networks. *IEEE J Biomed Heal Inform.* 2018;22:1218–1226
26. "PCR – Irma – image retrieval in medical antigens." [Online]. Available: https://www.irma-project.org/category/pcr/.
27. "University of Michigan," *University of Michigan Health System*. [Online]. Available: https://www.med.umich.edu/mss/. [Accessed: 31-Mar-2023]
28. L. Shen, L. R. Margolies, J. H. Rothstein, E. Fluder, R. McBride, and W. Sieh, "Deep learning to improve breast cancer detection on screening mammography," *Scientific Reports*, vol. 9, no. 1, pp. 1–12, 2019.
29. M. F. Ak, "A comparative analysis of breast cancer detection and diagnosis using data visualization and machine learning applications," *Healthcare*, vol. 8(2), p. 111, 2020.
30. Q. Hu, H. M. Whitney, and M. L. Giger, "A deep learning methodology for improved breast cancer diagnosis using multiparametric mri," *Scientific Reports*, vol. 10, no. 1, pp. 1–11, 2020.
31. S. Sharma, A. Aggarwal and T. Choudhury, "Breast Cancer Detection Using Machine Learning Algorithms," 2018 International Conference on Computational Techniques, Electronics and Mechanical Systems (CTEMS), Belgaum, India, 2018, pp. 114–118, doi: 10.1109/CTEMS.2018.8769187.
32. J. Wu and C. Hicks, "Breast cancer type classification using machine learning," *Journal of Personalized Medicine*, vol. 11, no. 2, p. 61, 2021.
33. S. J. Mambou, P. Maresova, O. Krejcar, A. Selamat, and K. Kuca, "Breast cancer detection using infrared thermal imaging and a deep learning model," *Sensors*, vol. 18, no. 9, p. 2799, 2018.

34. I. Daimiel Naranjo, P. Gibbs, J. S. Reiner, R. Lo Gullo, C. Sooknanan, S. B. Thakur, M. S. Jochelson, V. Sevilimedu, E. A. Morris, P. A. Baltzer, et al., "Radiomics and machine learning with multiparametric breast mri for improved diagnostic accuracy in breast cancer diagnosis," *Diagnostics*, vol. 11, no. 6, p. 919, 2021.
35. M. Masud, M. S. Hossain, H. Alhumyani, S. S. Alshamrani, O. Cheikhrouhou, S. Ibrahim, G. Muhammad, A. E. E. Rashed, and B. Gupta, "Pre-trained convolutional neural networks for breast cancer detection using ultrasound images," *ACM Transactions on Internet Technology (TOIT)*, vol. 21, no. 4, pp. 1–17, 2021.
36. T. Kavitha, P. P. Mathai, C. Karthikeyan, M. Ashok, R. Kohar, J. Avanija, and S. Neelakandan, "Deep learning based capsule neural network model for breast cancer diagnosis using mammogram images," *Interdisciplinary Sciences: Computational Life Sciences*, vol. 14, no. 1, pp. 113–129, 2022.
37. N. Chouhan, A. Khan, J. Z. Shah, M. Hussnain, and M. W. Khan, "Deep convolutional neural network and emotional learning based breast cancer detection using digital mammography," *Computers in Biology and Medicine*, vol. 132, p. 104318, 2021.
38. K. Tajane, S. Sheth, R. Satale, T. Tumbare, and O. Panchal, "Breast cancer detection using machine learning algorithms," in: J. S. Raj, Y. Shi, D. Pelusi, and V. Emilia Balas (Eds.), *Intelligent Sustainable Systems*, pp. 347–355. Springer: Berlin, Germany, 2022.
39. A. Rasool, C. Bunterngchit, L. Tiejian, M. R. Islam, Q. Qu, and Q. Jiang, "Improved machine learning-based predictive models for breast cancer diagnosis," *International Journal of Environmental Research and Public Health*, vol. 19, no. 6, p. 3211, 2022.
40. D. Chowdhury, A. Das, A. Dey, S. Sarkar, A. D. Dwivedi, R. Rao Mukkamala, and L. Murmu, "Abcandroid: A cloud integrated android App for noninvasive early breast cancer detection using transfer learning," *Sensors*, vol. 22, no. 3, p. 832, 2022.
41. E. A. Mohamed, E. A. Rashed, T. Gaber, and O. Karam, "Deep learning model for fully automated breast cancer detection system from thermograms," *PLoS One*, vol. 17, no. 1, p. e0262349, 2022.
42. A. Pillai, A. Nizam, M. Joshee, A. Pinto, and S. Chavan, "Breast cancer detection in mammograms using deep learning," in: B. Iyer, D. Ghosh, and V. Emilia Balas (Eds.), *Applied Information Processing Systems*, pp. 121–127. Springer: Berlin, Germany, 2022.
43. K. Jabeen, M. A. Khan, M. Alhaisoni, U. Tariq, Y.-D. Zhang, A. Hamza, A. Mickus, and R. Damaševičius, "Breast cancer classification from ultrasound images using probability-based optimal deep learning feature fusion," *Sensors*, vol. 22, no. 3, p. 807, 2022.
44. M. A. Jabbar, "Breast cancer data classification using ensemble machine learning," *Engineering and Applied Science Research*, vol. 48, no. 1, pp. 65–72, 2021.
45. M. Gupta and B. Gupta, "A Comparative Study of Breast Cancer Diagnosis Using Supervised Machine Learning Techniques," *2018 Second International Conference on Computing Methodologies and Communication (ICCMC)*, Erode, India, 2018, pp. 997–1002, doi: 10.1109/ICCMC.2018.8487537.

46. L.-Q. Zhou, X.-L. Wu, S.-Y. Huang, G.-G. Wu, H.-R. Ye, Q. Wei, L.-Y. Bao, Y.-B. Deng, X.-R. Li, X.-W. Cui, et al., “Lymph node metastasis prediction from primary breast cancer us images using deep learning,” *Radiology*, vol. 294, no. 1, pp. 19–28, 2020.
47. A. Bhattacherjee, S. Roy, S. Paul, P. Roy, N. Kausar, and N. Dey, “Classification approach for breast cancer detection using back propagation neural network: A study,” in *Deep Learning and Neural Networks: Concepts, Methodologies, Tools, and Applications*, pp. 1410–1421, IGI Global, 2020.
48. Z. Sha, L. Hu, and B. D. Rouyendegh, “Deep learning and optimization algorithms for automatic breast cancer detection,” *International Journal of Imaging Systems and Technology*, vol. 30, no. 2, pp. 495–506, 2020.
49. S. Eskreis-Winkler, N. Onishi, K. Pinker, J. S. Reiner, J. Kaplan, E. A. Morris, and E. J. Sutton, “Using deep learning to improve nonsystematic viewing of breast cancer on mri,” *Journal of Breast Imaging*, vol. 3, no. 2, pp. 201–207, 2021.
50. A. Bhardwaj and A. Tiwari, “Breast cancer diagnosis using genetically optimized neural network model,” *Expert Systems with Applications*, vol. 42, no. 10, pp. 4611–4620, 2015.
51. A. M. Abdel-Zaher and A. M. Eldeib, “Breast cancer classification using deep belief networks,” *Expert Systems with Applications*, vol. 46, pp. 139–144, 2016.
52. D. A. Ragab, M. Sharkas, S. Marshall, and J. Ren, “Breast cancer detection using deep convolutional neural networks and support vector machines,” *PeerJ*, vol. 7, p. e6201, 2019.
53. S. H. Kassani, P. H. Kassani, M. J. Wesolowski, K. A. Schneider and R. Deters, “Breast Cancer Diagnosis with Transfer Learning and Global Pooling,” *2019 International Conference on Information and Communication Technology Convergence (ICTC)*, Jeju, Korea (South), 2019, pp. 519–524, doi: 10.1109/ICTC46691.2019.8939878.
54. E. A. Bayrak, P. Kırcı, and T. Ensari, “Comparison of machine learning methods for breast cancer diagnosis,” in *2019 Scientific Meeting on Electrical-Electronics & Biomedical Engineering and Computer Science (EBBT)*, pp. 1–3, IEEE, 2019.
55. H. Dhahri, E. Al Maghayreh, A. Mahmood, W. Elkilani, and M. Faisal Nagi, “Automated breast cancer diagnosis based on machine learning algorithms,” *Journal of Healthcare Engineering*, vol. 2019, 2019.
56. A. Bhardwaj and A. Tiwari, “Breast cancer diagnosis using genetically optimized neural network model,” *Expert Systems with Applications*, vol. 42, no. 10, pp. 4611–4620, 2015.
57. M. M. Islam, H. Iqbal, M. R. Haque and M. K. Hasan, “Prediction of breast cancer using support vector machine and K-Nearest neighbors,” *2017 IEEE Region 10 Humanitarian Technology Conference (R10-HTC)*, Dhaka, Bangladesh, 2017, pp. 226–229, doi: 10.1109/R10-HTC.2017.8288944.
58. R. K. Samala, H.-P. Chan, L. M. Hadjiiski, K. Cha, and M. A. Helvie, “Deep-learning convolution neural network for computer-aided detection of microcalcifications in digital breast tomosynthesis,” in *Medical Imaging 2016: Computer-Aided Diagnosis*, vol. 9785, p. 97850Y, International Society for Optics and Photonics, 2016.
59. R. K. Samala, H.-P. Chan, L. Hadjiiski, M. A. Helvie, J. Wei, and K. Cha, “Mass detection in digital breast tomosynthesis: Deep convolutional neural network with transfer learning from mammography,” *Medical Physics*, vol. 43, no. 12, pp. 6654–6666, 2016.

60. D. H. Kim, S. T. Kim and Y. M. Ro, "Latent feature representation with 3-D multi-view deep convolutional neural network for bilateral analysis in digital breast tomosynthesis," *2016 IEEE International Conference on Acoustics, Speech and Signal Processing (ICASSP)*, Shanghai, China, 2016, pp. 927–931, doi: 10.1109/ICASSP.2016.7471811.
61. S. V. Fotin, Y. Yin, H. Haldankar, J. W. Hoffmeister, and S. Periaswamy, "Detection of soft tissue densities from digital breast tomosynthesis: comparison of conventional and deep learning approaches," in *Medical Imaging 2016: Computer-Aided Diagnosis*, vol. 9785, pp. 228–233, SPIE, 2016.
62. Z. Zhu, M. Harowicz, J. Zhang, A. Saha, L. J. Grimm, S. Hwang, and M. A. Mazurowski, "Deep learning-based features of breast mri for prediction of occult invasive disease following a diagnosis of ductal carcinoma in situ: preliminary data," in *Medical Imaging 2018: Computer-Aided Diagnosis*, vol. 10575, p. 105752W, International Society for Optics and Photonics, 2018.
63. R. K. Samala, H.-P. Chan, L. Hadjiiski, M. A. Helvie, C. Richter, and K. Cha, "Cross-domain and multi-task transfer learning of deep convolutional neural network for breast cancer diagnosis in digital breast tomosynthesis," in *Medical Imaging 2018: Computer-Aided Diagnosis*, vol. 10575, p. 105750Q, International Society for Optics and Photonics, 2018.
64. I. Reiser, R. Nishikawa, M. Giger, T. Wu, E. Rafferty, R. Moore, and D. Kopans, "Computerized mass detection for digital breast tomosynthesis directly from the projection images," *Medical Physics*, vol. 33, no. 2, pp. 482–491, 2006.
65. G. Van Schie, M. G. Wallis, K. Leifland, M. Danielsson, and N. Karssemeijer, "Mass detection in reconstructed digital breast tomosynthesis volumes with a computer-aided detection system trained on 2d mammograms," *Medical Physics*, vol. 40, no. 4, p. 041902, 2013.
66. H.-P. Chan, J. Wei, Y. Zhang, M. A. Helvie, R. H. Moore, B. Sahiner, L. Hadjiiski, and D. B. Kopans, "Computer-aided detection of masses in digital tomosynthesis mammography: Comparison of three approaches," *Medical Physics*, vol. 35, no. 9, pp. 4087–4095, 2008.
67. K. R. Mendel, H. Li, D. Sheth, and M. L. Giger, "Transfer learning with convolutional neural networks for lesion classification on clinical breast tomosynthesis," in *Medical Imaging 2018: Computer-Aided Diagnosis*, vol. 10575, p. 105750T, International Society for Optics and Photonics, 2018.
68. N. Antropova, B. Q. Huynh, and M. L. Giger, "A deep feature fusion methodology for breast cancer diagnosis demonstrated on three imaging modality datasets," *Medical Physics*, vol. 44, no. 10, pp. 5162–5171, 2017.
69. T. G. Debelee, M. Amirian, A. Ibenthal, G. Palm, and F. Schwenker, "Classification of mammograms using convolutional neural network based feature extraction," in *International Conference on Information and Communication Technology for Develoment for Africa*, pp. 89–98, Springer, 2017.
70. T. Kooi, G. Litjens, B. Van Ginneken, A. Gubern-Mérida, C. I. Sánchez, R. Mann, A. den Heeten, and N. Karssemeijer, "Large scale deep learning for computer aided detection of mammographic lesions," *Medical Image Analysis*, vol. 35, pp. 303–312, 2017.
71. S. M. Lawson, R. L. Clark, and R. F. Crouse, "Aero-optic performance of supersonic mixing layers," in *Window and Dome Technologies and Materials II*, vol. 1326, pp. 190–195, SPIE, 1990.

72. A. S. Becker, M. Mueller, E. Stoffel, M. Marcon, S. Ghafoor, and A. Boss, "Classification of breast cancer in ultrasound imaging using a generic deep learning analysis software: A pilot study," *The British Journal of Radiology*, vol. 91, p. 20170576, 2018.
73. M. H. Yap, M. Goyal, F. Osman, E. Ahmad, R. Martí, E. Denton, A. Juette, and R. Zwiggelaar, "End-to-end breast ultrasound lesions recognition with a deep learning approach," in *Medical Imaging 2018: Biomedical Applications in Molecular, Structural, and Functional Imaging*, vol. 10578, p. 1057819, International Society for Optics and Photonics, 2018.
74. S. Y. Shin, S. Lee, I. D. Yun, S. M. Kim, and K. M. Lee, "Joint weakly and semi-supervised deep learning for localization and classification of masses in breast ultrasound images," *IEEE Transactions on Medical Imaging*, vol. 38, no. 3, pp. 762–774, 2018.
75. J. Li, M. Fan, J. Zhang, and L. Li, "Discriminating between benign and malignant breast tumors using 3d convolutional neural network in dynamic contrast enhanced-mr images," in *Medical Imaging 2017: Imaging Informatics for Healthcare, Research, and Applications*, vol. 10138, p. 1013808, International Society for Optics and Photonics, 2017.
76. M. M. Jadoon, Q. Zhang, I. U. Haq, S. Butt, and A. Jadoon, "Three-class mammogram classification based on descriptive cnn features," *BioMed Research International*, vol. 2017, pp. 1–11, 2017.
77. M. Kallenberg, K. Petersen, M. Nielsen, A. Y. Ng, P. Diao, C. Igel, C. M. Vachon, K. Holland, R. R. Winkel, N. Karssemeijer, et al., "Unsupervised deep learning applied to breast density segmentation and mammographic risk scoring," *IEEE Transactions on Medical Imaging*, vol. 35, no. 5, pp. 1322–1331, 2016.
78. G. Palma, I. Bloch, and S. Muller, "Detection of masses and architectural distortions in digital breast tomosynthesis images using fuzzy and a contrario approaches," *Pattern Recognition*, vol. 47, no. 7, pp. 2467–2480, 2014.
79. M. Yousefi, A. Krzyzak, and C. Y. Suen, "Mass detection in digital breast tomosynthesis data using convolutional neural networks and multiple instance learning," *Computers in Biology and Medicine*, vol. 96, pp. 283–293, 2018.
80. L. Zou, S. Yu, T. Meng, Z. Zhang, X. Liang, and Y. Xie, "A technical review of convolutional neural network-based mammographic breast cancer diagnosis," *Computational and Mathematical Methods in Medicine*, vol. 2019, pp. 1–16, 2019.
81. A. Jalalian, S. B. Mashohor, H. R. Mahmud, M. I. B. Saripan, A. R. B. Ramli, and B. Karasfi, "Computer-aided detection/diagnosis of breast cancer in mammography and ultrasound: A review," *Clinical Imaging*, vol. 37, no. 3, pp. 420–426, 2013.
82. G. Meenalochini and S. Ramkumar, "Survey of machine learning algorithms for breast cancer detection using mammogram images," *Materials Today: Proceedings*, vol. 37, pp. 2738–2743, 2021.
83. B. ElOuassif, A. Idri, M. Hosni, and A. Abran, "Classification techniques in breast cancer diagnosis: A systematic literature review," *Computer Methods in Biomechanics and Biomedical Engineering: Imaging & Visualization*, vol. 9, no. 1, pp. 50–77, 2021.
84. X. Liu and Z. Zeng, "A new automatic mass detection method for breast cancer with false positive reduction," *Neurocomputing*, vol. 152, pp. 388–402, 2015.

85. Y. Jiménez-Gaona, M. J. Rodríguez-Álvarez, and V. Lakshminarayanan, "Deep-learning-based computer-aided systems for breast cancer imaging: A critical review," *Applied Sciences*, vol. 10, no. 22, p. 8298, 2020.
86. M. M. Altaf, "A hybrid deep learning model for breast cancer diagnosis based on transfer learning and pulse-coupled neural networks," *Mathematical Biosciences and Engineering*, vol. 18, no. 5, pp. 5029–5046, 2021.
87. D. Arefan, A. A. Mohamed, W. A. Berg, M. L. Zuley, J. H. Sumkin, and S. Wu, "Deep learning modeling using normal mammograms for predicting breast cancer risk," *Medical Physics*, vol. 47, no. 1, pp. 110–118, 2020.
88. A. Sivasangari, D. Deepa, T. Anandhi, S. C. Mana, R. Vignesh, and B. Keerthi Samhitha, "Deep learning modeling using normal mammograms for predicting breast cancer," in: S. Shakya, R. Bestak, R. Palanisamy, and K. A. Kamel (Eds.), *Mobile Computing and Sustainable Informatics*, pp. 411–422, Springer: Berlin, Germany, 2022.
89. G. Sanson, J. Welton, E. Vellone, A. Cocchieri, M. Maurici, M. Zega, R. Alvaro, and F. D'Agostino, "Enhancing the performance of predictive models for hospital mortality by adding nursing data," *International Journal of Medical Informatics*, vol. 125, pp. 79–85, 2019.
90. H. Li and M. L. Giger, "Artificial intelligence and interpretations in breast cancer imaging," in *Artificial Intelligence in Medicine*, pp. 291–308, Elsevier, 2021.
91. Y. Gu, J. Chi, J. Liu, L. Yang, B. Zhang, D. Yu, Y. Zhao, and X. Lu, "A survey of computer-aided diagnosis of lung nodules from ct scans using deep learning," *Computers in Biology and Medicine*, vol. 137, p. 104806, 2021.
92. J. Yanase and E. Triantaphyllou, "The seven key challenges for the future of computer-aided diagnosis in medicine," *International Journal of Medical Informatics*, vol. 129, pp. 413–422, 2019.

Chapter 17

Complex dynamical interplay of health, climate and conflicts with data-driven approach

Syed Shariq Husain
OP Jindal Global University

CONTENTS

17.1 INTRODUCTION

Humans have the tendency to form groups and prefer to coordinate with others for collective action. The settlement pattern has emerged from simple patches to huge and complex pattern of living spaces defined in terms of nations, languages, ethnicity and geography, common heritage or ideologies. The tendency to coordinate and act collectively provides the opportunity to defend the common threat and has also been a key cause for the rapid development of human society. This tendency to cooperate not only interacts with the immediate relatives but extends to the dimensions of unrelated individuals [45]. Also, the driving force of evolution takes part within this system of interaction and interplay. This gives rise to varying interactions among different individuals and is responsible for

DOI: 10.1201/9781003368342-17

certain interesting patterns emerging from such phenomena. Here, phenomena of segregation can be observed in different forms including race, class, gender, caste, religious or political ideology, etc. [53, 54]. In a social system, the complex level of interactions often is linked with the positive and negative aspects of the dimension of human social behaviour. These, together with the convolution of several factors, play a deep role in the complexity of social system. Therefore, to capture the pattern and model the complexity of human social behaviour a wide range of aspects and parameters may be taken into account viz, bonding, jealousy, greed, sacrifice, conflicts and war, resources and justice, etc. [45].

From time to time, the entire globe has seen various conflicts, war and epidemics, which not only resulted in loss of lives but also lead to cascading failure of various sectors due to inter-dependency upon multiple factors. Unlike normal social phenomena, anti-social phenomena are very different and depict complicated characteristics stemming from various deeply interwoven interactions. The interactions taking part among the agents of such anti-social activities may or may not be same, but the drivers or agents of such activities are less in numbers. In a formal manner, often a conflict is defined as an activity that results from the interaction between conscious but may not necessarily rational beings having their interests mutually inconsistent with each other. Human civilization has always been affected with the violent activities resulting from conflicts and these anti-social phenomena. In accordance with reference Lahr et al. [37], the case of inter-group violence, considered as one of the earlier recorded conflicts, took place in eastern Africa around 10,000 years ago in which attempts were made to seize resources and caused the killings of dozens of people [37]. Following the development of human civilization and further witnessing the industrial revolution [42], there has been a shift in lifestyle and attitudes towards living. It is pertinent to quote that here materialism-driven, self-centric humans have adopted the notions of racial superiority and discrimination on contrary to the fundamental values of human rights. In addition to the sociological explanation and Marxian explanation of class struggle, recently with the availability of high volumes of data, and techniques from artificial intelligence and physics can shed light on the spread and formation, structure and dynamics of such phenomena. Here physicists and computer scientists attempt to capture the underlying patterns with the empirical observation, and develop mathematical model, which may lead to better prediction and risk assessment close to the reliable confidence interval. Hence, the interdisciplinary field of "Sociophysics" not only captures the patterns of large-scale statistical measurement of social variables but also takes into account multiple indicators for more precise observations [1, 8, 9, 51].

Moreover, the impact of climate change, river and delta discharges, disaster, armed conflicts, epidemics, pandemics and its responses, the adoption or switching off [10] certain idea or policy measures, mobility patterns and rescue operations through these approaches have the potential to better manage the situation and respond. Such tools and techniques through empirical data enables to precisely measure the ocean currents and winds, landscape and its type, water resource management, etc., and offer better insights to monitor such systems and its impact on humans.

Empirical evidence have depicted that following Industrial revolution, the use of fossil fuels increased manifold times. This along with rapid growth in urbanization, reduced green cover have contributed towards climate change and deteriorating weather conditions [47]. The situation can be well understood in terms of the theory of the tragedy of the commons, which is a situation in which members or individual users, having free access to resources which is shared in society without any well-defined governing rules for the access and use, act independently according to their self-interest and, not in accordance with the common good of all other users, results in depletion of the resource due to their uncoordinated action [25]. The application of tragedy of commons extends to atmosphere and climate, ocean and resources, etc. Moreover, harmful radiations and depleted ozone cover have worsened the situation [3]. This is evident through climate change conditions that impact almost everyday with its growing and increasingly pervasive effects [58], e.g., wildfires in Australia, cyclones in the Indian Ocean, droughts in Sahel region of Africa, floods in part of South Asia and rising sea levels in the Pacific. It is becoming increasingly apparent that, in addition to, being an environmental challenge, climate change also has dramatic impact on people, as lives are lost, habitats are destroyed, and communities are displaced. In some circumstances, climate change can even pose threat to peace and security.

Unprecedented number of people have been displaced by the humanitarian crises for example arm conflicts and terrorism in Syria, Iraq and parts of Africa, devastating natural disasters, like hurricanes, namely

Matthew in Haiti, Jamaica and Bahamas and disease outbreaks such as Ebola in West Africa, and Zika in Latin America and global pandemic Covid-19.

It is not just coincidence that many countries that are vulnerable to climate change are often vulnerable to conflict. Majority of UN peace operations are often in countries considered most affected by climate change. These regions act as climate change hotspots and consist of Sudan, Somalia, Mali, Congo, etc. However, climate change does not directly cause conflicts, but it links this to risk factors and acts as a *"stress multiplier"*; for example, it can intensify competition over natural tangible resources including water and agricultural resources that tend to drive food prices up and as a result has a tendency to increase geopolitical tensions or trigger conflicts.

Various socioeconomic aspects have been studied through the lens of resource mismanagement and conflicts. Out of many indicators, it has been observed that more often there is an economic cost associated with conflicts, whereas it is also linked with the colonial past and other factors too. For example, Debraj Ray et al. have established that conflicts are often triggered by economic factors that may be over due to mismanagement of resources, schizophrenic resources and its hold and governance in relation to different ethnicities [49]. Resource dynamics and path dependence involve several explanations and take into consideration how extraction was carried out with respect to land tenure rights, the dynamics of structural and sectoral change for labour markets where ethnic or racial division exists against immigrants, candidacy of potential business resources against usage of agrarian land. Such interconnection between multiple variables creates a complex behaviour, for example, conflicts in several communities or sects with different ethnicities in various parts of Africa and Asia and conflicts in Darfur, Rwanda is among some of the many instances [49]. Frey et al. [17] have established that arm conflicts and terrorism, etc., not only affect the common masses who faced the direct consequences, but there comes with it an indirect cost related to it. This often has affected upon the economy. The major segment or sectors of the economy that are impacted, include GDP, FDI-Foreign Direct Investment, tourism sectors, infrastructure losses. Not only this, but it also has-short term cost which is for humanitarian aid and rehabilitation and long-term cost to re-establish the infrastructural damage and for healing up of the affected sectors. In loose terms, it could

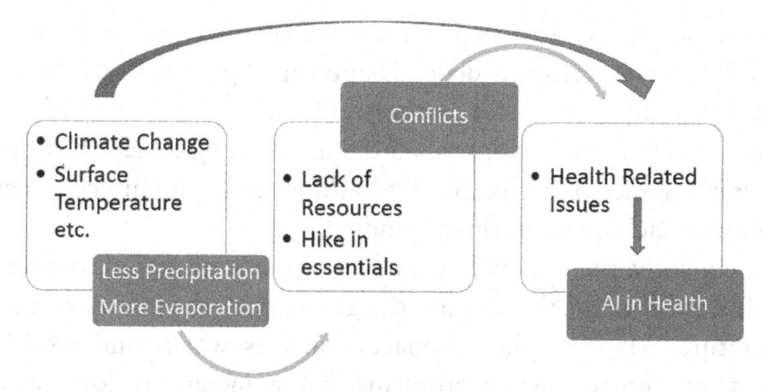

Figure 17.1 Schematic diagram representing the 'possible' pathway depicting the influence of climate change to health issues via conflicts and humanitarian crises. However, there may exist many possibilities including micro-level interaction among different actors and local socioeconomic condition playing its role in such complex dynamical system. Also, due to local socioeconomic and sociopolitical conditions and various type of interactions involved, conflicts are not always climate change-driven. But conflict give birth to several medical emergencies.

be observed that the impact of climate change results in higher surface temperature, anomaly in rainfall, cyclones and storms, wildfire and other extreme events, etc. For example, due to higher surface temperature and anomaly in rainfall, there is lesser amount of precipitation which result in shortage of water resources, which if not covered by alternative means, may influence the agriculture and other related sectors. This, in turn, triggers the food prices due to lesser yield and has the tendency to boil the situation and may cause the conflicts (Figure 17.1). Following the consequences, of conflicts some other crime happens to take place alongside ongoing conflicts. Furthermore, as a result of these armed conflicts or extreme event on the affected population, "Pandora's box of trouble" is opened. With it comes the health-related issues for the affected population in addition to mass migration and shelter in rescue camps. The population is not only affected by direct impact of conflicts like wounds and injuries escaping death, they are often prone to PTSD–Post Traumatic Stress Disorder especially the kids of affected wartorn families, lack of basic amenities and emergency first aid due to infrastructural damage which may result in various health issues [35].

Accordingly, in compliance with WHO, *"health is not merely the absence of disease, infirmity or physical fitness but is considered as the state of complete physical, mental and social well-being"*. The variation in life expectancy is suggestive of the variability of health and in WHO framework it depends upon the "genetics", "behaviour", "environmental and physical influences", "medical care" and "social factors" which are deeply interconnected. Challenges identified by Fadi et al., in the Lancet [41] specifically in the Arab region are conflicts and war, stigma, lack of institutional funding.

Consequently, the ongoing climate change is anticipated to have considerable effect on health around the globe, with the effects rising with temperature. Many of these impacts, such as water- and food-borne diseases, are already major problems in low-income regions. Another vulnerability could be increase in malnutrition, as a result of extreme weather events like drought. The crucial factor responsible here is decrease in yields of major crops due to the physiological tolerance limits of plants in hot regions[6, 46, 60].

In addition to this, humanitarian crises are a major and growing contributor to ill health and vulnerability worldwide. The impact of such events on health and health systems can undermine decades of social development and present a number of challenges for public health. Effective health responses in proper settings are required for such situations. Major sufferers are low-income household or nations that are deeply hit by such humanitarian crises at different scales respectively. Armed conflicts causes, injuries, displacement and death, but it continues to affect people's health even after the front lines have moved. It devastates essential health services, disrupts medical supplies, forces medical staff to flee and leaves the national immune system broken when deadly diseases arrive and affect the entire system. In a direct effect of climate change and global health there exist a likelihood of range enhancement of existing diseases and emergence of new disease. For instance, the malaria vector, 'Anopheles' may increase the total number of annual cases and likely to spread to the new regions. These are also the potential carrier of other related diseases like dengue, chikungunya, yellow fever in addition to malaria. Change in climatic conditions can lead to extreme weather conditions, resulting in heavy rainfalls, floods and elevated temperatures poses the threat of enteric diseases and thereby bringing forward the risk of food-borne diseases and malnutrition [59]. One such example is related with gastrointestinal disease in humans due to contaminated poultry by Compylobacter in Europe. In a study conducted by Kovats et al. it has been reported that increase in seasonal temperature results in increasing trends of human infected with Campylobacter [50].

The impact upon low income and less developed countries is often observed despite lesser contribution toward global warming. The overlap of the health condition with climate and in some region its interplay with conflicts brings forward the presence of diseases and medical condition. The climate-sensitive, conflict-sensitive and climate-conflict-sensitive outcomes and diseases comprise heat stress, heat stroke causing mortality or morbidity, particulate matter or air pollution-related diseases, disease transmission through toxic or vector-affected water bodies, wounds, injuries, affected mental condition and post-traumatic stress disorder, malnutrition and migration of population and refugee camps [44]. AI informed data-driven studies can help monitor the impact of climate and weather conditions, landscape monitoring including soil pH, moisture and nutrients content to assure better yield and thereby reducing the risk of conflicts, health emergency and medical condition. Hence, AI and data has the potential to provide deep insight and better understand such systemic studies, assess the risk and recommend policies.

As of now, the emergence of artificial intelligence and machine learning on centre stage for various applications is playing a pivotal role across different disciplines. The employ-ability of mathematical and computational techniques result in better informed systems that can be marked and through this the existing abnormalities can be identified. The wide ranging applications of such tools have potential to capture the abnormalities, early detection of diseases and identification of key regulators in healthcare domain. Not only this, the detection of pre-cursor to such happenings is made possible through early warning signals or early detection of several events; for example, the early detection of floods due to heavy rainfall made possible to save lives, minimizes the impact of disease spread post such mishappenings, has saved infrastructural damage and reduces the stress on economy by cutting the cost (of first aid) [12, 34].

17.2 DATA SCIENCE AND COMPUTATIONAL METHODS

Data science in broad terms is an interdisciplinary field that employs the use of various tools and techniques from different disciplines to deal with structured and unstructured data to extract meaningful information. The field integrates/disseminate knowledge from different perspectives and incorporate systemic thinking and complexity theory. Computational methods on voluminous amount of real world data have the potential to provide deeper insights and better policy recommendations. Statistical techniques and machine learning methods are playing a crucial role in dealing with the large amount of data generated nowadays on regular basis [52].

As an illustration to the data-driven studies, in this chapter, we analyse different datasets publicly available. Here, we have used (i) the world happiness data for different countries, (ii) conflicts and terrorism data and (iii) the surface temperature data for different countries is considered. Following the data cleaning and processing, this data is analysed with some computational techniques to demonstrate the ability of data science and provide the glimpse of machine learning techniques mentioned in this chapter.

17.2.1 Data-driven analyses

To perform a concrete analyses in a data-driven dynamical system and ask appropriate questions, it is often required to prepare and know about the structured or unstructured data. Following this, the process of data cleaning and processing is performed subject to requirement. The data taken into consideration is World Happiness data for the year 2015–2017, GDELT for ethnic conflicts and GTD for terrorism data, whereas surface temperature data for various countries is utilized for the studies. The data consist of several indicators having columns as happiness score, ranks, economy in terms of GDP, freedom in lifestyle, health in terms of life expectancy, etc. Similarly, for GTD type of attacks, source and targets of attack, lat and long, location, modus operandi, etc. Also, GDELT data after processing consists of yearwise data in relation to different countries. Surface temperature data consist of country wise surface temperature [22, 23]. Here in Figure 17.2, the result displays the countries having least happiness score or the ten most unhappiest countries of the world for the years 2015 – 2017, respectively. It is pertinent to note that in these plots, the countries are Afghanistan, Rwanda, Syria, Central African Republic and Yemen out of others. Surprisingly, the countries with poor score are also the wartorn, terror or conflict-affected regions of the world [29]. The variation of Happiness score with economy in terms of GDP is displayed by the *left* plot Figure 17.3 for two different years. Similarly, the variation of Happiness score with health through life expectancy is depicted in Figure 17.3. It is

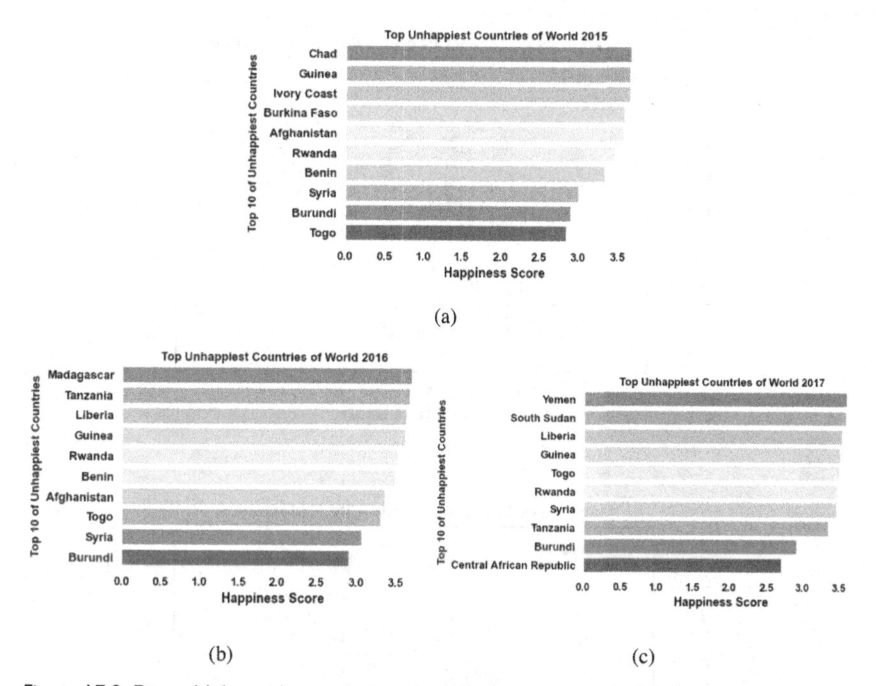

Figure 17.2 Figure(s) here shows the ten least happy countries of the World for the year 2015, 2016, 2017 respectively. (a) Least happy countries for the year 2015, (b) Least happy countries for the year 2016, and (c) Least happy countries for the year 2017. (Data source(s) consist of World Happiness Report for the respective years [63].)

important to note that here the happiest countries appear towards the right extreme of the plot, whereas the affected and least happy nations are near the left part of the plot. The data here is plotted for two consecutive years. Happiness score, in turn, depends on many parameters and is suggestive or reflective of the overall health of a country, e.g., health, GDP or economy, freedom in life choices, etc. Computing various statistics related to these provide more precise analysis and deeper understandings. Following this, more relevant and appropriate questions could be asked to uncover the relational patterns through data-driven machine learning methods. Implementation of such techniques often resorts to the type of research question asked and the type of data to use computational and mathematical techniques and artificial intelligence. Further inquiring and computing the data results in capturing the three-dimensional variation and interplay of the health, economy and happiness data. Close examination of the plot indicates the appearance of

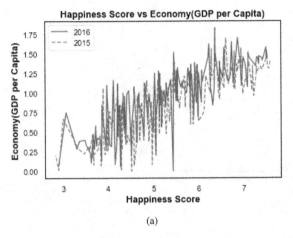

(a)

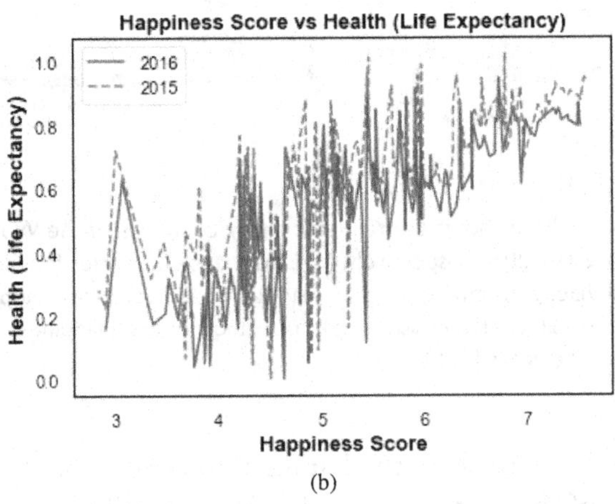

(b)

Figure 17.3 Panel (a) shows the variability of the Happiness score with the Economy in terms of GDP per capita. Panel (b) shows the variation of Happiness score against Health in terms of Life Expectancy. Here, solid line curve depicts the values for the year 2016 while dashed(–) denotes the values for the year 2015.

happiest countries at the right part of the figure, whereas the least happy countries are towards the left part of the plot. Computed fit may be taken as a tool that guides to understand that countries on the lowest point on the surface towards the left side is indicative of the least happy countries and less life expectancy. Various socioeconomic conditions are also responsible for such situation. This indicates that these affected countries are vulnerable toward the triggering of conflict or climate-sensitive conflict. In addition, the terror affected nations face various problems due to infrastructural damage, non-availability of medical

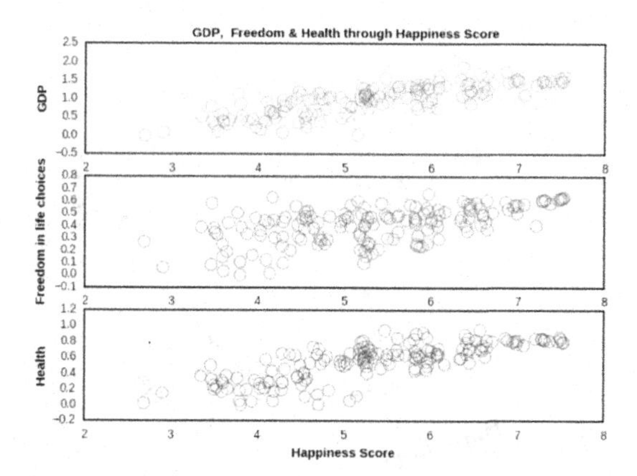

(a) The trend of variation of GDP, Freedom in life choices, & Health in relation to Happiness score.

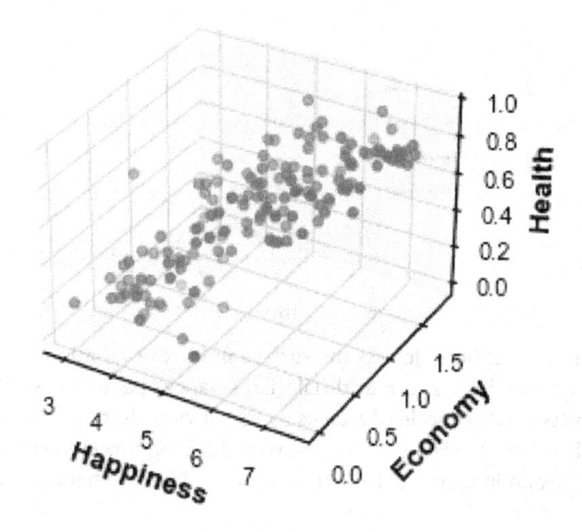

(b) Here it is clearly visible that Happiness score varies with Health. Hence, it is evident that Countries with least scores for happiness are affected by various health related issues e.g., lack of medical services and infrastructural unavailability etc.

Figure 17.4 Panel (a) represent the plots for factor varying with Happiness score(s). Panel (b) represent the 3D variation of Happiness score with Economy and Health. Here, it is important to note that the affected Countries which have least score can be observed near left bottom of the 3D plot.

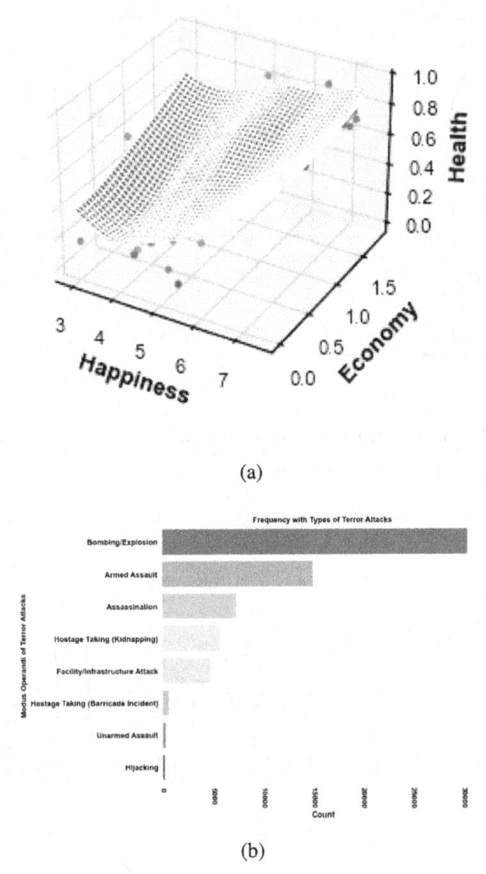

Figure 17.5 The figure(s) here depicts the surface fit for the variation in, Happiness Score, Economy(GDP), and Health(Life Expectancy) parameters. The adjacent plot depicts various mode of attacks by terror organisations. (a) Surface Fit for the variability of the Happiness score with the Economy in terms of GDP per capita and health in terms of life expectancy. (b) Modus operandi of different terror organisations.

practitioner and absence of front line staffs for medical emergencies (Figure 17.4). Figure 17.5b depicts the various modes of attacks by various organization(s)(also reported in Ref. [30]). The plot captures that throughout years the favourite *modus operandi* is bombing and explosions by the source organisation(s). It is followed by armed assault, kidnapping and infrastructure attack. Keeping the nature of attack in consideration and the components involved, *first aid* measure should be taken. In such situation machine learning-based first aid, medication recommendation, may provide additional layer of insights for such highly undesired events. The world map shows the variation of happiness scores and average surface temperature as shown by the figure(s). There comes a wide range of factors responsible for the ongoing situation in the region. The web of various factors interplaying together such as climatic conditions, ethnicity, land and natural resources management, drought, famine, ongoing conflicts, infrastructural damage, affected economic conditions are often seen as the obstruction towards attaining stability. However, in systemic view, some of the factors are giving rise to certain situation and feedback loops often keeps them (Figure 17.6).

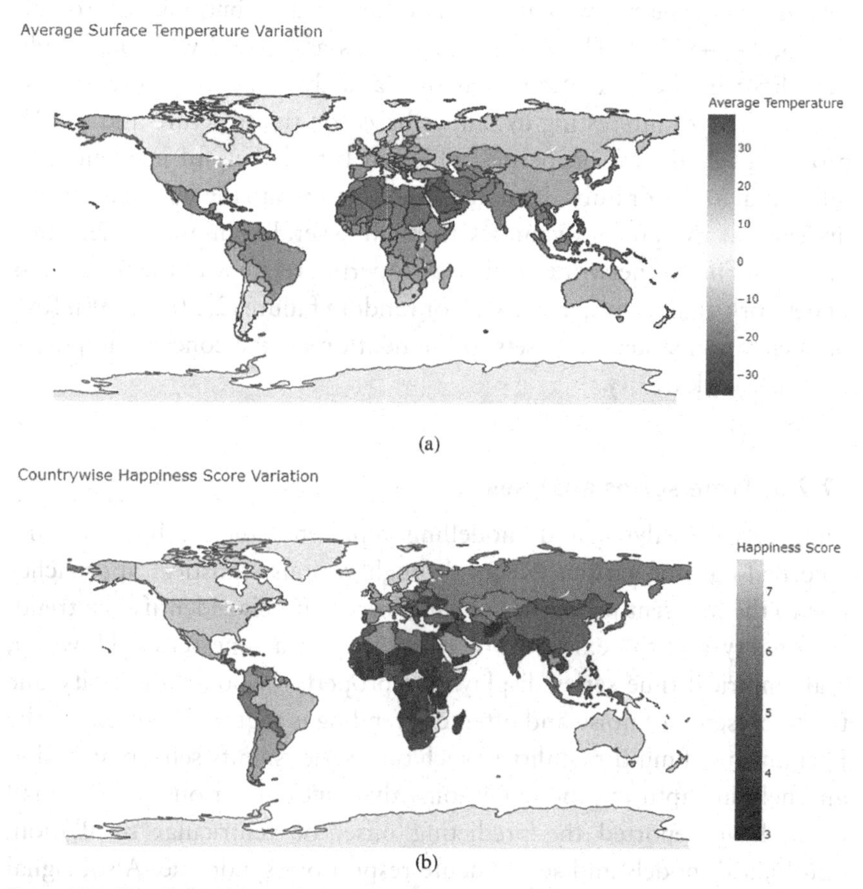

Figure 17.6 The figure(s) here depicts (a) Heatmap in terms of Average Surface Temperature Variability. (b) The heatmap for Happiness Score.

17.2.2 Complex networks

Beginning from the classic Konigsberg problem of seven bridges of Königsberg in Kaliningrad, Russia, graph theory [15, 62] journeyed through various disciplines including Sociology, Biology, Epidemiology, etc. It has entered into the analysis of gene regulatory networks, metabolic pathways, human sexual interactions and recently into network medicines [4, 16, 27, 33, 39, 43]. A network is composed of nodes and edges in which nodes represent an actor or entity whereas the edges are symbolic of type of interactions or relation involved. There are class of networks namely, random, small world and scale-free graphs respectively that depicts different distributions accordingly [5, 13, 14, 48, 61]. The various properties associated with the graphs shed light in the formation, structure and dynamics. These networks are reflective of interesting dynamics based on the structure and exhibit prominent statistical properties which in turn is helpful in identifying influential nodes or hubs. It enables us to better map the interactions and understand the group dynamics through several community detection methods. Further network resilience properties relate with the robustness of network against targeted attack or random failure [2, 20, 30, 38]. Recommendation system also sets its foundation on the concepts imported from network theory.

17.2.3 Time series analyses

Time series analyses and modelling represents the dealing of daily recorded data of various events through various statistical approaches due to the inherent properties of times series. It helps identify the trend, seasonality and the existence of periodicity in a time series. However, real empirical time series displays the property of non-stationarity due to the presence of noise and often de-trending is required. Moreover, the phenomena of multifractality in such time series signify self-organisation and help in capturing the undergoing dynamics at various scales. Small et al. have reported the predicting onset of ventricular fibrillation, ontological models and severe acute respiratory syndrome. Also, signal analysis is often employed to detect mental disorder and helps in detection and diagnosis of such patients. The use of complex network theory in recent days in the study of time series analysis is shown to be of great importance across varying disciplines like health, finance, climate, computational-neuroscience and ECG/EEG analyses. To unravel the dynamics of nonlinear time series for a system several methods and techniques from nonlinear dynamics, modelling and quantification measures are proposed. Implementation of such methods for real world data finds potential for deep understanding and relational pattern of these systems. In some domains, the findings and estimations are important, however, the methods need more precise and controlled testing to be clinically significant. As time series of real world data is noisy, it is sometimes cast into complex networks and statistical properties of it are explored. This often results in different dynamics due to differences in topological structures. One application of such technique shed light to differentiate the cardiogram of sinus rhythm for healthy volunteers and coronary care patients through statistical properties [36, 55–57].

17.3 MACHINE LEARNING METHODS

As mentioned, data plays a crucial role to use AI-inspired techniques to get insights and identify the relational patterns. Choosing a machine learning algorithm depends upon the data under consideration and the objective of the problem. Broad classification includes supervised, unsupervised and reinforcement learning. For a supervised learning in a dataset, to implement ML dependent variables are referred as labels whereas independent variables are considered as features. Combination of sufficient amount of data with proper ML algorithm brings forward a model connecting such features and labels. Following this the random subset of data is considered as training and test and hence chosen model is built and tested. Then new data points can be estimated through this model under consideration. After hyper-tuning the parameters during the training by algorithm, this model is calibrated. The most common example of the supervised learning is associated with regressions and depending upon the data-type linear or polynomial regression can be employed into use whereas for classification logistic regression, k-NN(k-Nearest Neighbour), support vector machine or decision trees can be resorted upon. For unsupervised learning, the potential choice of techniques is related to clustering and dimensionality reduction in which for former K-means clustering is the most popular method wherein for latter LDA(Linear Discriminant Analysis), PCA(Principle Component

Analysis), ICA(Independent Component Analysis), SVD(Singular Value Decomposition) are often implemented. However, in addition to these, there exist several subclasses as reinforcement learning and neural nets and deep learning [7, 19, 24, 26, 40].

These methods play key role in assisting to uncover many interesting patterns and are prominently used. For instance [24] have used machine learning methods to forecast PTSD. In a wide range of data-driven research activities, clustering and dimensionality reduction approaches are often used. The clustering approach uses a distance metric to calculate the distances between the points in the given data. The returned values are then used to project or group similar points. The dimensional reduction approach is frequently used to visualize high-dimensional data by projecting it into a low-dimensional embedding space. A widely used kernel-based approach is the support vector machine. It projects the input space onto a higher-dimensional feature space using a kernel function. Following this, a linear regression is then performed in the modified space. Here, the training is expressed as a convex quadratic optimization problem. This is further solved using efficient optimization algorithm approach. The success of this approach is determined by the kernel type and hyperparameters chosen. Another concept is $k-nearest\ neighbours$ which deals with the classification and regression. The approach selects k closest input points in the training data and delivers the prediction as the average of k outputs. Commonly used metrics is distance with respect to data characteristics, e.g., Euclidean distance and hamming distance. However, choice of k depends upon the data. Decision tree is another approach implemented for classification and regression as a type of recursive partitioning approach. It divides the multidimensional input space associated with training points into regions in a recursive manner, so that inputs with similar results are grouped together. A bunch of "if-else" rules emerges from the division. It is depicted as branching where at the end of each rule, an average of the output values is computed and preserved for each region. The decision tree uses the "if-else" rule to return the preserved value as the projected value on introducing a new testing point. Random forest is a bootstrap aggregating or "bagging" technique that takes random subsamples of the training dataset and creates a decision tree for each of them. This collection of decision trees are averaged to get the predicted value. Gradient boosting techniques possess many similarities with random forest. The main idea is to construct each tree in such a manner so as to minimize the error of the previous tree [26].

17.3.1 Artificial neural network

Artificial neural networks are interconnected group of various nodes. These are inspired by the simplification of neurons of a brain, where each node is representative of an artificial neuron. Deep neural networks [7], are a type of artificial neural network. These are distinguished by stacked layers, in which symbolically, an arrow represents a connection from the output of one artificial neuron to the input of another. In it, layers are made up of a number of units which receives input from previous layers. These are then collected in a weighted linear mode and are processed via a "nonlinear" function. The training points are fed to the first layer, and the predictions are obtained from the last layer. During the training phase, the weights of the stacked layers are adjusted to reduce the prediction error on the training data. To accomplish the objective, the stochastic gradient descent optimization approach is commonly considered. It computes the gradients of the objective function in the network to update the weights.

17.4 IMAGE ANALYTICS

Machine learning is finding its application across various disciplines from applied engineering problems to real world challenges. It helps in capturing important patterns, artefact detection and extracting meaningful information from various types of data. Nowadays, captured digital images usually possess no differences with its source. As a result, the principle of pattern recognition obtained from machine learning can play a key role in the identification of various diseases.On account of digital nature of images being processed, machine learning allows a wider range of algorithms that can be implemented to the input data or pixels. Implementing machine learning techniques for pattern recognition indicates the presence of abnormalities in the affected region, thereby confirming the diseased region. Different classifiers may be trained using linear discriminative analysis, support vector machine, and random forest techniques as reported by Zarinabad et al. Pattern recognition model has the potential for early detection, more precise evaluation and suitable drug recommendations. The image analytics through artificial intelligence can also be implemented for mapping vegetation and water bodies obtained from satellite imagery or photogrammetry data. The presence of various indices, for example $NDVI$, which is a dimensionless index and is defined as "*The ratio of the reflective difference of the visible & near-infrared region to the sum of the visible & near-infrared region*".

$$\text{NDVI} = \frac{\text{NIR} - \text{Red}}{\text{NIR} + \text{Red}} \tag{17.1}$$

Here, NIR and Red represent the spectral reflectance in the visible (Red and near-infrared region (NIR), respectively. It gives important indication of green cover and vegetation and has the potential to assess agricultural farmland. It is also used for hydrological purposes. The value of it varies from 1.0 to −1.0, where a positive value is an indicator of green vegetation.

Besides, NDVI (Normalized Difference Vegetation Index), other prominent indices are EVI (Enhanced Vegetation Index), NDWI (Normalized Difference Water Index), etc., which aids in better capturing insights of such studies and may help and guide in preventing mishappenings, reducing the risk, and providing evidence informed policy recommendation. The course of time lead toward the introduction of artificial neural networks in this domain. Following this, deep neural networks are new entrants that employed machine learning models in the field of image analytic and natural language processing [21, 64].

17.5 NATURAL LANGUAGE PROCESSING

The use of social media not only helped to get connected with others but also nowadays playing an important role in various aspects of human lives. Not only does it help in spreading information but also help local bodies and agencies to react and provide support in times of needs that may include the events associated with heavy rain or flooding, etc. With the growing use of Twitter, there are many instances where officials have responded to the situation that struck citizens. Also, these social media data is often used for sentiment analysis. Natural language processing provide application in translation, in extracting keywords and thereby provides policy recommendation.

With the recent advancement of computing tools, advanced algorithms, vast amount of data from different domains, more precise and application-oriented studies can be performed with accuracy. The area of natural language processing incorporates various tools for extracting information from structured and unstructured data sources. This can catalyze the way of viewing by scientists and policy makers to model and plan conservation interventions on various natural resources. Also, text analysis of social media posts also shows the existence of provoking texts that act as a pretext for conflicts and clashes. Keeping a focus on Australia, Jakubowicz et al., have performed a series of studies regarding online racism, targets and victims. These findings have the potential to pinpoint policy recommendations to safeguard the interest of targeted communities through regulatory agencies and government involvement with civil and criminal law in relation to the usage and code of conduct at cyberspace [31, 32]. Data science approaches are often used in many industries, such as fraud detection in monetary or banking transactions, monitoring faults during production and intelligent alerts in faults diagnosis, healthcare sectors, etc. These could be employed to monitor and analyse different conservation projects with time series data available through various means e.g. monitoring soil nutrient, presence of toxic levels, water quality, pH, etc., in order to avoid the undesired outcomes that may trigger environment damage or harm human health. This is achieved through different means and methods to tap and analyse the data.

Apart from this, the unstructured clinical record and the patient feedback after a visit to medical practitioner may provide insights into the patient experience. These responses can act as valuable piece of information which usually is not available in the structured record. This may shed light in understanding the underlying phenomena arising from the various responses and help mapping it based on the NLP-driven keywords or phrase identification. This will further inform healthcare practitioner for healthcare decisions and diagnosis and confronts the interplaying complexity at various scales with different factors including treatment, drugs, nutrients, diets, surroundings or locations. As a result, such application-oriented NLP, employing data mining in healthcare and sentiment analysis, has a potential to provide better informed systems for decision-making and thereby assist government, public and private organizations in delivering more efficient care to the deserving and affected patients.

17.6 RECOMMENDATION SYSTEM

A recommendation system is a type of information filtering system that enables to forecast the use depending upon the preference of an item. Simply it is an algorithm that provides suggestions in many cases depending upon the relevance of the product or article in terms of some characteristics. Recommender systems are algorithms that propose appropriate objects to users in a variety of disciplines, such as friend recommendation in social networking, product recommendation in online purchasing and text-based medicine recommendations. The methods are divided into two categories, viz; collaborative filtering and content-based methods. To generate fresh recommendations, collaborative approaches for a recommender system employs the method that is completely dependent on past interactions between users and products. The so-called "user-item interactions matrix" stores these interactions. The key idea that governs collaborative approaches is that previous user-item interactions are adequate to predict future user-item interactions. However, for the other i.e., "content based", the idea utilizes content-based methods in order to try to build a model, depending upon the available "features". These features play a pivotal role to explain the observed user-item interactions. These tools open a new gateway towards precise and speedy matching suggestion in different domains including healthcare sector [28].

17.7 CHALLENGES

Through data with algorithms computers have the ability to interpret review and recommend solutions to complex health-related or medical issues. With the help of analysis of data through artificial intelligence, the diagnosis can be much faster, precise and and results in more precise predictability. Computational methods enable to analyse the influence of parameters like climate change or humanitarian crises through various means and its impact on health and natural resources. Different types of data including satellite images and photogrammetry provide important insights in understanding and analyses. Real-time data from different domains e.g., pollutant concentrations, particluate matter and other often help in assessing its impact on different aspects of health like lungs and breathing-related disorders. These approach also result in reduction of costs. Artificial intelligence has the potential to develop intelligent medications where *AI* will be used to precisely assess the space and time of the affected cells of patient. In such cases, patient with complicated pathologies may be treated efficiently with artificial intelligence-assisted algorithms and robots closer to more confidence interval. The scope of *tele-medicine* may emerge from the use of artificial intelligence and machine learning methodologies. It is defined as the practice of getting counselling and prescription for diagnosis in virtual mode, where remotely distant patient and doctor can be brought together through recommending algorithms depending upon the query and specialization of patient and doctor. Here data analysis, family history and lifestyle habits through proper algorithms can assist in tracking, monitoring and providing insights for medications. Also, for a densely populated country like India, where equal distribution of healthcare facilities is a big challenge. According to the statistics the observations are: efficient health infrastructure and skilled medical professionals are mostly centred in big urban centres where as majority of population is widely distributed across the country. Here, the concept of tele-medicine can play a pivotal role and may have promising effects. Machine learning and statistical methods are implemented to reduce trial and errors and introduce more reliable models in the field of drug development, thereby cutting the cost and efforts by an appreciable amount. Monitoring medical responses efficiently and accurately through machine learning models efficiently cuts the time consumption. Nevertheless, the vast amount of covid data treated with such machine learning methods shed light in terms of formation, to keep track of genetic mutation of virus and the mechanism in order to develop vaccines. However, privacy, security and biases in data-driven studies with artificial intelligence is one of the obstructions [11, 18].

17.8 CONCLUDING REMARKS

This chapter aims to make an attempt to explore the variability between ethnic conflicts/terrorism, climate variability, its influence upon health and to develop an analytical framework in addition to literature review that could guide in making use of the combination of methods and complexity approach. The computational approaches to real world data in this not only help to understand clinical challenges but also provide insights to prevent such mishappenings. The artificial intelligence and machine learning approaches enable to predict and anticipate the healthcare requirements in post war and conflict settings. It also facilitates in development of precise and novel treatments. Data-inspired modelling has the potential to estimate the healthcare burden for more effective intervention. Higher values of economy and health as depicted in Figure 17.4b is suggestive of improved happiness score and the interplay of these variables is indicative of the overall health of a country. The interplay of climate and conflicts results in various health problems i.e., infectious disease, non-communicable diseases, maternal and children health and malnutrition. Conflicts triggered mental health are post-traumatic stress disorder, insomnia, anxiety and depression. It has many long-term consequences including susceptibility to infectious and chronic diseases; for example, outbreaks of cholera in conflict-affected Yemen, and acinobacter in war-affected Iraq. Moreover, UN Network on racial discrimination & protection of minorities framework should be practiced for the protection of any existing, ethnic, linguistic and religious minor group in order to prevent the ethnicities in falling prey in such crises zone.

The network facilitates to understand the "interactions" and reveals about the undergoing dynamics. The human responses in dynamical situation often dictate/guide the emergence as the system evolves. Different responses when mapped result in the emergence of communities in a network on account of this. The adoption of new policy measures for sustainability and well-being of society can be facilitated further through innovation diffusion mechanism. Therefore, the primary aim of the article is to implement the artificial intelligence and complexity-inspired approaches to novel interdisciplinary settings and thereby promoting research that can provide deep insights and help in understandings of such complex issues which could guide for policy recommendations.

ACKNOWLEDGEMENT(S)

The author would like to thank Mr. S. F. Husain for his valuable support, critical discussions and inputs. The author also thanks S. Dini, A. Verma and A. Gupta.

REFERENCES

[1] Abergel, F., Aoyama, H., Chakrabarti, B. K., Chakraborti, A., Deo, N., Raina, D., & Vodenska, I. (Eds.). (2017). *Econophysics and Sociophysics: Recent Progress and Future Directions*. Switzerland, Cham: Springer International Publishing.

[2] Albert, R., Jeong, H., & Barabási, A. L. (2000). Error and attack tolerance of complex networks. *Nature*, 406(6794), 378–382.

[3] Bais, A. F., McKenzie, R. L., Bernhard, G., Aucamp, P. J., Ilyas, M., Madronich, S., & Tourpali, K. (2015). Ozone depletion and climate change: impacts on UV radiation. *Photochemical & Photobiological Sciences*, 14(1), 19–52.

[4] Barthélemy, M., Barrat, A., Pastor-Satorras, R., & Vespignani, A. (2004). Velocity and hierarchical spread of epidemic outbreaks in scale-free networks. *Physical Review Letters*, 92(17), 178701.

[5] Barabási, A. L., & Albert, R. (1999). Emergence of scaling in random networks. *Science*, 286(5439), 509–512.

[6] Bita, C., & Gerats, T. (2013). Plant tolerance to high temperature in a changing environment: scientific fundamentals and production of heat stress-tolerant crops. *Frontiers in Plant Science*, 4, 273.

[7] Bengio, Y., Goodfellow, I., & Courville, A. (2017). *Deep Learning* (Vol. 1). Cambridge, MA: MIT Press.

[8] Castellano, C., Fortunato, S., & Loreto, V. (2009). Statistical physics of social dynamics. *Reviews of Modern Physics*, 81(2), 591.

[9] Chakrabarti, B. K., Chakraborti, A., & Chatterjee, A. (Eds.). (2006). *Econophysics and Sociophysics: Trends and Perspectives*. Hoboken, NJ: John Wiley & Sons.

[10] Chakraborti, A., Husain, S. S., & Whitmeyer, J. (2018). A model for innovation diffusion with intergroup suppression. arXiv preprint arXiv:1802.08943, submitted to Eds. Chakraborti et al., *Quantum Decision Theory and Complexity Modelling in Economics and Public Policy* (Cham: Springer).

[11] Cohen, I. G., & Mello, M. M. (2019). Big data, big tech, and protecting patient privacy. *JAMA*, 322(12), 1141–1142.

[12] Dunn, J., & Balaprakash, P. (Eds.). (2021). *Data Science Applied to Sustainability Analysis*. Amsterdam, Netherlands: Elsevier.

[13] Renyi, E. (1959). On random graph. *Publicationes Mathematicate*, 6, 290–297.

[14] Erdős, P., & Rényi, A. (1960). On the evolution of random graphs. *Publication of the Mathematical Institute of the Hungarian Academy of Sciences*, 5(1), 17–60.

[15] Euler, L. (1741). Solutio problematis ad geometriam situs pertinentis. *Commentarii Academiae Scientiarum Petropolitanae*, 8, 128–140.

[16] Freeman, L. C. (1978). Centrality in social networks conceptual clarification. *Social Networks*, 1(3), 215–239.

[17] Frey, B. S., Luechinger, S., & Stutzer, A. (2007). Calculating tragedy: Assessing the costs of terrorism. *Journal of Economic Surveys*, 21(1), 1–24.

[18] Froomkin, A. M., Kerr, I., & Pineau, J. (2019). When AIs outperform doctors: confronting the challenges of a tort-induced over-reliance on machine learning. *Arizona State Law Journal*, 61, 33.

[19] Ghahramani, Z. (2015). Probabilistic machine learning and artificial intelligence. *Nature*, 521(7553), 452–459.

[20] Girvan, M., & Newman, M. E. (2002). Community structure in social and biological networks. *Proceedings of the National Academy of Sciences*, 99(12), 7821–7826.

[21] Groten, S. M. E. (1993). NDVI-crop monitoring and early yield assessment of Burkina Faso. *Remote Sensing*, 14(8), 1495–1515.

[22] GDELT: The global database of events, language and tone (gdelt) (2016). www.gdeltproject.org/

[23] Global terrorism database (gtd)-codebook: Inclusion criteria and variables, as on 3 jan, 2013, https://www.start.umd.edu/gtd/downloads/codebook.pdf (2018) https://www.start.umd.edu/gtd/contact/ (2018)

[24] Galatzer-Levy, I. R., Karstoft, K. I., Statnikov, A., & Shalev, A. Y. (2014). Quantitative forecasting of PTSD from early trauma responses: A machine learning application. *Journal of Psychiatric Research*, 59, 68–76.

[25] Hardin, G. (1968). The tragedy of the commons. *Science*, 162 (3859): 1243–1248.

[26] Hastie, T., Tibshirani, R., & Friedman, J. H. (2009). *The Elements of Statistical Learning: Data Mining, Inference, and Prediction* (Vol. 2, pp. 1–758). New York: Springer.

[27] Hempel, S., Koseska, A., Nikoloski, Z., & Kurths, J. (2011). Unraveling gene regulatory networks from time-resolved gene expression data–a measures comparison study. *BMC Bioinformatics*, 12(1), 1–26.

[28] Hirschberg, J., & Manning, C. D. (2015). Advances in natural language processing. *Science*, 349(6245), 261–266.

[29] Husain, S. S., & Sharma, K. (2019). Dynamical evolution of anti-social phenomena: A data science approach. In: F. Abergel, B. K. Chakrabarti, A. Chakraborti, N. Deo, & K. Sharma (Eds.), *New Perspectives and Challenges in Econophysics and Sociophysics*, (pp. 241–255). Cham: Springer.

[30] Husain, S. S., Sharma, K., Kukreti, V., & Chakraborti, A. (2020). Identifying the global terror hubs and vulnerable motifs using complex network dynamics. *Physica A: Statistical Mechanics and Its Applications*, 540, 123113.

[31] Jakubowicz, A., Dunn, K., Mason, G., Paradies, Y., Bliuc, A. M., Bahfen, N., & Connelly, K. (2017). *Cyber Racism and Community Resilience*. Cham: Palgrave Macmillan.

[32] Jakubowicz, A. (2018). Algorithms of hate: How the Internet facilitates the spread of racism and how public policy might help stem the impact. *Journal and Proceedings of the Royal Society of New South Wales*, Vol. 151, No. 467/468, pp. 69–81.

[33] Jeong, H., Tombor, B., Albert, R., Oltvai, Z. N., & Barabási, A. L. (2000). The large-scale organization of metabolic networks. *Nature*, 407(6804), 651–654.

[34] Jongman, B., Wagemaker, J., Romero, B. R., & De Perez, E. C. (2015). Early flood detection for rapid humanitarian response: Harnessing near real-time satellite and Twitter signals. *ISPRS International Journal of Geo-Information*, 4(4), 2246–2266.

[35] Kadir, A., Shenoda, S., Goldhagen, J., Pitterman, S., Suchdev, P. S., Chan, K. J., & Arnold, L. D. (2018). The effects of armed conflict on children. *Pediatrics*, 142(6).

[36] Kantz, H., & Schreiber, T. (2004). *Nonlinear Time Series Analysis*, (Vol. 7). Cambridge: Cambridge University Press.

[37] Lahr, M. M., Rivera, F., Power, R. K., Mounier, A., Copsey, B., Crivellaro, F., ... & Foley, R. A. (2016). Inter-group violence among early Holocene hunter-gatherers of West Turkana, Kenya. *Nature*, 529(7586), 394–398.
[38] Lancichinetti, A., & Fortunato, S. (2009). Community detection algorithms: A comparative analysis. *Physical Review E*, 80(5), 056117.
[39] Liljeros, F., Edling, C. R., & Amaral, L. A. N. (2003). Sexual networks: implications for the transmission of sexually transmitted infections. *Microbes and Infection*, 5(2), 189–196.
[40] LeCun, Y., Bengio, Y., & Hinton, G. (2015). Deep learning. *Nature*, 521(7553), 436–444.
[41] Maalouf, F. T., Alamiri, B., Atweh, S., Becker, A. E., Cheour, M., Darwish, H., Ghandour, L.A., Ghuloum, S., Hamze, M., Karam, E., & Khoury, B. (2019). Mental health research in the Arab region: Challenges and call for action. *The Lancet Psychiatry*, 6(11), 961–966.
[42] More, C. (2002). *Understanding the Industrial Revolution*. Oxfordshire, England: Routledge.
[43] NacuS., Critchley-Thorne, R., Lee, P., & Holmes, S. (2007). Gene expression network analysis and applications to immunology. *Bioinformatics*, 23(7), 850–858.
[44] Patz, J. A. & Olson, S. H. (2006). Climate change and health: Global to local influences on disease risk. *Annals of Tropical Medicine & Parasitology*, 100(5–6), 535–549.
[45] Perc, M., Jordan, J. J., Rand, D. G., Wang, Z., Boccaletti, S., & Szolnoki, A. (2017). Statistical physics of human cooperation. *Physics Reports*, 687, 1–51.
[46] Phalkey, R. K., Aranda-Jan, C., Marx, S., Höfle, B., & Sauerborn, R. (2015). Systematic review of current efforts to quantify the impacts of climate change on undernutrition. *Proceedings of the National Academy of Sciences*, 112(33), E4522–E4529.
[47] Pirani, S. (2018). *Burning up: A Global History of Fossil Fuel Consumption*. London: Pluto Press.
[48] Posfai, M., & Barabási, A. L. (2016). *Network Science*. Cambridge: Cambridge University Press.
[49] Ray, D., & Esteban, J. (2017). Conflict and development. *Annual Review of Economics*, 9, 263–293.
[50] Sari Kovats, R., Edwards, S. J., Charron, D., Cowden, J., D'Souza, R. M., Ebi, K. L., & Schmid, H. (2005). Climate variability and campylobacter infection: An international study. *International Journal of Biometeorology*, 49(4), 207–214.
[51] Sen, P., & Chakrabarti, B. K. (2014). *Sociophysics: An Introduction*. Cary, NC: Oxford University Press.
[52] Schatz, B. R. (2000). Learning by text or context? [Review of the book *The Social Life of Information*, by J. S. Brown & P. Duguid]. *Science*, 290, 1304.
[53] Schelling, T. C. (1969). Models of segregation. *The American Economic Review*, 59(2), 488–493.
[54] Schelling, T. C. (1971). Dynamic models of segregation. *Journal of Mathematical Sociology*, 1(2), 143–186.
[55] Small, M. (2005). *Applied Nonlinear Time Series Analysis: Applications in Physics, Physiology and Finance*, (Vol. 52). Singapore: World Scientific.

[56] Scheffer, M., Bascompte, J., Brock, W. A., Brovkin, V., Carpenter, S. R., Dakos, V., ... & Sugihara, G. (2009). Early-warning signals for critical transitions. *Nature*, 461(7260), 53–59.
[57] Scheffer, M. (2020). *Critical Transitions in Nature and Society*. Princeton, NJ: Princeton University Press.
[58] Stott, P. (2016). How climate change affects extreme weather events. *Science*, 352(6293), 1517–1518.
[59] Thomas, K. M., Charron, D. F., Waltner-Toews, D., Schuster, C., Maarouf, A. R., & Holt, J. D. (2006). A role of high impact weather events in waterborne disease outbreaks in Canada, 1975–2001. *International Journal of Environmental Health Research*, 16(03), 167–180.
[60] Wahid, A., Gelani, S., Ashraf, M., & Foolad, M. R. (2007). Heat tolerance in plants: An overview. *Environmental and Experimental Botany*, 61(3), 199–223.
[61] Watts, D. J., & Strogatz, S. H. (1998). Collective dynamics of 'small-world' networks. *Nature*, 393(6684), 440–442.
[62] Wilson, R. J. (1986). An eulerian trail through Königsberg. *Journal of Graph Theory*, 10(3), 265–275.
[63] World Happiness Report (2016). https://worldhappiness.report/ed/2016/.
[64] Zarinabad, N., Abernethy, L. J., Avula, S., Davies, N. P., Rodriguez Gutierrez, D., Jaspan, T., & Peet, A. (2018). Application of pattern recognition techniques for classification of pediatric brain tumors by in vivo 3T 1H-MR spectroscopy: A multi-center study. *Magnetic Resonance in Medicine*, 79(4), 2359–2366.

Index

Printed in the United States
by Baker & Taylor Publisher Services

Printed in the United States
by Baker & Taylor Publisher Services